# Syphilis in Shakespeare's England

Johannes Fabricius

Jessica Kingsley Publishers
London and Bristol, Pennsylvania

First published in the United Kingdom in 1994 by
Jessica Kingsley Publishers Ltd
116 Pentonville Road
London N1 9JB, England
and
1900 Frost Road, Suite 101
Bristol, PA 19007, U S A

Copyright © 1994 Johannes Fabricius

Denne afhandling er af Det sundhedsvidenskabelige fakultet ved Københavns universitet antaget til offentligt at forsvares for den medicinske doktorgrad.
København, den 6. januar 1994
Ove Noren dekan
Forsvaret finder sted på Medicinsk Historisk Museum
Bredgade 62, København, fredag den 2. september 1994, kl. 14.00.

**Library of Congress Cataloging in Publication Data**

A CIP catalogue record for this book is available from the Library of Congress

**British Library Cataloguing in Publication Data**

A CIP catalogue record for this book is available from the British Library

ISBN 1-85302-270-5 PB

Printed and Bound in Great Britain by
Biddles Ltd., Guildford and King's Lynn

# CONTENTS

IN MEMORY OF
KIRSTEN FABRICIUS
(1948–1991)

# Acknowledgements

Many colleagues have contributed their help and encouragement during the five years of the study which this volume describes. Among those who have worked with me directly on this research I particularly wish to express my appreciation and gratitude for their invaluable help to Professor, dr. med. Axel Perdrup; Professor, dr. med. et phil. Egill Snorrason; Professor, dr. phil. Helmer Kofod; Kai Bent-Hansen, M.D.; Michael Waugh, M.D. of the University of Leeds School of Medicine; Professor A.J.H. Rains of the Royal Society of Medicine; Professor Harrison T. Meserole of Texas A&M University; Poul Aagaard Christiansen of the Danish National Library of Science and Medicine, Copenhagen; and John Symons and Robin Price of the Wellcome Institute for the History of Medicine.

My particular thanks also go to Professor, med. dr. Bengt I. Lindskog who has been an untold help and support to me, as has also his experienced and wise counsel. I am further indebted to my late friend, dr. phil. Vagn Lundgaard Simonsen for his keen interest in my work at its very beginning and for his valuable suggestions and criticisms. I also wish to record the encouragement and financial aid so kindly given to me by my late friend Mr. Andreas Simonsen, just as I specifically want to thank my friend and relative Mr. Paul J.A. Fabricius for writing out for me his considered comments and criticisms, which have been of great value to me.

I am particularly grateful to Miss Wendy Share, M.A., who once more undertook to correct an English manuscript of mine. Help so kind, disinterested, timely and effective as this is a gift that touches the heart. I am similarly grateful to Mrs. Inger Lise Franke whose patience, care and accuracy carried the manuscript from the writer's hands to the printer's.

My debt to others is heavy: among my friends above all to Mr. Finn Blytmann who helped me on my way at every stage of a long journey by his inexhaustible obligingness and resourcefulness in dealing with a variety of difficulties and problems. Finally, I wish to express my sincere appreciation and gratitude to the Carlsberg Foundation, Copenhagen, which made it possible for me to study a variety of sources and books in England during my five years of research. Part of the financial costs involved in printing the book has been borne by the Danish Medical Research Council and the Danish Research Council for the Humanities, to which institutions my profoundest thanks are due.

In the middle of this work I lost my wife, Mrs. Kirsten Fabricius, to whose memory I dedicate this book with love.

*Hillerød, July 1994.*
*Johannes Fabricius*

# ILLUSTRATIONS

# PREFACE

Christ as *salvator mundi*, or 'Saviour of the World', adorns the title-page of Joseph Grünpeck's *Tractatus de pestilentiali scorra sive mala de franczos* (Augsburg, 1496), which is the earliest dated book on syphilis (Figure 1). Christ's troubled expression and compassionate gesture reflect one of the most shocking experiences of European history: the invasion at the close of the Middle Ages of a venereal plague sweeping, within a few years, over the entire Continent and corrupting the blood of Renaissance man.

The numerous records on the Continent of the event and the space devoted to it by a large number of medical scholars are matched by a corresponding meagreness of records and studies in England. This discrepancy is so conspicuous that one is left with the impression that the disease never crossed the Channel. At the end of the 16th century, Shakespeare praised divine providence for having protected his native country with a ring of waves. 'This precious stone set in the silver sea, Which serves it in the office of a wall,' he chanted in *Richard II*, while in the same work he also compared his beloved island to a 'fortress built by Nature for herself Against infection and the hand of war' (2,1:46–7;43–4).

England as a country blessed by a state of 'splendid isolation' even in medical matters permeates scholarly accounts of the kingdom in Tudor and Stuart times and seems to suggest that 'the pox', as syphilis was called in England, never really posed a serious threat to that country. A couple of examples will serve to illustrate this point. In 1911, the noted Shakespearean scholar John Dover Wilson published a rich collection of 16th and 17th century sources describing *Life in Shakespeare's England*. A remarkable feature of this survey is the absence of any sources describing prostitution, brothels and venereal diseases – as though they had no part in life in Shakespearean England. In 1977, similarly, Lawrence Stone, a sociologist at Princeton University, published his monumental and classic study *The Family, Sex and Marriage in England 1500–1800*. Stone concludes that 'The greatest risk from promiscuous sexual activity…was clearly gonorrhoea…On the other hand, syphilis does not seem to have been a serious threat. The ubiquity of gonorrhoea and the rarity of syphilis seems to have been an established feature of England at least by the late sixteenth century' (Stone, 1988, p.599).

Do the accounts of Wilson and Stone actually reflect the impact of syphilis on England at the time? In order to examine this question, the author of this study has made a search of virtually every relevant record which has survived from the period 1495–1650. Scholarly contributions to the subject have also been consulted but strange as it may sound to students of medical history, this particular field presents a 'black hole' – to use an image from astrophysics. Social historian F.G. Emmison in

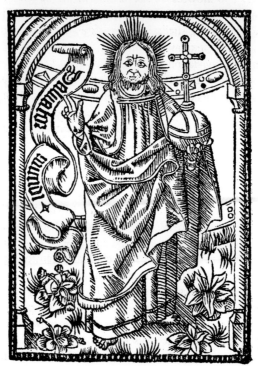

Figure 1. Title-page of Grünpeck's syphilis treatise, 1496.

1973 summed up the vacuum thus: 'There is virtually no authoritative modern history of venereal diseases in England' (p.31).

Charles Creighton's *A History of Epidemics in Britain* (1891) is the only book which deals with the subject at any length, and even here the author's contribution is limited to the eighth chapter of his book, where 15 pages deal strictly with the subject of syphilis in England. Creighton presents the reader with a score of references from contemporary chroniclers and religious reformers, translators of foreign literature on the subject, notices in official documents, and, finally, relevant passages in the medical literature of the time, such as William Bullein's *Bulwarke of Defence* (1562) and *Dialogue of the Fever Pestilence* (1562), Thomas Gale's *Certain Works of Chirurgerie* (1563), John Jones's *Dyall of Agues* (1566), John Banister's *A Needefull New and Necessarie Treatise of Chyrurgerie* (1577), John Read's *A Most Excellent and*

*Compendious Method of Curing Wounds* (1588), Peter Lowe's *An Easie, Certaine and Perfect Method to Cure and Prevent the Spanish Sicknes* (1596), and William Clowes's *A Short and Profitable Treatise Teaching the Cure of the Disease Called Morbus Gallicus by Unctions* (1579).

Creighton's list of medical authors is not complete, however, and his medical passages are not quoted in full, just as his analysis of them does not exhaust their full range of information. When, for instance, William Clowes mentions 'rogues and vagabondes' and 'lewd alehowses' as key factors in the dissemination of syphilis, this information does not prompt Creighton to an examination of this group of the population, its size and habits; similarly, the proliferation of alehouses in the 16th and 17th centuries is left unexamined.

Creighton's limited material on syphilis in England, however, was nevertheless sufficient to make him realize 'what its prevalence and its serious effects on the public health must have been continuously in the generations before [the Restoration period], and most of all in the generation which experienced the full force of it as an epidemic' (Creighton, 1891, p.428). Creighton clearly entertained no illusions about Tudor and Stuart England as an island protected by 'the silver sea' against syphilitic infection.

For all its shortcomings, Creighton's contribution cut the first sod and still remains a valuable starting point for the student of the subject. What has appeared since Creighton's work reveals his importance, for Michael A. Waugh's excellent survey of *Venereal Diseases in Sixteenth-Century England* (1973, pp.192–99) is built almost entirely on Creighton's material and adds little new to the subject. It is to Waugh's credit, however, that he has drawn scholarly attention to the 'cornucopia of writings on venereal diseases [that] can be found in the daily records, court books (Emmison), and belletristic works of those times' (p.192). Waugh, in this connection, mentions J.D. Rolleston's *Venereal Disease in Literature* (1934, pp.147–82), in which Shakespeare provides the source for most of the quotations, while Rolleston himself draws attention to other notable sources such as the plays of George Chapman, Francis Beaumont, John Fletcher, Ben Jonson, John Webster, Philip Massinger, and John Ford.

It is Shakespeare's allusions to syphilis which have also, more than those of any other author, been most fully covered by medical scholars such as J.C. Bucknill in his monograph *The Medical Knowledge of Shakespeare* (1860), J.W.L. Crossfill's *Classified Medical References in the Works of Shakespeare* (1954–7, vols.40–3), Francis R. Packard's *References to Syphilis in the Plays of Shakespeare* (1924, pp.194–200), and C. Whitney Wolfe's *Shakespeare Refers to Syphilis* (1960, pp.112–4). Frankie Rubinstein's *A Dictionary of Shakespeare's Sexual Puns and Their Significance* (1984) contains several references to venereal disease, and G.W. Bentley's dissertation *Shakespeare and the New Disease: the Dramatic Function of Syphilis in Troilus and Cressida, Measure for Measure, and Timon of Athens* (1989) examines Shakespeare's references to syphilis from a literary point of view – as images of corruption, decay and degeneration which help to give unity and dramatic structure to the tragedies he has focused on. References to syphilis in the plays of Shakespeare's contemporaries, on the other hand, have been covered only minimally by medical scholars, and so a systematic examination of this area is a much-needed task and one that has been undertaken in the present study, which also examines the morality plays and interludes that precede Elizabethan drama. Preliminary studies in this field include Gordon Williams's two short but valuable articles *A Sample of Elizabethan Sexual Periphrasis* (1968, pp.94–101) and *An Elizabethan Disease* (1971, pp.43–57), and Paul G. Brewster's excellent *A Note on the "Winchester Goose" and Kindred Topics* (1958, pp.483–91).

In addition to the references to syphilis in the dramatic literature of the 16th and 17th centuries, important information is to be found in the prose works of Shakespeare's contemporaries, notably the pamphlets of Robert Greene, Thomas Nashe, George Whetstone, Samuel Rowlands, and Thomas Dekker. (The methodological problems involved in drawing upon these pamphlets for medical and social information are treated on pp.109–24.) The fact is that these pamphlets represent a mixture of facts and fiction, just as they present a satirical and moralistic, even Puritanical, attitude toward syphilis to the reader.

Additional sources include the writings of the social reformers of the period, such as Thomas More, Simon Fish, Robert Crowley, John Howes, Henry Chettle, John Awdeley and Thomas Harman. Valuable information is also to be obtained from such theological writers as John Fisher, Thomas Becon, Hugh Latimer, John Bale, and Thomas Fuller, and from historians such as Bernard André, Robert Fabyan, Charles Wriothesley, William Camden, John Stow, Ralph Holinshed, and William Harrison. Of particular interest are the private literary sources such as letters, reports and diaries dealing with prominent persons of the times.

The political documents that have been consulted by the author of the present study include *The Statutes of the Realm* (1817–19) (vols. 3–5), *Acts of the Privy Council* (1890–1905) (edited by J.R. Dasent), *Calendar of State Papers, Domestic* (1856–72) (edited by R. Lemon and E. Green), *Tudor Royal Proclamations* (1964–69) and *Stuart Royal Proclamations* (1973–83) (both edited by P.L. Hughes and J.F. Larkin).

The sources collected by R.H. Tawney and E. Powers in *Tudor Economic Documents* (1924) especially provide important information on the economic and social conditions of the period.

The secular and ecclesiastical court books of the time are of further interest and include the *Middlesex County Records* (1886–88) (edited by J.C. Jeaffreson), and the records from the *Essex Archdeaconries* (1973) (quoted by F.G. Emmison), and the *Somerset Court* (quoted by G.R. Quaife) (see pp.264–8).

Last but not least, the author has consulted the entire medical literature of the period, which means the inclusion of a number of authors not mentioned by Creighton, notably, Thomas Vicary, Thomas Moulton, Andrew Boord, John Banister (*Collected Works*), John Woodall, John Hester, John Cotta, and Joseph Binns.

Unfortunately, none of the medical authors of the period provides data which would allow for a statistical analysis of the prevalence of syphilis in the English population. The difficulties of diagnosis in an age that confused syphilis and gonorrhea, which was without the Wassermann test, and which tended to cover up occurences of syphilis, the 'foul disease', make such a task impossible. It is true that in 1662 the father of modern statistics and demography, John Graunt, made an attempt to assess the prevalence of syphilis in the London population on the basis of statistical material collected during the first half of the 17th century. Significantly, however, he despaired of the task because the shame attached to syphilis resulted

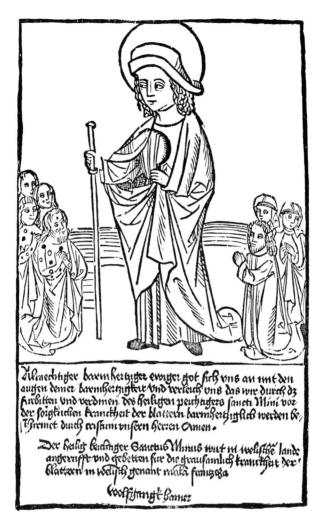

Figure 2. The above flyleaf, possibly the oldest pictorial rendering of the venereal plague in Europe, was produced in about 1495 by the woodcarver Wolfgang Hamer, who worked in Nuremberg from 1480 to 1490 (Sudhoff, 1912, Tafel. XIX). The woodcut shows a group of syphilitic men and women kneeling in front of St. Minus, one of the patron saints of the sufferers of the French disease. The text consists of the syphilitics' prayer to the saint and finishes with an explanatory note by Wolfgang Hamer: "'Almighty, merciful and eternal God, look upon us with the eyes of your mercy and grant us that we, through the prayers and merits of our patron, Saint Minus, will be mercifully protected by our Lord Christ against the horrible disease of the blisters. Amen." In the Romance countries, patron Saint Minus is implored for help against the cruel disease of the blisters, called in Romance languages the French disease. Wolfgang Hamer.'

in its being chronically underreported (see pp.29–30). The sources dealing with syphilis in England, then, allow for conclusions which describe the disease medically though not statistically, whereas the same sources allow for conclusions regarding the psychological impact of the disease on the individual and also for conclusions concerning the impact of syphilis on the social, economic, political, religious, and cultural spheres of the English nation in the 16th and 17th centuries.

In concluding our survey of sources, we should like to note that the present study includes a complete pictorial record of syphilis on the Continent and in England, and all the pictures are analyzed in depth by the texts accompanying the woodcuts and engravings.

There could be no better starting point for a study of *Syphilis in Shakespeare's England* than to examine the origin of the term 'syphilis'. Where did the name come from, and how did the disease arise and spread across the entire planet as a venereal plague that is still with us? An attempt is made to answer these questions in our next chapter, which also provides a survey of the European background to the syphilitic epidemic against which the English Experience must be viewed if it is to be fully understood.

# 1

# THE SINISTER SHEPHERD

In 1530 the Veronese physician Girolamo Fracastoro (c. 1478–1553) published a poem called *Syphilis sive morbus gallicus* ('Syphilis or the French Disease') (Fracastoro, 1988, pp.26–95).* In the poem, Fracastoro invented a famous myth of how a 'bold Leader' (III, 104) – 'The bravest Youth that ever stemm'd the Main' (III, 105) – sailed westward from Spain, past Anthylia, Hagia, Ammerie and Gyane, to Ophir, 'a mighty Island in the Middle of the Sea' (III, 119–20). The Spanish leader (probably Columbus) and his shipmates rejoiced in the wonders of the New World and, during their explorations of its virginal regions, they happened one day to shoot some beautiful birds in 'Ophir' which belonged to the Sun-God. On this occasion one of the birds that escaped the Spaniards' massacre uttered a prophecy of dire ills:

> Nor end your sufferings here; a strange Disease,
> And most obscene, shall on your Bodies seize. (III, 189–90)

Before the Spanish leader and his shipmates left Ophir, they had the chance to observe a crowd of scabby and pimply aborigines conducting a propitiary service to the Sun-God:

> A cloud of Grief o'er ev'ry Face was spread,
> All languish'd with the same obscene Disease,
> And years, not Strength distinguisht the Degrees;
> Dire flames upon their Vitals fed within,
> Whiles Sores and crusted Filth prophan'd their Skin.
> At last the Priest in snowy Robes array'd,
> The Boughs of healing Guiacum display'd,
> Which (dipt in living Streams) he shook around
> To purge, for holy Rites the tainted Ground.
> An Heifer then before the Altar slew,
> A Swain stood near on whom the Bloud he threw;
> Then to the Sun began his mystick Song,
> And streight was seconded by all the Throng.
> Both Swine and Heifers now by thousands bleed,
> And Natives on their roasted Entrails feed. (III, 238–47)

---

* The English translation by Nahum Tate (1686) is quoted after the reproduction in Dryden's *Examen poeticum* (London, 1693), pp.1 84.

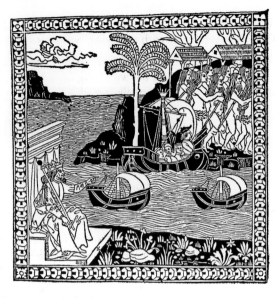

Figure 3. Columbus lands 1492 with his caravels on a West Indian island, which is 'annexed' by the Spanish king (left). The woodcut adorns a Florentine edition 1493 of Columbus's letter describing his discovery of the New World. Girolamo Fracastoro's poem *Syphilis* (1530) suggests the medical consequences of the event:

> Say, Goddess, to what Cause we shall at last
> Assign this Plague, unknown to Ages past;
> If from the Western Climes 'twas wafted o'er,
> When daring Spaniards left their Native shore;
> Resolv'd beyond th' Atlantick to descry,
> Conjectur'd Worlds, or in the search to dye. (I, 32–7)

The Spanish leader correctly guessed that the natives' disease was identical with 'The strange Disease that on our Troops shou'd fall' (III, 251–2) according to the prophecy of the holy bird. He therefore made inquiries about the disease and the rites performed in connection with it, and the native prince obligingly answered the Spaniard's questions. He finally went on to tell him the strange story of the origin of the plague, and the discovery of guaiac as a cure.

> A Shepherd once (distrust not ancient Fame)
> Possest these Downs, and *Syphilus* his Name. (III, 288–90)[*]

He kept the flocks of King Alcithoos, and one year the drought was so extreme that the cattle perished for want of water. So incensed was Syphilus that he shouted blasphemous insults at the Sun-God, deciding from henceforth to offer no sacrifices to him, but to worship King Alcithoos instead. The shepherd won all the people to his way, and the king was overjoyed and

> Proclaim[ed] Himself in Earth's low sphere to be
> The only and sufficient Deity. (III, 319–20)

---

[*] The name has no origin in classical mythology, and this also applies to the name of the king of the island, Alcithoos. A widely accepted explanation, however, is that Fracastoro took the name Syphilus from the tale in Ovid's *Metamorphoses* of Sipylus, the son of Niobe, who was slain by Apollo, the Sun-God, because Niobe had insulted Latona, Apollo's mother, by boasting that she had 12 children to Latona's meagre two (Ovid, 1961, p.153). The style of Fracastoro's didactic poem and Latin hexametres is probably inspired by Lucretius's *De Rerum Natura* and Virgil's *Georgica*.

But King Alcithoos had failed to take into account the reaction of the offended
Sun-God, who retaliated with terrifying swiftness and power:

> Th'all-seeing Sun no longer could sustain
> These practices, but with enrag'd Disdain
> Darts forth such pestilent malignant Beams,
> As shed Infection on Air, Earth and Streams;
> From whence this Malady its birth receiv'd,
> And first th'offending Syphilus was griev'd,
> Who rais'd forbidden Altars on the Hill,
> And Victims bloud with impious Hands did spill;
> He first wore Buboes dreadfull to the sight,
> First felt strange Pains and sleepless past the Night;
> From him the Malady receiv'd its name. (III, 321–32)

When the disease rose to epidemic proportions, the Sun-God was appealed to and,
after proper sacrifices had been made to him, the God ordered two of his female
deities, Juno and Tellus, to send the people a sacred tree, the guaiacum, as a cure for
the disease. The Spanish sailors learned from the natives how to prepare the remedy,
and 'not forgetfull of their Country's good' (III, 397), freighted their largest ships
with the rich wood.

> *Iberian* Coasts, you first were happy made
> With this rich Plant, and wonder'd at its Aid;
> Known now to *France* and neighbouring *Germany*,
> Cold *Scythian* Coasts and temp'rate *Italy*,
> To *Europe's* Bounds all bless the vital Tree. (III, 401–4)

After the Spanish sailors had learned this legend about the origin of the disease with
which they had been threatened by the bird of the Sun-God, they set sail for their
homeland. But it was too late; they had all caught the disease and, on their return,
they spread it throughout Europe.

## THE GREAT CONTROVERSY

Albrecht Dürer's woodcut reproduced in Figure 4 adorns a broadsheet entitled
*Vaticinium*, or 'prophetic poem'. It was written by the town physician of Nuremberg,
Dietrich Uelzen (*floruit* 1486–96), who here described the new plague in what is
probably the first printed article on syphilis. The Zodiac above the man is inscribed
with the year of the great conjunction between Saturn and Jupiter in the sign of
Scorpio and the house of Mars – an astrological event which was widely regarded
as having inaugurated the new plague (see Figure 9).

Dürer's figure of the syphilitic has often been confused with that of a leper –
and he appears as such in certain works. The confusion is due to the fact that the
papular lesions of syphilis may simulate the nodular lesions of leprosy. Right down
to modern times, gonorrhea, leprosy and syphilis were confused by medical
observers, who allowed such wholly different diseases to go undifferentiated (see
pp.255–61).

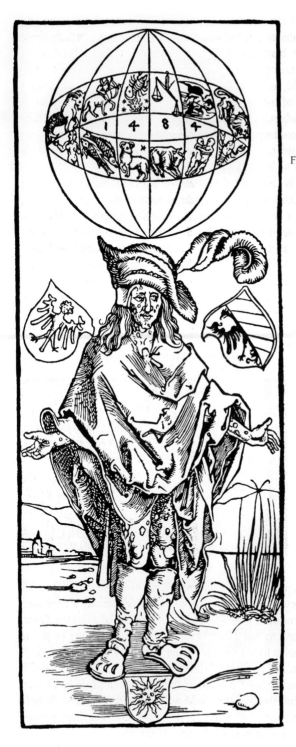

Figure 4. The woodcut of a syphilitic is one of the oldest pictorial renderings of the new disease in Europe. It derives from the hand of Albrecht Dürer (1471–1528) and it is dated August 1, 1496. Dürer later visited Italy from which he wrote a letter on August 18, 1506, asking his prior 'to pray to God for my protection, particularly against the French [pocks], for I know nothing that I dread more since nearly everybody has them. They devour many people, so that they simply die of them' (Fuchs, 1843, p.336).

Syphilis is a systemic disease caused by the spirochete *Treponema pallidum*, usually transmitted through sexual contact but occasionally occurring congenitally from infection in the mother. The historical origin of venereal syphilis is obscure. Indisputable reference to it in European literature occurred only after the return of Columbus from the New World, and a widely held theory of a New World origin was supported when evidence of treponematosis was found in the skeletal remains of pre-Columbian American Indians. On the other hand, 'leprosy' in Europe before 1500 was considered highly contagious, was associated with sexual contact, had hereditary features, and was said to respond to mercury treatment; therefore, it is likely that many cases thought to be leprosy were actually syphilis.

The medical world is still divided over this question: some scholars support the Columbian or New World Theory, while others adhere to the Unitarian or African Theory. According to the latter, syphilis, yaws and the other treponematoses are manifestations of a single disease, the treponemal disease or treponematosis, which is said to have been spread by races emigrating voluntarily from Africa and later forced by the slave trade. The theory postulates that the disease has existed since ancient times and maintains that descriptions of conditions identical with syphilis occur in the Old Testament and in classical and medieval literature. Finally, the theory assumes that a torpid strain of *Treponema pallidum* mutated at the end of the 15th century and became virulent in the wake of the unusual movements of populations in the Age of Discovery.

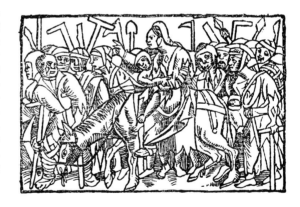

Figure 5. A Rabelaisian poem entitled *The Triumph of the High and Mighty Dame Syphilis* was published by an anonymous author at Lyons in 1539. The poem's final woodcut of a series of 38 shows 'the baggage' or impedimenta of Dame Syphilis's triumphal procession with its diseased and crippled soldiers and a whore riding on a horse with her child – a figure symbolizing the 'infecting Venus' (Montaiglon, 1874, emblema XLVII).

Historical sources show that syphilis was spread by sailors and soldiers at the end of the 15th century, just as they seem to indicate that the disease was a new one and, to all appearances, first introduced into Spain by the explorers of America. From here the disease was transmitted to the army of Charles VIII of France (*regnebat* 1483–98) by Spanish mercenaries in his service. When, in 1494, the French king crossed the Alps to assert by force of arms his claim to the throne of Naples, syphilis was brought into Italy, where an epidemic occurred during the siege of Naples in early 1495. The plague did what the Italians could not and compelled the French to evacuate the city. In the spring of 1495 the army was in undisciplined retreat from Italy, carrying with it the new disease to the rest of Europe.

The unmitigated intensity of the great syphilitic epidemic in Europe at the end of the 15th century is probably explained by several factors. It is likely that the strain of *Treponema pallidum* then operating was more virulent than that now encountered, just as a disease is frequently at its most virulent during the exponential phase of an epidemic. Second, there was very likely no 'herd immunity' to syphilis among 15th-century Europeans, who may have succumbed finally to the phenomenon of 'disease synergy'. The Oslo Study showed that syphilis produced a mortality rate in excess of that which was directly attributable to the disease itself (Gjestland, 1955, pp.343–55).

Malnutrition and intercurrent illness probably exacerbated syphilis, and since these were prevalent among armies of earlier times, many more men were often lost to disease than to battle. The poorly provisioned 15th-century armies were at particular risk and as such became an important vector for the pan-continental spread of syphilis.

## THE SERPENTINE DISEASE

Girolamo Fracastoro was one of the four great syphilographers of the 16th century, the three others being the physicians Ruy Diaz de Isla (1462–1542), Francisco Lopez de Villalobos (c. 1473–1550), and Giovanni de Vigo (1450–1525). Diaz de Isla was close to the events since he worked on the Iberian peninsula at the time when Columbus's crew returned from their American expedition. Between 1510 and 1521 he wrote a book which was published in 1539 at Seville under the title *Tractado contra el Mal Serpentino: que vulgarmente en España es llamado Bubas* ('Treatise against the Serpentine Disease, which in Spain is commonly called the Buboes'). In his first chapter on *The Serpentine Disease* he treats of its origin:

> 'It has pleased Divine Justice to give and send us unknown afflictions, never seen or recognized or found in medical books, such as this *serpentine disease*. The which turned up and was observed in Spain in the year of Our Lord 1493 in the city of Barcelona, which city was infected and in consequence all Europe and the universe in all known and communicable regions; the which disease had its origin and birth once and for all in the island now called Hispaniola [Haiti], as has been determined by wide and infallible experience. And as this island was discovered by the Admiral Don Cristobal Colon [Christopher Columbus], at that time holding conversation and communication with the people thereof, and as the disease is contagious, it easily laid hold of them and presently was seen in the fleet itself. And as it was a disease never seen nor known by the Spaniards, although they felt pains and other effects of the aforesaid malady, they attributed it to the hardships of the sea, or to other causes according to the fancy of each of them. At the time the said Admiral Don Cristobal Colon arrived in Spain the Catholic Sovereigns were in the city of Barcelona. And when they went to give an account of their voyage and their discoveries, straightway the city began to be infected and the said disease began to spread, as was later seen by wide experience; and as the disease was not known and was so frightful, those who observed it had resort to much fasting and prayer and charity that Our Lord might keep them from falling prey to such a disease. And in the following year, 1494, the Most Christian King, Charles of France, who at that time was reigning, collected a great host and marched into Italy, and when he entered the country with his army, many Spaniards infected with this disease were with him,

and immediately the camp was infected with the said malady; and the French, as they did not know what it was, thought that it came from the atmosphere of that country. The French called it the *Disease of Naples*. And the Italians and Neapolitans, as they had never been acquainted with such a disease, called it the *French Disease*. From that time on as it continued to spread, they gave it a name, each one according to his opinion as to how the disease had its origin. In Castilia they called it *Bubas*, and in Portugal the *Castilian Disease*, and in Portuguese India the Indians called it the *Portuguese Disease*. Just as we here used to speak of pains, tumors, and ulcers as buboes, the Indians of Hispaniola formerly called this disease *Guaynaras, hipas, taybas* and *iças*. I call it the *Serpentine Disease of the Island of Hispaniola*...because according to its loathsomeness I do not know anything to which I could more naturally compare it than to the serpent. For as the serpent is abominable, terrifying and horrible, so is this disease abominable, terrifying and horrible. A grave disease that separates and corrupts the flesh and breaks and rots the bones and disrupts and contracts the sinews, and consequently I give it that name.' (Bloch, 1901–11, pp. 180–1, 306–7. Trans. J. Fabricius)

## THE POISONOUS SERPENT OF SYPHILITIC INFECTION

Figure 6. Four hundred years after Diaz de Isla published his treatise against *The Serpentine Disease*, a Danish artist created this poster. The inscription reads: 'Warning: venereal diseases are more common and more malicious than ever.' The poster was published against syphilis and gonorrhea, which had exploded among the population after the German occupation of Denmark in 1940. The serpentine symbol for syphilis commonly used by Diaz de Isla and the Danish artist Anton Hansen (1891–1960) was probably an unconscious echo of the serpentine drama with which the Bible opens. In the Garden of Eden, Eve was tempted by the Serpent and so brought about the Fall of Adam: 'And the eyes of them both were opened, and they knew that they were naked...And Adam knew Eve his wife; and she conceived, and bare Cain' (Genesis 3:7; 4:1). The biblical Serpent's association with nakedness and sexuality, temptation and fall, crime and punishment, made it an apt symbol for the new venereal disease in Europe. In the work of two of the greatest poets of European culture, Shakespeare and Goethe, the serpent emerges as their metaphorical expression for the dreaded disease and its poisonous effects. In a collection of poems entitled *Römische Elegien* (1795), Johann Wolfgang von Goethe (1749–1832) describes his Bohemian life and amorous experiences in Rome during the years 1788–90. In the second of four elegies which he never ventured to publish, Goethe voices his fears that the

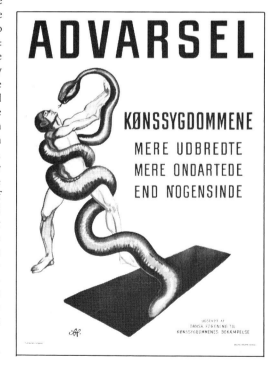

syphilitic serpent may sting him in the course of his sexual exploits:

> Doch welch ein feindlicher Gott hat uns im Zorne die neue
> Ungeheure Geburt giftigen Schlammes gesandt?
> Überall schleicht er sich ein, und in den lieblichsten Gärtchen
> Lauert tückisch der Wurm, packt den Geniessenden an.
> Sei mir, hesperischer Drache, gegrüsst, du zeigtest dich mutig,
> Du verteidigtest kühn goldener Äpfel Besitz!
> Aber dieser verteidiget nichts – und wo er sich findet,
> Sind die Gärten, die Frucht keiner Verteidigung wert.
> Heimlich krümmet er sich im Busche, besudelt die Quellen,
> Geifert, wandelt in Gift Amors belebenden Tau.
>
> …
>
> Eins nur fleh ich im stillen, an euch, ihr Grazien, wend ich
> Dieses heisse Gebet tief aus dem Busen herauf:
> Schützet immer mein kleines, mein artiges Gärtchen, entfernet
> Jegliches Übel von mir; reichet mir Amor die Hand,
> Oh! So gebet mir stets, sobald ich dem Schelmen vertraue,
> Ohne Sorgen und Furcht, ohne Gefahr den Genuss. (Goethe, 1949, pp.223–6)[*]

The poem presents love and syphilitic infection in the same metaphorical setting as Shakespeare's *Hamlet* (1,5:35–91), where a similar catastrophe lies in wait for King Hamlet while he is 'sleeping in my orchard' (1,5:35). Here a 'serpent' (1,5:36,39) stings him in the shape of Claudius – a 'treacherous, lecherous, kindless villain' (2,2:576–7) who has seduced and 'whored' (5,2:64) the former King's wife in a *drame à trois* which has poisonous consequences for all the partners involved (see pp.46 and 231–3). 'Let heaven requite it with the serpent's curse' (4,2:16), cries Emilia in a bawdy context in *Othello* when denouncing Desdemona's slanderer, Iago – 'hell gnaw his bones' (4,2:138). Another English poet availing himself of serpentine imagery in describing 'the pox' is the satirist Samuel Rowlands (1570?–1630?). In *The Letting of Humours Blood in the Head-Vaine* (1600), he describes the return of a countryman with the 'French disease':

> This Gentleman hath serued long in Fraunce,
> And is returned filthy full of French,
> In single combat, being hurt by chaunce,
> As he was closely foyling at a Wench:
> Yet hot alarmes he hath endur'd good store,
> But neuer in like pockie heate before.
>
> He had no sooner drawne, and ventred ny-her,
> Intending onely but to haue a bout,
> When she his Flaske and Touch-boxe set on fyer,
> And till this hower the burning is not out.
> Iudge, was not valour in this Martiall wight,
> That with a spit-fier Serpent so durst fight.
>
> 　　　　　　　　　　　　　　(Rowlands, 1880, vol.1, p.15)

---

[*]　　O, what an inimical god has spitefully sent us / This novel, monstrous birth of poisonous dregs?/ Everywhere it sneaks in, and in the loveliest gardens / The treacherous serpent hides, waiting for pleasure-loving couples. / I greet thee, Hesperian dragon, who showed thy courage / When boldly defending the golden apples in the paradisical Garden. / But this dragon defends nothing, and where it lurks, / The gardens and their fruits are not worth protection. / In secret it crouches in the bush, defiling the sources, / Changing to poison with its foam Cupid's life-giving dew…
For one thing only I pray – to you Graces / I send up from my bosom my most ardent prayer:/ Protect for ever my little, pleasant garden; and take away / Every evil disease from me. And when Cupid gives me his hand, / O, so grant me always whenever I trust the little rogue / His offered delights without worry, fear or danger. (Translation by J. Fabricius)

## THE SYPHILITIC EPIDEMIC AS A DIVINE PUNISHMENT

More than a quarter of a century before Fracastoro and Diaz de Isla published their works on syphilis, a Spanish doctor named Francisco Lopez de Villalobos wrote a long poem on the same disease. Because the syphilitic pustules in Spain were called *bubas*, Villalobos entitled his poem *Tratado sobre las pestiferas bubas* and had it published in 1498 in Salamanca. Here he stated that the illness had started in 1494 and that it was a new and extremely contagious disease. Villalobos's description of the ravages of the new disease rivals Diaz de Isla's description of the horrors of 'The Serpentine Disease':

> III
> It was a pestilence ne'er to be found at all
> In verse or in prose, in science or in story,
> So evil and perverse and cruel past control,
> Exceedingly contagious, and in filth so prodigal,
> So strong to hold its own, there is little got of glory;
> And it makes one dark in feature and obscure in countenance,
> Hunchback'd and indisposed, and seldom much at ease,
> And it makes one pained and crippled in such sort as never was,
> A scoundrel sort of thing, which also doth commence
> In the rascalliest place that a man has. (Major, 1939, p.18)

Unlike a number of other diseases which more commonly struck the poor, syphilis in no way spared the great and was therefore particularly suited to be viewed as due to God's wrath. In several stanzas Villalobos voices his belief, in common with the doctors and priests of his age, that the plague was sent by an angry God in punishment of the many sins committed by man. In stanza IV he states the opinion of some theologians as to the supervention of the new disease, while in stanza VIII he gives the opinion of another class of theologians:

> IV
> Theologians pretend the cause of it doth lie
> In certain new-found sins that are rife in Christendom.
> Oh! Providence divine, oh! judgement from on high!
> Which ever hast in store a perfect penalty.
> Howe'er we go astray, our folly is brought home.

> VIII
> But some to luxury, and all of wanton sense,
> To which the world is giv'n do refer the same.
> The ailment, say they, is a just and proper sentence;
> According to the sin so is the repentance,
> And the part that suffers most is the part most to blame.
> (Major, 1939, p.19)

## THE HIGH CONTAGIOUSNESS OF THE 'POX'

One of the eyewitnesses of the first wave of the epidemic of syphilis in Europe was the Italian physician Giovanni de Vigo, who became the private physician of Pope

Julius II in 1503. In 1514 he published in Rome his famous work *Practica copiosa in arte chirurgica*, which sums up all the surgical learning of his time and was so successful that it ran to 52 editions. In the fifth chapter of the volume, entitled 'De morbo gallico', he explored the new disease (see pp.67–9), at the same time as he reminded the reader of its most dreaded aspect: 'It was and it is still, as stated before, a contagious disease, and in particular through coitus: the copulation of a man with an unclean woman, or vice versa' (Vigo, 1520, p.73).

Soon it was discovered, however, that other means of transmission were possible. The public baths of medieval towns, the barbers' shops, the drinking cups shared in homes and taverns, and the custom of kissing were all found to be dangerous and infectious. In Erasmus's colloquy *A Marriage in Name Only* (1523), Gabriel informs Petronius that 'the disease is transmitted not by one means alone but spreads to other persons by a kiss, by conversation, by touch, by having a little drink together' (Erasmus, 1965, p.410).

In another of Erasmus's colloquies, *Inns* (1523), William tells Bertulf: 'Twenty-five years ago nothing was more customary among us than public steam baths. Now these are cold everywhere, for the new scab has taught us to let them alone' (Erasmus, 1965, p.150).

The new disease soon became so common that it appeared to Shakespeare as something inevitable. In *2 Henry IV*, Falstaff says:

> 'A man can no more separate age and covetousness that he can part young limbs and lechery. But the gout galls the one and the pox pinches the other…A pox of this gout! Or a gout of this pox! For the one or the other plays the rogue with my great toe.' (1,2:229–32;244–6)

Widespread dread of the numerous sources of infection, combined with exaggerated ideas of the contagiousness of the 'pox', caused enlightened men like Erasmus to protest against the customs of the time and to call for radical public measures. In *A Marriage in Name Only*, Gabriel tells Petronius:

GAB.   This disease is simply slow but sure death, or rather burial. Victims are wrapped like corpses in cloths and unguents.

PET.   Very true. At least so deadly a disease as this should have been treated with the same care as leprosy. But if this is too much to ask, no one should let his beard be cut, or else everybody should act as his own barber.

GAB.   What if everyone kept his mouth shut?

PET.   They'd spread the disease through the nose.

GAB.   There's a remedy for that trouble, too.

PET.   What?

GAB.   Let them imitate the alchemists: wear a mask that admits light through glass windows and allows you to breathe through mouth and nose by means of a tube extending from the mask over your shoulders and down your back.

PET.   Fine, if there were nothing to fear from contact with fingers, sheets, combs, and scissors.

GAB.   Then it would be best to let your beard grow to your knees.

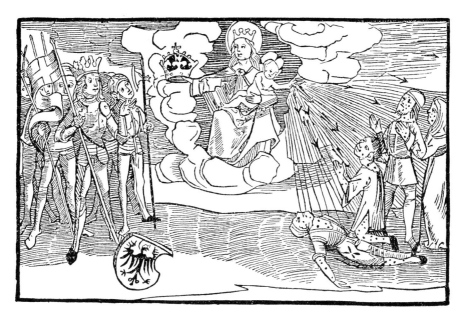

Figure 7. In September 1496, the German professor of jurisprudence Sebastian Brant (1457–1521), author
of the didactic-satiric poem *The Ship of Fools* (1494), published a flyleaf at Basel with the title *Eulogium
de pestilentialis scorra sive mala de Franzos*. The flyleaf was adorned with the above woodcut and it described
in poetic form the skin symptoms of the 'French disease'. Like the Frisian poet-physician Dietrich
Uelzen, Sebastian Brant presumed the cause of the new plague to be in the stars, but he also connected
it with the 'mortal sin' (*exitiale Nephas*) whose time for expiation had now come. Probably Brant was
here drawing attention to the same crime which the Holy Roman Emperor Maximilian (*regnebat
1493–1519*) shortly afterwards emphasized in his *Edict against the Blasphemous*, issued on February 1,
1497. It is the earliest known German state document on syphilis, and it shows that the new disease
had spread to the whole of Germany by 1495–96. The Edict summoned the inhabitants of the Holy
Roman Empire 'to avoid all blasphemies and oaths uttered in the name of God and his holiest members'
(Haustein, 1930, p.319). In former times, such 'maltreatment' (*misshandtlung*) of God had had dire
consequences, 'and in our own time', the Edict went on, 'it is evident that all sorts of plagues and
punishments have ensued, especially now with the serious diseases and curses on men that are called
the evil blisters (*bösen blattern*), which mankind has never known nor heard of. We think them expressions
of God's proper justice' (p.319). The woodcut on Brant's flyleaf expresses a similar view, the Queen of
Heaven holding out the crown to Maximilian, while the Christ Child shoots his fatal arrows against
the syphilitic sinners on Earth.

PET.   Evidently. In the next place, make a law that the same man may not be both
        barber and surgeon.

GAB.   You'd reduce the barbers to starvation.

PET.   Let them cut costs and raise prices a little.

GAB.   Passed.

PET.    Then make a law to prohibit the common drinking cup.

GAB.    England would hardly stand for that!

PET.    And don't let two share the same bed unless they're husband and wife.

GAB.    Accepted.

PET.    Furthermore, don't permit a guest at an inn to sleep in sheets anyone else has slept in.

GAB.    What will you do with the Germans, who wash theirs barely twice a year?

PET.    Let them get after the washerwomen. Moreover, abolish the custom, no matter how ancient, of greeting with a kiss.

GAB.    Not even in church?

PET.    Let everyone put his hand against the board.[*]

GAB.    What about conversation?

PET.    Avoid the Homeric advice to 'bend the head near', and let the listener in turn close his lips tight.

GAB.    The Twelve Tablets would scarcely suffice for these laws.
        (Erasmus, 1965, pp.411–12)

Erasmus's observations reveal his understanding of the extragenital means of transmission of syphilis and also his dawning awareness of the mechanisms of infection. These were later described by his great contemporary Girolamo Fracastoro, who in 1546 outlined his conception of epidemic diseases in *De contagione et contagiosis morbis*. Here he stated that each is caused by a different type of rapidly multiplying minute body, and that these bodies are transferred from the infector to the infected in three ways: by direct contact; by indirect contact with carriers such as soiled clothing and linen; and by transmission through the air. Fracastoro's theory of micro-organisms as a possible cause of disease was the first scientific statement of the true nature of contagion, infection, disease germs, and modes of disease transmission and, significantly, his revolutionary contribution to medicine grew out of his studies of the new venereal disease, to which he gave the name syphilis (see pp.1–3).

## THE POISONED KISS AND BREATH

The profound way in which the new venereal epidemic affected social customs and manners is nowhere more apparent than in its poisoning of the general custom of touching with the lips as a sign of love or as a greeting. This affective gesture presented a real danger, since the secondary lesions of syphilis, especially the ones in moist areas such as the lips and the mouth, teem with spirochetes and are the most contagious of all the sores in the commoner treponematoses. Especially in England, the kissing custom seems to have been widely practised and hence to have been a source of venereal infection. The German merchant Samuel Kiechel, visiting England in 1585, says that 'when a foreigner or an inhabitant goes to a citizen's house on business, or is invited as a guest, and having entered therein, he is received

---

[*]   A small tablet or plaque kissed by the celebrant at Mass and then by each of the worshippers.

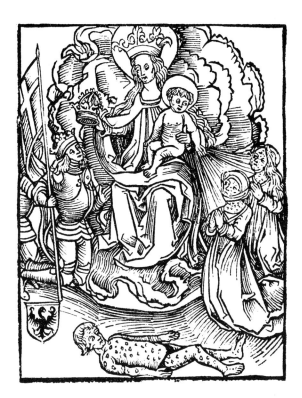

Figure 8. In 1496, there appeared at Augsburg the first dated book on syphilis, printed in November in a Latin and, on December 17, in a German edition under the titles *Tractatus de pestilentiali scorra sive mala de franczos* and *Ein hübscher Tractat von dem Ursprung des Bösen Franzos*, both by the publisher Hans Schauer. The author was Joseph Grünpeck (c. 1473-c. 1550), a layman who later contracted syphilis himself. His book is strongly influenced by Sebastian Brant's poem which it reproduces in full, commenting on it and discussing at length the astrological facts and their causal relation to the new plague (see Figure 9). Grünpeck describes the terrible scourge that is syphilis and gives directions for avoiding it, and (in the Latin edition) various cures for the 'wild warts' (*die wilden wartzen*). He recommends that sufferers consult a physician, but also refers the patient to mercurial inunction as a remedy, and to a gargle to combat stomatitis which occurs as a side-effect of mercurial chemotherapy. The woodcut of the title-page is strongly inspired by the illustration of Sebastian Brant's poem (Figure 7).

by the master of the house, the lady, or the daughter, and by them welcomed (*willkommen heisst*), – as it is termed in their language – he has even a right to take them by the arm and to kiss them (*zu küssen*), which is the custom of the country; and if any one does not do so, it is regarded and imputed as ignorance and ill-breeding on his part. The same custom is also observed in the Netherlands' (Rye, 1967, p.90).

Another foreign merchant, Alessandro Magno, visiting London in 1562, observed that 'Many of the young women gather outside Moorgate and play with young lads, even though they do not know them. Often, during these games, the women are thrown to the ground by the young men who only allow them to get up after they have kissed them. They kiss each other a lot. If a stranger enters a house and does not first of all kiss the mistress on the lips, they think him badly brought up' (Magno, 1983, p.144; see also Camden, 1975, pp.164–5).

Middleton's play *Women Beware Women* (1657) testifies to the dangers of this custom. 'You make your lip so strange', says Leantio during a quarrel with his newly-wed wife, Bianca, who answers him:

> Is there no kindness betwixt man and wife,
> Unless they make a pigeon-house of friendship,
> And be still billing? 'tis the idlest fondness
> That ever was invented, and 'tis pity
> It's grown a fashion for poor gentlewomen;
> There's many a disease kiss'd in a year by't,
> And a French curtsy made to't: alas, sir! (3,1:158–65)

In addition to kissing, Erasmus, at the end of *A Marriage in Name Only*, hints at breathing as an agent of syphilitic infection. This idea of the airborne transmission of the new contagion was later established as a scientific fact by Fracastoro. In *De contagione* he stated his conviction that the air 'was the source of this disease' (Fracastoro, 1930, p.149), and that the air had become 'putrefied' because of the detrimental conjunction of Saturn, Jupiter, and Mars in 1484 (Figure 9). 'We may believe that when that conjunction of heavenly bodies occurred', he finished his ominous reasoning, 'it drew forth an immense amount of vapours. These mingled with the air and were agitated in diverse ways and directions, until finally they induced a foul putrefaction, and the germs from it were carried to us' (p.151). In similar fashion, concluded Fracastoro, the foul breath of the syphilized person became the carrier of putrefied germs and an agent of disease transmission.

In England this popular but erroneous conception of syphilitic infection was used as a political weapon in the anti-cleric nobles' attempt to overthrow the King's Lord Chancellor, Thomas Wolsey (1475?–1530). One of the charges against the ambitious and arrogant Cardinal was that he had intended to kill King Henry VIII (*regnebat* 1509–47) by infecting him with his own 'foul and contagious disease'. In the Articles of Arraignment of Wolsey in the House of Peers, the sixth charge was: 'The same Lord Cardinall, knowing himself to have the foul and contagious disease of the great pox, broken out upon him in divers places of his body, came daily to your Grace [the King], rowning in your ear, and blowing upon your most noble Grace with his perilous and infective breath, to the marvellous danger of your Highness. And when he was once healed of them, he made your Grace believe that his disease was an impostume in his head, and of none other thing' (Edward, 1649, p.267).

By the time Francis Bacon (1561–1626) wrote his famous essays and treatises, it appears that enlightened men had arrived at a more realistic opinion of syphilitic infection and its ways of transmission. In his natural history *Sylva Sylvarum* (1627), the English philosopher and scientist included syphilis among those 'infectious diseases' that 'are merely in the humours, and not in the spirits, breath, or exhalations; and therefore they never infect but by touch only; and such a touch also as cometh within the *epidermis*; as the venom of the French pox, and the biting of a mad dog' (Bacon, 1857–74, vol.2, p.439).

Still, the origin of syphilis remained a mystery to the inquiring minds of the Renaissance, who advanced a number of ingenious theories to meet the challenge. While Fracastoro, Villalobos, Uelzen, Brant, Grünpeck, Stäber, Gilino, Torella, Pintor and Almenar assumed an astrological origin of the disease, Manardus, Leoniceno, Aquila and Matthioli postulated its origin from leprosy. Francis Bacon, who was convinced of 'the venomous quality of man's flesh' (Bacon, 1857–74, vol.2, p.347), especially in its putrefied stage, endorsed what was perhaps the most fantastic theory of all. 'The French,' he wrote in *Sylva Sylvarum*,

> 'do report, that at the siege of Naples [in 1495] there were certain wicked merchants that barrelled up man's flesh (of some that had been lately slain in Barbary) and sold it for tunney; and that upon that foul and high nourishment was the original of that disease. Which may well be; for that it is certain that the cannibals in the West Indies eat man's flesh; and the West Indies were full of the pocks when they were first discovered.' (pp.347–8)

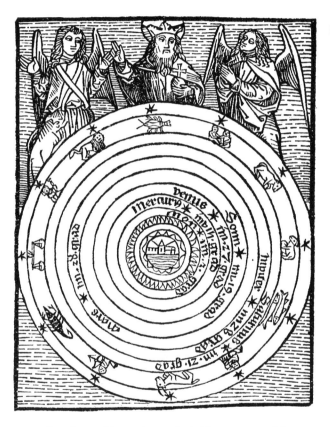

Figure 9. The woodcut from Joseph Grünpeck's treatise on syphilis *Tractatus de pestilentiali scorra sive mala de franczos* (Nuremberg, 1496) provides a geocentric representation of the universe which shows the relevant positions of the planets at the creation of the world. The inexorable mechanism of this celestial clock, asserts Grünpeck, led to the great conjunction in 1484 of Saturn and Jupiter in the sign of the Scorpion. A venereal plague had to result from this event since Scorpio rules the genitals, while Jupiter signifies expansion and Saturn death. The divine will behind the fatal cosmic and medical events is symbolized by the figures at the top of the woodcut. A second interesting astrological interpretation of the time was advanced by Pedro Pintor (1423–1503), private physician to Pope Alexander VI Borgia, who, in a treatise on syphilis entitled *De morbo foetido et occulto, his temporibus affligente* (Rome, 1500), predicted that the French disease would disappear with the changing position of the planets in the Zodiac: 'We believe that this disease will continue until Saturn is in the Bull, and that consequently it will terminate in the year 1500' (Vorberg, 1924, p.99).

In *A Marriage in Name Only* (1523), Erasmus renders the story of a 'young nobleman' named Pompilius who is 'a reprobate whoremonger' (Erasmus, 1965, pp.403, 406) and prematurely aged because of his hideous disease, like the soldier in *The Soldier and the Carthusian*. In the colloquy, Erasmus strongly attacks a married couple who allow their daughter of sixteen to be married to the syphilitic Pompilius. The case affords Erasmus an opportunity for giving his unsparing denunciation of parents who allow a daughter to marry a diseased man, and leads him to appeal to the authorities to establish some sort of registration before a marriage licence is given. 'It is amazing', concludes Petronius, 'that princes, whose duty it is to look out for the commonwealth, at least in matters pertaining to the person – and in this regard nothing is more important than sound health – don't devise some remedy for this situation. So huge a plague has filled a large part of the globe – and yet they go on snoring as if it made no difference at all' (pp.408–9).

After Erasmus's observations, we can appreciate better the passage in his friend Thomas More's *Utopia* (1516) which assures us that in Utopia an affianced pair are shown to each other naked to prevent ignorance or deception about the health of the future partner. 'In the choice of wives they carefully follow a custom which seemed to us foolish and absurd', More relates. 'Before marriage some responsible and honourable woman, either a virgin or a widow, presents the woman naked to her suitor and after that some upright man presents the suitor naked to the woman' (More, 1968, vol.1, p.413).

Another interesting feature in Utopia is the way in which its inhabitants are restrained from promiscuity: 'If a man (or woman) is convicted of an illicit affair before marriage, he is severely punished and marriage is denied him for his whole life, unless a prince's pardon remits the punishment' (p.413). As to married couples, More goes on, the Utopians 'punish adulterers with the severest bondage. If both parties are married, they are divorced, and the injured persons may be married to one another or to someone else…If anybody commits adultery a second time, his punishment is death' (p.414).

Erasmus's observations and More's proposals in *Utopia* reflect a dramatic change of public opinion in regard to sexual customs and regulations, and strongly contrast with the promiscuous manners and liberal mores of the late Middle Ages. This change, which highlights the connection between microbes and morals, we shall study at closer range in our next section.

In the period between 1450 and 1550, Western European civilization burst the shackles of the Middle Ages and, with the Renaissance, introduced a number of revolutionary changes in philosophy and science, art and religion, technology and communication. The invention of printing, the discovery of America and of a water route to the Far East, the heliocentric arrangement of the solar system, the development of Renaissance art, the beginnings of modern physics and medicine, and the Protestant Reformation all occurred within this short period of time. A galaxy of names marks these cultural achievements, which are among the most significant events in history: Gutenberg, Columbus, Vasco da Gama, Magellan, Copernicus, Michelangelo, Leonardo da Vinci, Paracelsus, Fracastoro, Vesalius, Luther, and Calvin.

The ships that left the European seaports to open up the world to the West inaugurated the Age of Discovery, which greatly stimulated commerce and economy in Western Europe and gave rise to a prosperous class of merchants, shipowners, and industrialists in the growing cities. The new spirit of adventure and conquest was set against a permissive society which enjoyed a freedom between the sexes not realized since antiquity. The bath houses at the end of the 15th century in which men and women bathed naked together are a monument to this sexual freedom of Renaissance man, which was reflected in a widespread promiscuity at all levels of society. Even the clergy participated in these liberal mores, with the popes of the Renaissance giving the lead.

Then came the syphilitic shock, at the moment when the Renaissance was beginning to unfold its petals into full bloom. The epidemic proportions of the new plague and the virulence of its effects turned the promiscuous habits of the time into a mortal danger. The bath houses were the first to suffer, and their closure was followed by restrictive measures directed against prostitutes and brothels in all cities of Europe (see pp.57–61).

Soon the microbes of the Renaissance had repercussions also in the field of religion and morals, where theologians such as Martin Luther (1483–1546) and Jean Calvin (1509–64) steered the development of Protestant ethics in the direction of sexual puritanism. Both reformers glorified marriage as a divine institution and violently denounced sexuality outside marriage. At a time when syphilis was raging all over Germany, Luther held a 'Sermon on Marriage' (*Predigt vom ehelichen Leben*), 1522, in which he thundered: 'Now it rests with the secular sword and the authorities to kill the adulterer, for he who breaks his marriage has already severed himself from life and is to be regarded as a dead human being...And in those places where the authorities are weak and negligent and do not kill, the adulterer may move on to another far country and propose to women if he cannot resist the temptation. However, to avoid such a bad example, it would be better if one made short work of him and killed him' (*aber es were besser, todt todt mit yhm, umb bösses exempels willen zu meyden*) (Luther, 1907, p.289).

In Geneva, Switzerland, Calvin reformed the city along the lines of moral austerity that later came to be labelled 'Puritan'. Dancing was regarded as a diabolical incitement to lust and was prohibited together with drama and music. The numerous taverns and brothels in the city were closed and prostitution ruthlessly suppressed. To Calvin's Scottish pupil, John Knox (1502–72), the city appeared as 'a perfect school of Christ', and when Calvinism spread to England and Scotland, the Puritans clamoured for the introduction of measures similar to those that Calvin had instituted in Geneva. In Elizabethan England, for example, Puritan extremists such as Philip Stubbes and Thomas Lupton agitated for capital punishment to stop 'whoredom' and the spread of the venereal plague. In *The Anatomie of Abuses* (1583), Philip Stubbes fulminated:

'I would wish that the man or woman who are certainly known without all scruple or doubt to have committed the horrible fact of whoredom, adultery, incest or fornication either should drink a full draught of *Moyses* cup, that is, taste of present death; or else, if that be thought too severe (for in evil, men will be more merciful than the Author of mercy himself, but in goodness, farewell mercy) then would God they might be cauterized and seared with a hot iron on the cheek, forehead, or some other part of their body that might be seen, to the end [that] the honest and chaste Christians might be discerned from the adulterous Children of Satan. But alas, this vice (with the rest) wants such due punishment as God his Word does command to be executed thereupon.' (Stubbes, 1877–9, p.99)

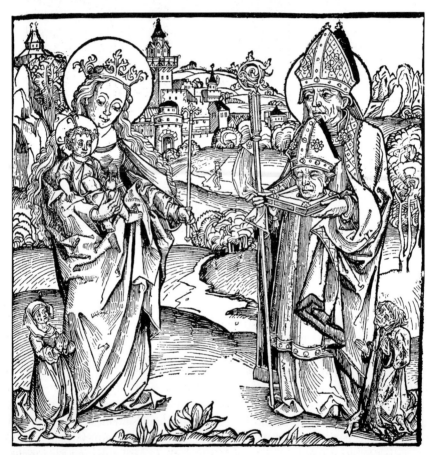

Figure 10. In this woodcut by the German artist Georg Stuchs, yet another French saint is appealed to by sufferers of the French disease. St. Denis (Dionysius) (right) was the first bishop of Paris and the patron saint of France, executed about 258 AD during a persecution of Christians under Emperor Valerianus. According to legend, St. Denis, after his beheading on Montmartre (*Mons martyrium*), walked with his head in his hand to the abbey at St. Denis. On the Nuremberg flyleaf published c. 1496, he is implored by a syphilitic man and woman kneeling before him and the Holy Virgin with the Child: 'Protect me against the horrible disease which is called the French disease and for which you in France have healed a great number of Christians' (Sudhoff, 1912, Tafel XX. The prayer to St. Denis is printed under the picture).

Figure 11. The condemnation of promiscuity and the elevation of premarital chastity were also expressed by contemporary artists. The woodcut shows the Wedding of Youth and Cleanness in Stephen Hawes's (1475–1523?) allegorical poem, the *Example of Virtue* (1509). The poem describes the transformation of Youth into the figure of Virtue after his struggle with a lady on a goat representing Sensuality and his conquest of a three-headed monster representing the World, the Flesh and the Devil. Having passed the test, Virtue is rewarded by the King of

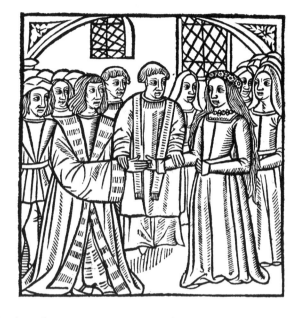

Love, who gives him his daughter Cleanness in marriage. In Hawes's vision, 'Saynt Ierome' himself performs the ceremony (above), accompanied by tolling bells, organ music and the song of angels, coming 'down from heuen hye' (Hawes, 1974, p.60).

'If that I could paint out foule lecherie In her deformed shape and loathsome plight', another English poet wrote about 1600, in reference to 'the French disease',

> Or if I could paint spotlesse Chastitie,
> In her true portraiture and colours bright,
> I thinke no maid would euer proue an whore,
> But euerie maid would chastitie adore. (Lane, 1876, p.133)

'He that stealyth is hanged', observed another Puritan, Henry Brinklow (d. 1546), 'and why ought not he also to be hanged that commytteth adultery?' (Brinklow, 1874, p.18).

Such suggestions from the Puritan quarter may give an indication of the serious threat to public health posed by promiscuity and prostitution. Morals were clearly affected by the new venereal scourge, and there is evidence that enlightened men reasoned along the same lines as Erasmus and More, Luther and Calvin. In England, for example, the leading humanist and clerical reformer John Colet (1467?–1519), a close friend of Erasmus's, emphasized the necessity of premarital chastity because of the dangers of syphilitic infection incurred through promiscuous living, or 'misuse of the flesh', as the clergyman phrased it. In a sermon held some time before his death in 1519, Colet gave the youth of his parish, congregated in St. Paul's Cathedral, 'A ryght fruitfull monicion'. 'If thou be laye and vnmaryed', he admonished his youngsters, 'kepe the[e] clene vnto the tyme thou be maryed. And remember the sore and terrible punysshement of Noes flood, and of the terryble fyre and brymstone, and sore punysshement of Sodom and Gomor, don to man for misusying of the flesshe. And in especyall, call to remembraunce the meruailous and horryble punysshment of the abhominable great pockes, dayly apperynge to our sightes, growynge in and vpon mannes flesshe; the whiche soore punysshement, euery thynge well remembred, can not be thought but principally for the inordinate misuse of the fleshe' (Lupton, 1909, pp.307–8).

## THE FATAL MICROBES OF THE RENAISSANCE

The extreme contagiousness of the 'pox' during the first wave of the syphilitic epidemic in Europe was due to the way in which the spirochete *Treponema pallidum* moves from host to host via the skin and the mucous membranes of the mouth and the sex organs. The treponemal spirochete is a close-coiled, slender and regular spiral organism which propels itself by rotating and changing its shape. Once the spirochetes have penetrated a break in the skin – the tiniest scratch is enough – or a moist body surface, they divide every 30 *hours*, rather than in the 20 or 30 *minutes* in which most disease bacteria divide. The growth rate of the treponematoses is therefore considerably slower than that of other diseases. It is estimated that several hundred spirochetes are usually present during the transmitting event, whether it is venereal or not. Some of them fail to get through and die in the attempt; and, depending on the stage of the disease in the source, some may not survive after they get through. However, when the infection comes from an early, active stage of the disease, the spirochetes are able to escape initial host defence and to go on multiplying themselves in the organism. This is the highest degree of infectiousness we know.

The low degree of immunity in the population of Renaissance Europe and the sexual means of transmission of syphilis, combined with its non-venereal possibilities of transmission, soon turned the new disease into a devastating plague. A syphilitic barber, an infected cup or towel, or a kiss from a diseased person were enough to pass on the disease. Contemporary sources amply convey the horror which the 'pox' inspired in all quarters of the population, while also testifying to the hysteria to which fears of contamination led. 'It proceeds also by lying in vncleane lynnen', wrote the Scottish surgeon Peter Lowe (1550?–1612?), 'by wearing the garments of them which are infected, and by lying with such as haue any spyces of it. So that we see many by that meanes infected, without any company of women. Moreouer, it proceedes also by sucking the Nurse any way diseased with this sicknes, by drinking after them which haue Vlcers in their throat, by kissing or receiuing the breath of such as are infected, and by sitting on the priuie after them, & sometimes by treading bare-footed on the spettle of those which haue beene long corrupted' (Lowe, 1596, sig.B2$^r$).[*]

---

[*] 'It happeneth also a man to be infected by sweat', another syphilographer, Phillipp Hermann, wrote in *An Excellent Treatise Teaching How to Cure the French Pockes* (1590), 'and that commeth by lying with another, for when one man lieth with another that is infected, and the same doo sweat sore, hee must needes be infected with the venome of his sweate. But this infection dooth not alwaies chaunce, for if the person infected haue had it a long time, and that it doth not appeare outwardly, but lyeth hidden inwardlie, he dooth not infect so sore, nor so soone as those that are but newlie infected with it. Therefore let euery man take heede, that he doo not lye with them whom he knoweth not, for that it is very dangerous' (Hermann, 1590, p.3).

The fatal microbes of the Renaissance particularly affected the relations between the sexes, where they introduced a hitherto unknown element of anxiety, suspicion and circumspection. Shakespeare's *The Comedy of Errors* (1592–3) provides a glimpse of this new situation in the way the marital conflict between Antipholus and Adriana is presented. The source of their bitter quarrelling is Antipholus's promiscuous leanings and secret attraction to prostitutes, which makes it increasingly difficult for him to 'keep fair quarter with his bed' (2,1:108). In the heated dialogue of the play's second act, Adriana makes it clear to her husband that his behaviour presents a danger also to her, plainly telling him that she will be 'possessed with an adulterate blot, My blood…mingled with the crime of lust' (2,2:140–1) if he succumbs to the temptations of Ephesus:

> For if we two be one, and thou play false,
> I do digest the poison of thy flesh,
> Being strumpeted by thy contagion.
> Keep then fair league and truce with thy true bed,
> I live unstained, thou undishonoured. (2,2:142–6)

The fact that Adriana's anxieties were shared by many of her sisters in Tudor and Stuart England appears from a variety of sources (below and p.90). One of them is a verse in the broadsheet ballad *A Marry'd Woman's Case* from 1609, in which it is stated:

> A Woman that's to a Whoremonger wed is in a most desperate Case.
> She scarce dares to perform her Dutie in Bed with one of Condition so base:
> For sometimes he's bitten with Turnbull-street Fleas –
> the Poxe or some other infectious Disease
> and yett, to her Perill, his Lust she must please.
> Oh! Thus lives a woman that's married. (Burford, 1990, p.141)

'I dare not lye with him, he is so rank a Whoremaster', Rhodope says of her husband, Bartello, in Beaumont and Fletcher's *Women Pleased* (c. 1620) – an anxious confession to which Lopez, her lover, replies:

LOPEZ        And that's a dangerous point.

RHODOPE   Upon my conscience, Sir,
                   He would stick a thousand base diseases on me…

LOPEZ        I am sound Lady.

RHODOPE   That's it that makes me love ye.

LOPEZ        Let's kiss again then.

RHODOPE   Do, do.

'Do, the Devil', comments Rhodope's jealous husband, who has happened to overhear their conversation, 'And the grand Pox do with ye' (4,3:292).

Needles to say, a poxed husband or wife could infect the whole family, a danger which was particularly present among the lower classes of the population with their cramped living conditions and poor hygiene. In Norwich, for example, the keeper of St. Bennet's gates lazarhouse dealt over the two years following her husband's death in the 1620s with a range of serious medical cases, including two of the French pox, one of them involving a whole family (Pelling, 1985, p.128). Similarly, the keeper of St. Stephen's gates lazarhouse in Norwich was involved in contracts with the city for up to £3 for keeping the sick poor, which included a woman and four children with syphilis (p.129).

## THE DANGERS OF BREAST FEEDING

Perhaps the most tragic way in which the new disease could be passed on was that of a mother infecting her unborn child. Nearly all of the early syphilographers saw and recorded syphilitic disease in infants and young children. Like Peter Lowe, they also discovered that syphilitic nurses could pass on the infection. The monthly nurse, wet-nurse and children's nurse were a common part of the establishment of the higher social classes, and Roger Finlay's study of the demography of London (1580–1650) has demonstrated that infants from wealthier parishes were sent out of London to be nursed in country parishes (Finlay, 1981, pp.146–8). As further demonstrated by Valerie Fildes, wet-nursing in the 16th and 17th centuries was practised on such a scale that it can be classed as a cottage industry (Fildes, 1988, pp.142–73).*

Physicians gradually found out that not only could a nurse with syphilis infect her sucking child, but a syphilitic baby could also infect a healthy nurse. The London physician William Clowes (1544–1604), surgeon to St. Bartholomew's Hospital and a contemporary of Shakespeare's, recorded tragic examples of both such cases in his book *A Briefe and Necessary Treatise, Touching the Cure of the Disease Now Usually Called Lues Venerea, by Unctions and Other Approoued Waies of Curing* (1596). In describing the case of a 12-year-old girl with syphilis, Clowes wondered whether she had been infected through her parents or else

> 'was infected, as diuers are, by sucking the corrupt milke of some infected nurse, of whom I haue cured many, for such milke is ingendred of infected blood, and I may not here in conscience ouerpasse, to forewarne thee good Reader, of such lewde and filthie nurses: for that in the yeere 1583, it chanced that three young children, all borne in this citie of London, all of one parish, or very neere togither, and being of honest parentage, were put to nurse, the one in the countrie, and the other two were nursed in this citie of London: but whithin lesse than halfe a yeere, they were all three brought home to their parents and freends, greeuously infected with this great and odious disease, by their wicked and filthy nurses: Then their parents seeing them thus miserably spoiled and consumed with extreme paines, and great breaking out upon their bodies, and being so yoong, sicke and weake, vnpossible to be weaned, were forced, as nature doth binde, to seeke by all meanes possible to preserue these poore seely [innocent] infants, which else had died most pitifully. To be breefe, ere euer those children could be cured, they had infected fiue sundry good and honest nurses.' (Clowes, 1596, pp.151–2)**

---

\*   For evidence of the practice in literature, see Thomas Middleton: *A Chaste Maid in Cheapside* (1639) (2,2:15–6;162–4;176). The Elizabethan mathematician and court-astrologer John Dee (1527–1608) was typical in employing wet-nurses for his children. They were paid at the rate of 6 shillings per month, and their charges regularly involved the cost of candles and soap (Dee, 1842, pp.14–17).

\*\*  Because of the dangers of passing on a syphilitic infection to suckling babies, the practice of employing wet-nurses came under increasing criticism during the Renaissance. The Elizabethan novelist and dramatist John Lyly (c. 1554–1606) provided the less medical but more popular view that 'a newe vessell will long time sauour of that lyquor that is first powred into it, and the infant will euer smell of the Nurses manners

William Clowes's observations were evidently of a quite recent date, for half a
century earlier a fatal quack cure for syphilis was recommended by Thomas Paynel,
a canon of Merton Abbey who was known primarily for his translations of foreign
medical treatises. In 'A remedy for the frenche pockes', appended to his translation
*A Moche Profitable Treatise against the Pestilence* (1534), he advised syphilitics to keep
a certain diet, to use pills of purgation, to anoint the body with 'oyle made of swete
almandes, and with terpentine', and finally to practise Roman Charity in order to
get rid of the pox: 'They which be infected with this sycknes…must drynke euery
mornynge womans mylke, and sucke it from the dugge, for that is most conuenient…who so wyll vse this thynge euery mornyng fastyng, shall by the grace of god
recouer his helthe, and so I praye god he may' (Paynel, 1534, sig. Biii$^{r-v}$).

Sources describing syphilis in children are extremely rare, but the Paracelsian
practitioner John Hester (*floruit* 1594) provides one af the few examples in his
treatise *The Pearle of Practise* (1594), in which he speaks of having treated 'A young
child foure yeares old that was grieuouslie tormented with the French disease, hauing
extreme payne in his bodie, and being full of sores' (Hester, 1594, p.14).

Yet another source refers to the syphilitic babies that were born to prostitutes,
whose trade exposed them to the ever-present danger of unwanted pregnancies. 'Let
me persuade you to forsake all harlots, Worse than the deadliest poisons', Bellafronte
tells four libertines in Dekker's *The Honest Whore*:

> They're seldom blest with fruit; for ere it blossoms,
> Many a worm confounds it.
> They have no issue but foul ugly ones,
> That run along with them, e'en to their graves:
> For 'stead of children they breed rank diseases,
> And all you gallants can bestow on them
> Is that French Infant, which ne'er acts but speaks. (3,3:49–50;53–9)

Bellafronte might have instanced the four new-born children of Henry VIII and
Catherine of Aragon who died shortly after birth, which was just as well.

## THE 'SENILE' FRENCH DISEASE

By the time that Clowes wrote his treatise on syphilis, the disease had lost much of
its original severity and extent. In 1546, Girolamo Fracastoro asserted in *De
contagione* that it looked 'as if the contagion had now entered on its old age'
(Fracastoro, 1930, p.155). A contemporary and ally of Clowes's, the surgeon John
Read (*floruit* 1588), emphasized the stark contrast between the original symptoms
of the disease and those he knew from his own practice. In 1588, Read published
a volume of translations entitled *A Most Excellent and Compendious Method of Curing
Woundes* (1588), which partly included the Latin manuscript of the English surgeon
John Arderne (*floruit* 1370), on the cure of fistulas, and partly the treatise on wounds

---

hauing tasted of hir milke. Therefore lette the mother as often as she shal beholde those two fountaynes of
milke, as it were of their owne accorde flowing and swelling with lycour, remember that shee is admonished
of nature, yea commaunded of dutie, to cherishe hir owne childe, with hir owne teates…the Lionnesse nurseth
hir whelpes, the Rauen cherisheth hir birdes, the Uiper hir broode, and shall a woman cast away hir babe?'
(Lyly, 1902, vol.1, p.265).

by the Spanish surgeon Francisco Arcaeus (c.1493-c.1573). In this volume, Read quotes the latter for a description of the *morbus gallicus* on its first appearance:

> 'This french disease did bring with it a kinde of vniuersall Skabbe, oftentimes with ring wormes, with the foulnes of all the body called *Vitiligo* and *Alopecia*, running sores in the head called *Acores*, and werts of both sortes, and many times with flegmatick or melancholick swellings, or vlcers corrosiue, filthie and cancrouse, and also running ouer the body together with putrifiyng of the bone, & many times also accompained with al kinde of griefe, with feuers consumptiues, and with many other differences of diseases.' (Read, 1588, fol.58ʳ)

This is not how the disease appeared in his day, John Read emphasizes in his 'Annotations of the ix. Chapter' of Arcaeus's book. 'No man that carrieth but the name of a Phisition is or can bee ignorant or vnexpert in the cure of this disease', he says with confidence, 'The disease daylie dying and wearing away by the exquisite cure there of' (fol.59ᵛ).*

The fact that both Fracastoro and Read observed a notable mitigation of the constitutional effects of syphilis indicates that there had been an observable abatement of the disease both in extent and intensity within the first half of the 16th century, following its outbreak among the Italian soldiery in 1494–95.

It may be difficult to give an explanation of this change, which some physicians including Uelzen, Brant, and Fracastoro, attributed to astrological influences (see Figure 9). One of the more earthly causes is probably to be found in natural selection: the more fulminant forms of infection were dying out as the normal sorts of adjustment between host and parasite asserted themselves, that is, as milder strains of the spirochete displaced those that killed off their hosts too rapidly. Another cause may be found in such widespread infection of the European population that a certain 'herd immunity' was developed, with a corresponding mitigation of the original symptoms of the disease as a result. The rise of the standard of living in the 16th century may also have played a part in the weakening of the venereal plague, for malnutrition and intercurrent illness were found by the Oslo Study to have had an exacerbating effect on the symptoms of syphilis. 'We may also perceiue the furie of this disease to be partlie asswaged, and therefore not so terrible as it hath beene', wrote the Paracelsian syphilographer Phillipp Hermann with a sigh of relief in 1557, 'and the older it is, the feebler it becommeth' (Hermann, 1590, p.2).

## 'A SHAMEFULL DISEASE CALLED THE FRENCH POCKES'**

The shadow of syphilis fell upon every country in Europe and upon every country visited by its sailors and soldiers, just as it fell upon every sector of society, striking the young and vigorous, cutting their working days in half, and making their later

---

\* Read uses a number of distinctions that have played a great part in the modern pathology of syphilis. 'All the signes of this griefe must bee verie readilie discerned and distinguished', (fol.60ʳ) he admonishes his colleagues. 'First know wether the sicknesse be newelie taken, or haue beene of long continuance, howe farre it reacheth, and what partes it hath infected. Whether Nerues, bones, or ioyntes. Whether the paines bee milde or cruell, whether the substance of the corruption bee much or little. Whether hard, knottie, or gentle in handling. If inward, or outward. If the vlcers or whelkes be many, or with much paine, verie fewe appearing. Or if whether Pustulus matter or Gummie substance appeare' (fol.59ᵛ–60ʳ).

\*\* Bullein, 1562, *The Book of Compounds*, fol.xlviiʳ.

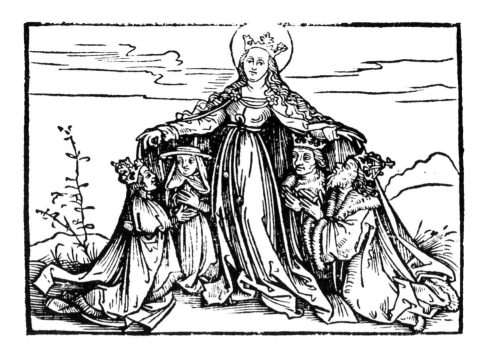

Figure 12. The cult of Mary was a prominent feature of late medieval Christianity, and in yet another woodcut (above), a prayer is sent to 'our most gracious mistress Mary to preserve us from the French disease' (caption). Two of the praying figures wear state crowns, the abbess a hat, and the fourth figure a papal crown. Syphilis knew no social distinctions and raged equally among the nobility, the royal houses and the Curia in Rome, where Pope Alexander VI Borgia (1492–1503) was himself a syphilitic, as was his successor, Pope Julius II (1503–13). The woodcut illustrates a Sapphic ode entitled *Mortilogus* (Augsburg, 1508) by Conrad Reitter, who was a prior of the Cistercian monastery at Donauwörth from 1509 to 1540. Reitter regards syphilis as nature's way of curbing human arrogance and teaching people a little humility. According to Reitter, contemporary Europe is a decadent civilization, especially in regard to sexual behaviour and religious observance, and syphilis is not only a satisfactory answer to the problems and hypocrisy of Renaissance society but also a necessary one. Enumerating all the perversions of a contemporary world, Reitter finds solace in 'the thundering revenger of crime who, lashing with a heavy scourge our grave sins, imparts to our transgressions a well-deserved punishment' (Vorberg, 1924, p.62).

life a time of suffering and misery. 'What sickness has ever traversed every part of Europe, Africa and Asia with equal speed?', Erasmus complained at the height of the syphilitic epidemic. 'What penetrates more quickly veins and bowels? What clings more tenaciously, what repels more vigorously the art and care of physicians? What passes more easily by contagion to another? What brings more cruel tortures?…This lues is a foul, cruel, contagious disease, dangerous to life, apt to remain in the system and to break out anew not otherwise than the gout' (Erasmus, 1926, vol.6, p.137). In these lines Erasmus touches upon an agonizing aspect of the *morbus gallicus*, one that made the disease an insidious one and part of a game of Russian roulette. Everyone knew how the disease began, but nobody knew how it would end. Some seemed to recover after the initial symptoms had disappeared, but others went on to develop a number of tormenting and ugly complications years later – deep scars on the skin and bones, perforation of the nose, paralysis of the legs, blindness, and even insanity. 'Lewdnesse fild him with reprochfull paine of that fowle evill which all men reprove', Edmund Spenser (1552–99) related in *The Faerie Queene* (1589) in reference to the pox, a disease, he added, 'That rots the marrow and consumes the braine' (1,4:231–3).

On top of such fears and anxieties came the moral opprobrium of syphilis which set it apart from all the other diseases suffered by man at the time. In England, for example, syphilis was uniformly referred to as the 'fowle disease' (Hester, 1594, p.59), a disease to be ashamed of and to hide from one's family and surroundings.

In Massinger's *A New Way to Pay Old Debts* (1633), the prodigal of the play, Frank Welborne, tries to cover up the unfortunate results of his adventures when 'lodg'd vpon the Banckside' (4,2:88). 'Thou were't my Surgeon', he tells one of his three creditors, 'you must tell no tales. Those days are done. I will pay you in priuate' (4,2:99–100).

An example of the collective repression of a scourge rivalling that of the bubonic plague may be found in the numerous popular euphemisms for syphilis. 'Men doe vse pretie termes for foule sores and call them by one name, when thei are another', William Bullein (d. 1576) complained in his *Bulwarke of Defence* (1562). 'It is nothing saie thei, but breaking out, or paines of the body, weakenesse of limmes, or a grene sicknes, through the obstruccion of the liuer. etc. with soche nicke names, whose very sure name is, the buttens of Napelles, *Gallicus morbus* comonlie called the Frenche poxe' (Bullein, 1562, *A Dialogue betwene Sorenes and Chyrurgie,* fol.ix$^v$).

Luckily for the bigoted, the satirists and the Puritans, victims of the French disease were frequently given away by an number of visible symptoms. In secondary syphilis, one of these is *alopecia*, or the thinning of the hair on the scalp, eyebrows, eyelashes and beard. 'Some patients lose their hair', observed Fracastoro in *De contagione*, 'that is, their beards, eyebrows, or the hair of the head, which makes them look monstrous and ridiculous' (Fracastoro, 1930, p.293). 'Last day I chaunst (in crossing of the streete) With *Diffilus* the Inkeeper to meete', Thomas Lodge (1558?–1625) quipped in his satire *A Fig for Momus* (1595):

> He wore a silken night-cap on his head,
> And lookt as if he had beene lately dead:
> I askt him how he far'd, not well (quoth he)
> An ague this two months hath troubled me;
> I let him passe: and laught to heare his skuce:
> For I knew well, he had the poxe by *Luce*:
> And wore his night-cappe ribbind at the eares,
> Because of late he swet away his heares. (Lodge, 1883, vol.3, pp.11–12)[*]

'The French Razor shaues off the haire of many of thy *Suburbians*', Westminster tells London in Thomas Dekker's *The Dead Tearme* (1608) (Dekker, 1884–6, vol.4, p.28),

---

[*]   Erasmus of Rotterdam used a similar device to hide the effects of his syphilis (Werthemann, 1930, passim; Cole, 1952, pp.529–31; Appelboom *et al.*, 1986, pp.1181–4).

while Samuel Rowlands in *The Knaue of Harts* (1612) relates the unpleasant consequences of a citizen's trip across the Thames to the suburbs of the south:

> This Gentleman, with Ores hath past the riuer,
> And very pockey newes he can deliuer:
> From Lambeth-Marsh he newly is transported,
> Where he hath beene most filthily consorted
> …
> And howsoeuer it may seeme disgrace,
> The poxe will pull away his Beard from's face:
> Nay, after that his chinne hath lost his pride,
> T'will put him to a Periwigge beside:
> But now he vowes whores bargaines very bare;
> For he hath try'd and found it to a haire. (Rowlands, 1880, vol.2, p.17)[*]

In *A Hundred and Fourteene Experiments and Cures of the Famous Physitian Philippus Aureolus Theophrastus Paracelsus…Collected by John Hester* (1596), the noted English iatrochemist presented the case of 'A certaine man [who] being long sicke of the pox had two tumours and an vlcer in his nose, at the which euerie day there came foorth great quantitie of stinking and filthie matter, in whose nose I cast this [mercurial] decoction with a siring' (Hester, 1596, p.7).

Hester here describes one of the most horrible lesions of syphilis, in which nasal and sometimes palate bones are destroyed by *gumma*, or gummy tumours, eating away the nose and in severe cases exposing the brain to the air. 'Why doth the Poxe so much affect to undermine the nose?', John Donne asked in his *Paradoxes and Problems* (1633), concluding that a sense of fitness and propriety is shown by nature when ending in one prominent member of the body what was begun in another prominent member. 'Beeing begot and bredd in the obscurest and secretest corner', he observed of the pox, and 'his Serpentine crawlings, and Insinuations bee[ing] not suspected nor seene, hee comes sooner to great place, and is abler to destroy the worthyest Member then a disease better borne. Perchance as mise defeate Elephants by gnawing theyr Proboscis, which is theyr nose, this wretched Indian Vermine practises to doe the same upon us' (Donne, 1980, p.40).

'Whores strike [men] with Cans, and glasses, and quart pots', observed the famous actor Nathan Field (1587–1620) in *Amends for Ladies* (1616), 'if they haue nothing by 'em they strike 'em with the Poxe, and you know that will lay ones nose as flat as a basket hilt Dagger' (3,4:69–75).

Another visible lesion of late or tertiary syphilis was described by the English satirist Barnabe Rich (1540?–1617), who rejoiced that victims of the 'foul disease' were not only stigmatized by alopecia and a sunken nose (with its concomitant alteration of the voice) but also by *tabes dorsalis* – a painful paralysis of the legs produced by degeneration of the posterior column of the spinal cord. Interspersed with the author's savage satire is interesting information about the usual cover-up of the pox and about social distinctions among the victims of syphilis, the upper classes sugaring over their misfortune by boasting of 'the gallant disease', while

---

[*]  cf. his 16th Epigram in *The Letting of Humours Blood* (1600), ibid., vol.1, p.22.

asserting that 'He shall not be accounted a Gentleman if that he doth not carry this marke of the pox about him' (Rich, 1617, p.25).

> 'I would I had now a Chaire with a backe, and a soft cushion, that I might set me downe to laugh at the whoremaster, but especially at him that they call *Senex Fornicator*, an old Fishmonger, that many yeares since ingrost the French pox, the which although he sometimes vseth to vent in secret among his friends; yet he will not so disfurnish himselfe, but that he will reserue sufficient for his owne store, and the rather to conceale his commoditie, in priuate, and would not haue it to be openly knowne, hee shelters them vnder strange titles; sometimes hee calls them the Gout, sometimes the Sciatica, and thus disguising them vnder these false applyed names, hee shamefully slandereth and belyeth the pocks.

> There be some others yet of a better disposition, that doth detest this fraudulent manner of dealing, that when they haue made some pretty shift to get the pocks, they do set them forth to open show, and finding them to be sociable, familiar, and conversant amongst Knights & Gentlemen, will grace them with a wrought night cap, yet not in any deceitfull manner, whereby to cousen his Maiesties subiects, but will so lay them open to euery mans view, that you shall see their true pictures in diuers parts of the face, but especially at the nose: he doth not so hide them, but you shall discerne them by his complexion, by his snuffling in his speach, by his very gate as he passeth and repasseth by you. If a Dogge doth chance to hit him ouer the shynnes with his taile, he cryes oh, and perhaps, raps out an oath or two.

> You shall neuer see him play any match at the Footeball, or to winne any wagers at running, or leaping; hee may sometimes dance the Measures, but these Corrantoes, and Scottish gigges, are out of his element: here is plaine dealing, and it should seeme these pox are honestly come by, when they are not hidden, but are thus laid open to euery mans view.' (p.25)

Yet another English source illuminates the complex of secretiveness, shame, malice, and bigotry surrounding the 'foul disease'. In *The Discoverie of Witchcraft* (1584), an Elizabethan justice of the peace, Reginald Scot (1538?–99), published a lurid case from the assizes held at Rochester in 1581. Here a vicar of Kent named John Ferral accused a woman named Margaret Simons of witchcraft, evidently because the clergyman was suffering from the symptoms of secondary syphilis, which in addition to a skin rash and alopecia may present with headache, malaise, fever, and a sore throat. The last symptom seems especially to have caused the vicar pain, and at the assizes he told the justices of the peace 'that alwaies in his parish church, when he desired to read most plainelie, his voice so failed him, as he could scant be heard at all. Which hee could impute, he said, to nothing else, but to hir inchantment' (Scot, 1930, Booke I, Chapter II, p.40).

'When I advertised the poore woman hereof', Reginald Scot relates, 'as being desirous to heare what she could saie for hir selfe; she told me, that in verie deed his voice did much faile him, speciallie when he strained himselfe to speake lowdest. How beit, she said that at all times his voice was hoarse and lowe: which thing I perceived to be true. But sir, said she, you shall understand, that this our vicar is diseased with such a kind of hoarsenesse, as divers of our neighbors in this parish, not long since, doubted that he had the French pox; & in that respect utterly refused to communicate with him: untill such time as (being therunto injoined by M.D. *Lewen* the Ordinarie) he had brought from *London* a certificat, under the hands of two physicians, that his hoarsenes proceeded from a disease in the lungs. Which certificat he published in the church, in the presence of the whole congregation: and by this meanes hee was cured or rather excused of the shame of his disease' (p.4).

'This I knowe to be true by the relation of divers honest men of that parish', Scot finishes his account,

> 'And truelie, if one of the Jurie had not beene wiser than the other, she had beene condemned thereupon, and upon other as ridiculous matters as this. For the name of a witch is so odious, and hir power so feared among the common people, that if the honestest bodie living chance to be arraigned therupon, she shall hardlie escape condemnation.' (p.4)*

## STATISTICS BLURRED BY THE COMMON COVER-UP

The shame attached to syphilis has led to its being chronically underreported and has made it difficult to estimate the prevalence or severity of the disease in any historical period. At the end of the Renaissance, an interesting account was recorded which may serve to demonstrate the way in which the existence of the 'foul disease' in England was still viewed *sub rosa* by the people of the Restoration period. The document testifies to the wide prevalence of syphilis and to its serious effect on public health in the generations before 1662.

In a pioneering book entitled *Natural and Political Observations Made upon the Bills of Mortality* (1662), the English captain John Graunt (1620–74) laid the foundations of modern statistics and demography. The 'bills of mortality' examined by Graunt were weekly records of deaths and baptisms dating back to the end of the 16th century – records that furnished him with raw material for his statistical and demographic studies. In search of regularities, Graunt made an assessment of the various causes of death in the London population over two separate periods, spanning the years 1629–36 and 1647–60 and covering 229,250 deaths. 'We finde one *Casualty* in our Bills, of which though there be daily talk, there is little effect', Graunt observed with an air of surprise in his 15th section,

> 'much like our abhorrence of *Toads*, and *Snakes*, as most poisonous Creatures, whereas few men dare say upon their own knowledge, they ever found harm by either; and this *Casualty* is the *French-Pox*, gotten, for the most part, not so much by the intemperate use of *Venery* (which rather causeth the *Gowt*) as of many common Women [prostitutes].

---

\* Another contemporary source possibly testifying to the connection between witch hunting and syphilis may be found in a sermon addressed by Bishop John Jewel (1522?–71) to Elizabeth I in 1559–60. Here the fanatic Calvinist clergyman urged immediate action against 'witches and sorcerers…[who] within these few last years are marvellously increased within this Your Grace's realm. These eyes have seen most evident and manifest marks of their wickedness. Your Grace's subjects pine away even unto death, their colour fadeth, their flesh rotteth, their speech is benumbed, their senses are bereft. Wherefore, Your poor subjects' most humble petition unto Your Highness is, that the laws touching such malefactors may be put in due execution' (Summers, 1958, p.116). This sermon was probably the occasion of a law passed in the fifth year of Elizabeth's reign, by which witchcraft was again made a felony, as it had been in the reign of Henry VIII.

In *Syphilis, Puritanism and Witch Hunts* (1990), Stanislav Andreski has postulated a connection between the Great Witch Craze in Western Europe and the syphilitic epidemic, but his chronological time-table does not bear closer scrutiny. The syphilitic epidemic culminated in the years between 1493 and 1530, while the Great Witch Craze culminated in the last two decades of the 16th century and the first two of the 17th century (Andreski, 1990, pp.21–84).

16. I say, the Bills of *Mortality* would take off these Bars, which keep some men within bounds, as to these extravagancies: for in the afore-mentioned 229250 we finde not above 392 to have died of the Pox…Now, forasmuch as it is not good to let the World be lulled into a security, and belief of Impunity by our Bills, which we intend shall not be onely as *Death's-head*, to put men in minde of their *Mortality*, but also as *Mercurial Statues* to point out the most dangerous ways that lead us into it, and misery. We shall therefore shew, that the *Pox* is not as the *Toads*, and *Snakes* afore-mentioned, but of a quite contrary nature, together with the reason why it appears otherwise

17. Foreasmuch as by the ordinary discourse of the world it seems a great part of men have, at one time, or other, had some *species* of this disease, I wondering why so few died of it, especially because I could not take that to be so harmless, whereof so many complained very fiercely; upon inquiry I found that those who died of it out of the Hospitals (especially that of *Kings-Land*, and the *Lock in Southwark*) were returned of *Ulcers*, and *Sores*. And in brief I found, that all mentioned to die of the *French-Pox* were returned by the *Clerks* of Saint *Giles's*, and Saint *Martin's in the Fields* onely; in which place I understood that most of the vilest, and most miserable houses of uncleanness were: from whence I concluded, that onely *hated* persons, and such, whose very *Noses* were eaten of[f], were reported by the *Searchers* [coroners] to have died of this too frequent *Maladie*'. (Graunt, 1662, pp.23–4)

A modern examination carried out by T.R. Forbes in 1971 confirmed the low figures that Graunt found in his material and whose reliability he so strongly suspected. In *Chronicle from Aldgate* (1971), Forbes examined the causes of 4,253 deaths as set down by the clerks of the Parish of St Botolph without Aldgate, London, from 1583 through 1599. 'French pox' or 'morbus gallicus' was given as a cause of death once in 1585, twice in 1587, and nine times in 1594–99, the total being 12 deaths out of 4,253 deaths. Also in this material it appears that many deaths from 'this too frequent malady' were not reported as such (Forbes, 1971, pp.105–6, 100–2).

The above figures may be compared to the casebook of the London surgeon Joseph Binns, which was examined by Lucinda McCray Beier in 1987. From 1633 through 1663, the doctor was consulted in 133 cases of syphilis or gonorrhea out of a total of 671 cases. Because of the numerous attempts at concealment recorded in Binns's casebook, McCray Beier thinks it possible that more of Binns's patients were syphilitic than the numbers given above indicate (McCray Beier, 1987, p.93).

In concluding this chapter, we emphasize the fact that among the majority of people syphilis carried its own stinging stigma, in that most of its victims had been promiscuous persons, or 'whore-masters'. Fears of social discrimination, religious condemnation, and personal rejection invariably induced sufferers of the pox to keep their disease to themselves, thus enduring on top of their physical ordeal what was probably the worst aspect of their condition, namely a sense of isolation and secret guilt. Already William Clowes alluded to 'those diseased persons which either for shame dare not bewray it, or for lacke of good Surgeons know not how to remedy it' (Clowes, 1596, p.150), and in *Hamlet* King Claudius presents a simile which perhaps belongs among the poet's most personal statements. 'But so much was our love', the King sighs with reference to the mad Prince,

> We would not understand what was most fit;
> But like the owner of a foul disease,

Figure 13. At the very time that the printing press was outgrowing its cradle, European civilization was brought face to face with syphilis. The novelty of copying from old manuscripts and old masters was wearing off, and the printing establishment quickly fixed on literature dealing with this newly recognized disease, so unorthodox in its manifestations and in its treatment. The numerous treatises devoted to syphilis between 1496 and 1500 attest to this great interest. The first book on the subject is probably Conrad Schellig's undated *In pustulas malas consilium* (Heidelberg, 1496), which was followed by Joseph Grünpeck's *Tractatus de pestilentiali scorra sive mala de franczos* and *Ein hübscher Tractat von dem Ursprung des Bösen Franzos* (Augsburg, 1496). Next came Nicolo Leoniceno's *Libellus de epidemia quam vulgo morbum Gallicum vocant* (Venice, 1497), Gaspare Torella's *Tractatus cum consiliis contra pudendagram seu morbum gallicum* (Rome, 1497), Johannes Widmann's *Tractatus de pustulis* (Rome, 1497), and Corradino Gilino's *De morbo quem Gallicum nuncupant* (Ferrara, 1497). The following year saw the publication

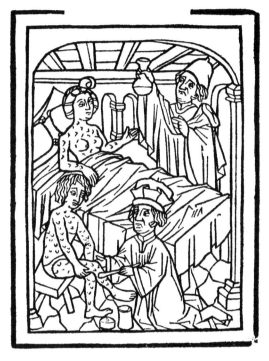

of Natale Montesauro's *De dispositionibus quas vulgares mal francoso appellant* (Verona, 1498), Antonio Scanaroli's *Disputatio utilis de morbo gallico* (Bologne, 1498), and Bartholomaeus Stäber's *A Malafranzos morbo gallorum praeservatio ac cura* (Vienna, 1498).*

The woodcut above adorns Stäber's treatise and shows a married couple infected with syphilis, the woman in bed and covered with bedclothes to the waist, the man sitting on a stool at the bedside, almost naked. Both patients are covered with skin lesions which appear to be those of pustular syphilides, the so-called 'wild warts' (*wilden wartzen*) and 'evil blisters' (*bösen blattern*) that were typical of the malign manifestations of the disease during its first outbreak in the 1490s. A doctor stands on one side, gravely examining a flask of urine, while the other kneels in front of the man, applying what is probably a mercurial unction to the patient's leg with a long spatula. Stäber was professor of medicine at the University of Vienna, where he became rector magnificus in 1490. After his death in 1506, he was buried in Stephansdom in the heart of the city. Stäber sees the skin symptoms featured in the woodcut as characteristic of the disease, but he fails to make other observations because his theoretical basis for understanding the disease is governed by the pathology of humours and astrological speculations.

---

* All the works mentioned are reprinted in Sudhoff, 1924.

> To keep it from divulging, let it feed
> Even on the pith of life. (4,1:19–23)

## CONCLUSION

The emergence of syphilis on the European scene at the end of the 15th century had a profound influence on the history of Western civilization during the Renaissance. According to the medical sources of the time, syphilis was experienced as a new disease whose venereal and non-venereal ways of transmission were recognized fairly quickly. This insight led to sensible preventive measures such as the closure of bath houses and brothels in the major cities of Europe, both establishments being found to be disseminating centres of syphilitic infection. Similarly, enlightened philosophers of the age called for hygienic and administrative measures to contain the venereal plague, with mandatory medical examination for everyone seeking a marriage license appearing as their most radical suggestion. (Almost five hundred years later, governments in the Western world are now being urged by similarly concerned citizens to require AIDS tests for couples seeking marriage licenses and to make it a criminal offence to engage in sex without disclosing one's diseased condition.)

Syphilis appears to have prompted a profound change in manners and morals during the Renaissance and to have led to a stressing of the desirability of monogamy, premarital chastity and absolute fidelity within marriage as the only safe position in both secular and religious matters.

From a medical–historical point of view, the advent of syphilis is an interesting subject because of the way in which the disease furthered the growth of modern medicine. The epidemic shocked the dormant medical mind of Western Europe into action and brought about a transition from magic to rational medicine. 'Syphilis is part of every branch of medicine', observed medical historian William Allen Pusey. 'It is an epitome of pathology, and the history of its progress since the beginning of the sixteenth century is the best illustration that we have of the evolution of the modern knowledge of medicine' (Pusey, 1933, p.3).

Fracastoro's observations on syphilis paved the way for his discovery of the mechanisms of infection, and Paracelsus's treatment of syphilis with mercury sparked the development of a revolutionary branch of medicine known as iatrochemistry, or biochemistry (see pp.12 and 255–6).

For these reasons, the appearance of syphilis on the European scene at the close of the Middle Ages is one of the most crucial events in modern history. The impact of the disease on almost every sphere of cultural life justifies renewed research for new avenues of understanding of this now classical field of medical–historical investigation.

# 2

# WONDER DRUGS FOR THE POX

With the 16th century began a huge outpouring of writings by the syphilographers. Their works are not only an index of activity in the study of syphilis, but also of the activity of medicine as a whole during this period. The literature of syphilis in the 16th century and the knowledge of the disease which it shows is of a surprising extent. These works include a complete description of all the skin manifestations of syphilis, with size, colour, character and location of the lesions. In addition, they include not only a description of what was long after recognized as the primary, secondary and tertiary effects of the disease, but also numerous descriptions of various cures. Since these cures failed to eradicate all of the spirochetes, the latent effects of the disease developed in spite of the treatment, and were then attributed not only to syphilis but to other causes.

Until the beginning of the 20th century, the treatment of syphilis was limited principally to mercury, which was given by mouth, by inunction, or by fumigation. Mercury in the treatment of syphilis is evident almost as early as the disease itself. The physicians Johannes Widmann (1497), Gaspare Torella (1497), Lopez de Villalobos (1498), Juan Almenar (1502), Giovanni de Vigo (1514), and Diaz de Isla (1539) were among the first Europeans who introduced it, but mercury had long been used by the Arabs in the treatment of scabies, psoriasis, leprosy and other skin diseases. It was known to the Oriental physicians as *Unguentum Saracenicum*, an ointment that contained a ninth part of mercury, and its wide use among the Arabs made it readily available in Europe when the new disease arrived.

The resolution of the syphilitic skin lesions after inunction with mercury gave the Arabian 'wonder drug' a wide application, and the treatment was joined to traditional theories of the origin of disease in an imbalance of the four humours – blood, phlegm, choler, and melancholy. According to the doctrine of the age, disease, including skin disease, was the outward manifestation of an internal alteration in the composition of the four humours, or in a disturbance of their relative proportions in the body. The indications for treatment were in accordance with these beliefs, and so diet and evacuation formed the basis of all therapy, although external application of medicaments were considered to be of importance in certain diseases, above all those related to dermatology. The treatments prescribed for syphilis by the physicians of the 16th century hence placed extreme emphasis on appropriate diets, exercises and purgatives, in addition to the use of mercury in a strength of one to forty. The quacks, however, rushing in blindly, used the ointment at once in strengths of up to one in eight and got quicker and more dramatic results. This forced the hands of the physicians, with disastrous consequences.

## THE QUICKSILVER CURE

The above aspects of mercurial chemotherapy may be studied in the syphilographic works of William Clowes, who can justly be called the first English venereologist. In 1596, Clowes presented himself as a decided advocate of 'quicksilver' in his book *A Briefe and Necessary Treatise, Touching the Cure of the Disease Now Usually Called Lues Venerea, by Unctions and Other Approoued Waies of Curing.*[*]

Figure 14. The engraving shows the title-page of *Venus Belegert en Ontset* (Amsterdam, 1685) by the famous Dutch physician Steven Blanckaert (1650–1702). The picture shows the treatment of syphilitic patients by mercurial fumigation (foreground) and mercurial inunction (centre). The man in the bed (background) is shown salivating as a result of mercurial chemotherapy – salivation indicating toxicity. The patient was anointed until salivation began, usually after four to five days. Paracelsus and his followers actually recommended that for chemotherapy to be effective three pints of saliva needed to be produced. At this dose poisoning was no doubt occurring, and Clowes testifies to later medical trends in which doses were gradually decreased in order to avoid toxic side effects. It was the application of the 'humoral' theory of mercurial action that was directly responsible for the enormous doses used by 16th-century physicians.

In the left foreground of the engraving is a patient in a tub – 'the powdering tub of infamy' as Shakespeare calls it in *Henry V* (2,1:79). Patients in these tubs were exposed to fumes from powder of cinnabar, a mercuric sulphide. The powder was thrown onto a hot-plate or chafing-dish and was volatilized, condensing as a powder on the patient's body. 'Sinaber which is vsed in fumes for the pox,' the noted surgeon John Woodall (1556?–1643) warned in *The Surgeons Mate* (1617), 'is a deadly medicine made halfe of quicksiluer, and halfe of brimstone by Art of fire: I meane by distillation. I know the abuse of these three recited [mercurial] medicines hath done vnspeakable harme in the common-wealth of England, and daily doth more and more, working the vtter infamy and destruction of many an innocent, man, woman, and child, which I would my wits or diligence knew to helpe' (Woodall, 1617, p.300).

In the foreground of the picture, an emaciated woman exhibits deep scars on her legs. These are the infamous gumma, which are the principal signs of later, or tertiary, syphilis. The gummy tumors, rubbery to the touch, are the result of localized skirmishes between the spirochetes and the body tissues, and they lead to the destruction of the skin, mucous membranes, and bones, leaving deep scars in their wake. They are aptly described by Clowes as 'bunchey nodes, & filthy abscessions or apostumes, with corruption of the bones of the head, called Talpa, and vpon the armes and legs called Tophus or Gommata, especially in old sicknesses, hauing their beginning of grosse and slimy fleame: and oftentimes I haue knowne these bones corrupted and rotten, and the flesh about it sound, nothing at all touched' (Clowes, 1596, p.154).

In addition to mercurial chemotherapy for syphilis, vegetable infusions, sulphur baths, hydrotherapeutic measures, and a variety of dietary and fasting cures were used by the doctors of the age.

---

[*]      This treatise was published as pp. 145–229 of the author's book *A Profitable and Necessarie Booke of Observations, for All Those That are Burned with Flame of Gun Powder, &c* (1596). All references are to this edition except for the passages quoted on pp. 108 and 110–12, which are taken from the 1579 edition of Clowes's treatise on syphilis. His first treatise on the subject appears to have been published previously in 1576, but no edition has survived. The revised edition of 1579 was published under the title *A Short and Profitable Treatise Touching the Cure of the Disease Called Morbus Gallicus by Unctions.*

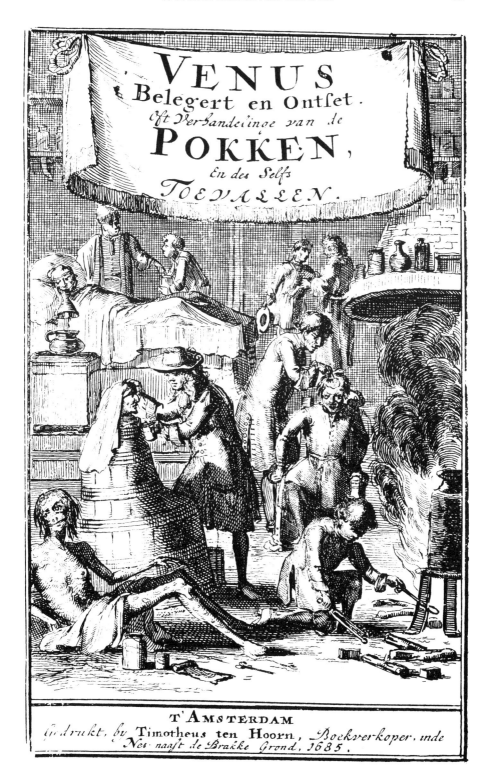

In his treatise on the topic, Clowes distinguishes three stages in the treatment of syphilis. 'The maner of cure (so far foorth as I meane in this short Treatise to deale with) consisteth of these parts, that is, of euacuation, diet, and use of unctions: euacuation is the first of these three to be used, namely purgings, letting of blood, and sweating' (Clowes, 1596, p.155).

In accordance with the doctors of his time, Clowes prescribes a certain diet for the patient, discouraging pork, salt meats, geese, ducks, fish, cheese, raw fruits and sweet wines while endorsing meats 'of easie digestion' such as 'weathers mutton, veale, lambe, and kid, being fed in drie grounds, yoong hares and rabbets, chickens, capons, hens, partriges, feasants, and birds of the woods and mountains' (pp.160–1).

Clowes finally arrives at the third part of his cure, namely 'the way and order of annointing with the unctions made of quicksiluer' (p.162). 'Let him be annointed against a good fire of coles', he opens his account of the mercury cure,

> 'and then they must rub or chafe it in well with their owne hands, if it be possible their strength will serue, and those parts or places that are to be annointed, are first the soles of the feete, and so up to the knees, also the thighes, buttocks, loines, and share bones, and likewise annoint both the armes, and under the arme holes, and the shoulder blades: but in any wise, as neere as you can, touch not the head, neither come neere any other principall parts with the unction, as the belly, for thereby truly I haue seene greeuous accidents to follow, and oftentimes death, as hereafter shall be declared. The annointing being thus finished, let a warme sheete be put round about the patient, and a double kercher well warmed, and bound about his head, and so couer him in his bed, with as many clothes as he is well able to beare: but if therewith he cannot sweate orderly, as you would desire, then applie to the soles of his feete, legs, thighes, and to both his sides, very hot bricks well wrapped in warme double clothes, or else bottels filled with very hot water.' (pp.162–3)

Having sweated for two or three hours, the patient, according to Clowes, must be relieved of his clothes and cooled in a gentle manner, after which the treatment must be repeated: 'He must be thus annointed and ordered, two or three daies togither or more, as you see occasion, untill the fluxe of flegmatike matter doth begin to flow from the mouth moderately, which doth happen commonly within two, three, or fower days, etc. [Figure 14 background]. Then cease from annointing, for otherwise it is very dangerous, as shall be declared' (p.163).

When the patient's 'gums, cheekes, toong and throte ranckle, ulcerate and swell', Clowes tells the doctor to 'wash and gargarise his mouth with new milke, wherein you may seeth a few violet leaues, and columbine leaues, and syrup of violets' (p.163). Clowes finally provides a recipe for 'A very good lotion' (p.164) with which the treatment may be terminated in a successful manner. At the same time, he issues a strong warning in connection with the quicksilver cure:

> 'Thus briefly haue I spoken of the manner of annointing, and the order of sweating, and the cure of the mouth: which with great foresight, care, and diligence is to be looked unto: for otherwise if it be neglected, then doth follow most commonly great and dangerous accidents, and this may come either by the disobedience and unrulines of the patient, or else through the ignorance or negligence of the Surgeon, not regarding the malice and sharpnesse of the fluxe, whereby it doth happen often times, that some haue beene eaten cleane through the cheeks, and also haue had their Vuula [uvula] therby taken away, by the means heereof they haue lost their

speeches and voices, others haue lost their teeth and mandible or iaw withall, insomuch they were neuer able afterward to receiue any food to sustaine them, but onely with a spoone untill their dying day. Therefore I am heere to aduertise thee good Reader, to be very wary of such carelesse and ignorant Surgeons, for those dangers and causes before spoken of.' (pp.164–5)[*]

Weighing the advantages and disadvantages of the quicksilver cure, Clowes finishes by warmly recommending it and stating that a drastic illness requires drastic methods: 'Extreme remedies are to be used aginst extreme diseases' (Clowes, 1596, p.170). 'Who would not feare the force, the pearcing and power reflexiue of Quicksiluer', his colleague John Read had asked eight years before in an annotation of Francisco Arcaeus's treatise on syphilis. 'And yet it is by experience well prooued, that many whose health was dispaired of, hath beene well recouered, by this extreme manner of curing' (Read, 1558, sig. 60ᵛ). Thinking, perhaps, of the same disease as Clowes and Read, in *Hamlet* Shakespeare has King Claudius observe that

> Diseases desperate grown
> By desperate appliance are relieved,
> Or not at all. (4,3:9–11)

## EFFICACY OF MERCURY CHEMOTHERAPY

Modern medicine has assessed the efficacy of the mercury cure in a variety of ways. Mercury was undoubtedly effective in clearing the cutaneous lesions of primary syphilis because of the relatively few spirochetes involved in the infection. However, it was ineffective in curing the infections of secondary syphilis, where a much larger number of active spirochetes is involved. On the other hand, mercury and heavy metal chemotherapy were undoubtedly of use in the treatment of the cutaneous lesions of tertiary syphilis. Here there are relatively few spirochetes, chronic inflammation, fibrosis and attempted healing by the body itself. Since mercury is a powerful antimitotic and anti-inflammatory agent, locally applied mercury probably aided healing and reduced gummas in a large number of cases (O'Shea, 1990, p.394). The great problem with mercury was its toxicity; stated in the simplest pharmacological terms, it had a very disadvantageous therapeutic ratio.

'Mercury is a fox', asserted John Woodall in *The Surgeons Mate* (1617), 'and will be too crafty for fooles, yea and will oft leaue them to their disgrace, when they relying vpon so vncertaine a medicine, promise health, and shall in stead of healing make their Patient worse then before…for euery horse-leech and bawd now vpon each trifle will procure a Mercuriall fluxe, yea many a pitifull one, whereby diuers innocent people are dangerously deluded, yea perpetually defamed and ruinated

---

[*] A court case against a surgeon in Kent brought before the Rochester Assizes on February 24, 1601, testifies to the dangers of mercurial treatment in unskilled hands: 'One Tristram Lyde a sourgeon, admitted to practise by the Archbishops lettres, was arraigned for killing divers women by annoyntinge them with quick-sylver,&c. Evidence [was] given that he would have caused the women to have stript themselves naked in his presence, and himselfe would have anoynted them; that he tooke upon him the cure, and departed because they would not give him more then their first agreement. He pleaded theire diseases were such as required that kinde of medicine; that it was there owne negligence, by taking cold in going abroade sooner then he prescribed; soe he was acquited. Sergeant Daniel sitting there as Judge sayd he knewe that there might be a purgacion by a fume' (Manningham, 1976, pp.53–4).

both of their good names, goods, healths and liues, and that without remedy. Methinks I could spend much time if I had it, euen in setting downe the good and bad things of quicksiluer, and yet I confesse I am too weak to describe the tenth part of his wonders' (Woodall, 1617, p.300). Taking his recourse to poetry, Woodall in an ode 'in praise of quicksiluer or Mercurie' sums up the efficacy of the silvery drug thus:

> The perfect cure proceeds from thee,
> For Pox, for Gout, for Leprosie,
> For scabs, for itch, of any sort,
> These cures with thee are but a sport. (p.301)[*]

## GUAIAC – THE WONDER DRUG FROM AMERICA

In the 16th century a second cure was applied to syphilis which came to rival that of the quicksilver cure. In the period between 1506 and 1516, Spanish sailors and travellers brought home from America the Indian wood *guaiacum*, which appears then to have circulated on the Iberian peninsula. The recipe of earliest date is that of a Spanish spicedealer which is dated June 22, 1516 (Munger, 1949, p.197).

In April 1519, the guaiac cure was introduced in Europe by the distinguished German humanist and poet-laureate Ulrich von Hutten (1488–1523). His *De guaiaci medicina et morbo gallico* (Mainz, 1519) dwelled at length on his own case of syphilis and subsequent cure by guaiac, whose manner of preparation and use as a decoction is described for the reader. *De guaiaci medicina* was greeted enthusiastically, and the book was reprinted not only in Latin but in many modern languages. Thus an English translation by Thomas Paynel appeared as early as 1533 in London. As a consequence, knowledge of the remedy spread across Europe, where popular opinion accorded it first place as a cure for syphilis. Von Hutten was followed eleven years later by Girolamo Fracastoro, who in the Third Book of his poem *Syphilis sive morbus gallicus* (1530) praised guaiac in an almost panegyric manner (see p.3).

Guaiac was embraced by the European doctors because of the toxic nature of the quicksilver treatment, where the curative dose and the poisonous dose were too close. Ulrich von Hutten in particular provided an eloquent description of the sufferings of syphilitic patients treated with mercury: the jaws, tongue, lips, and palate became ulcerated, the gums swelled, the teeth became loose and fell out, and saliva dribbled incessantly from the mouth. The breath became intolerably foetid, and the whole apartment where a patient was treated stank so unbearably that the stench, together with the most horrible gangrenous signs of mercurial poisoning, made death a lesser evil than the treatment.

It was in this context that guaiac arrived on the European scene, having secondary effects of a considerably milder nature than those of the quicksilver cure. *Guaiacum officinale L.* (zygophylloceae) is a tree which is found in the West Indies and on the north coast of South America. The tree was called *guaiacum* or *guaiacan* by the natives of Hispaniola (Munger, 1949, p.202). When the wood of the tree

---

[*]  For a modern and balanced discussion of mercury chemotherapy in the treatment of syphilis, see O'Shea, 1990, pp.392–5).

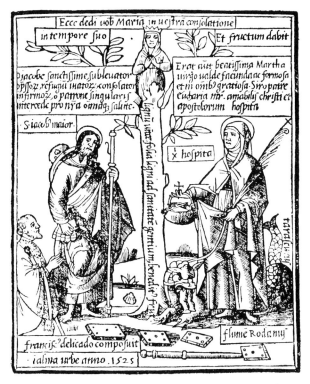

¶El modo de adoperare el legno de India occidentale:Salutifero remedio a ogni piaga z malincurabile.

Con gratia z priuilegio:per diece anni.

Figure 15. The woodcut above figures as the title-page of a pamphlet which 'Francisco Delicado composed in Rome in the year 1525'. The subject of the publication was the miraculous remedy for syphilis which the Spaniards had carried back from the New World and named guaiac after the Indians' term for the plant. The title of the pamphlet reads: 'Concerning the way in which the wood from the West Indies may be prepared. It is a curative remedy for every plague and every incurable malady'. *El modo de adoperare el legno* appeared at Venice, 1529, and it was published 'with grace and privilege for ten years' by Pope Clemens VII Medici (1523–1534). The Virgin Mary in the woodcut is identified with the guaiac tree, which bears the inscription: 'The tree of life; the leaves of the tree are for the health of the peoples; a blessed fruit.' At the top of the picture, the divine voice proclaims: 'Behold, I have given ye Mary for your consolation.' 'And in due time it [the tree] will bear fruit.'

Francisco Delicado (c. 1480-c. 1535), pictured in the woodcut, was an Italian clergyman of Spanish descent who had contracted syphilis at the beginning of the century. In the left foreground he is shown kneeling in front of 'St. James the Elder', who is depicted with his medieval symbols: Jacob's shell, the pilgrim's staff, and the pilgrim's hat – the latter flung over his shoulder. Around 1525 Francisco Delicado had undergone treatment for his disease at St. James Hospital in Rome, where he testified to having been cured by means of guaiac.[*]

[*] For an account of Francisco Delicado, see Fuchs, 1853, pp.193–204. See also Bloch, 1901–11, pp.35–43.

was introduced in Europe, no local name was known for it. The difficulty in naming the foreign wood is mentioned in von Hutten's letter to Willibald Pirckheimer (1470–1530), in which he confides to his friend his syphilitic condition and describes (in Latin) the new wonder-drug he has just encountered: 'I have the following news in regard to my health. The most important medicine comes from a wood, the correct name for which is still in doubt. Many are of the opinion that it resembles *Hebeno* [ebony], others that it resembles *Buxo* [boxwood]. That it is not *Hebenus* [ebony], we are certain' (Burckhard, 1717, p.49).

Like others of his day, von Hutten was confused by the extremely hard and heavy quality of guaiac which resembles that of ebony (Latin, *ebenus* or *hebenus*), and guaiac was often, therefore, referred to as *hebaeno* or *hebeno*. Similarly, Gonzalo Hernandes de Oviedo (1478–1557) in his *La historia natural y general de las Indias* (1535) notes that some people prefer to call guaiac the *ebony* (Munger, 1949, p.204).

In William Bullein's medical treatise *Bulleins Bulwarke of Defence againste all Sicknes, Sornes and Woundes* (1562), it is stated that 'Guaicum, or *Guaiacanum,* called *Lignum sanctum,* or the holy wodde or wodde of life, is of a kinde of *Ebenus'* (Bullein, 1562, *The Booke of Simples,* fol.lx$^r$).

## THE HOLY WOOD FROM THE NEW WORLD

The identification of guaiac and ebony appears throughout the medical literature of the time. Marshall Montgomery provides a number of examples (Montgomery, 1920, pp.23–4), and a particularly interesting one is found in a book of the learned Spanish physician Nicolas Monardes (1493–1588), published in 1565 as *Historia medicinal de las cosas, que se traën de las Indias occidentales.* The book was translated into English by John Frampton and published at London in 1580 as *Joyfull Newes out of the Newe Founde Worlde.* The work is cited by Sir Walter Raleigh in his book on *The*

---

'O James, most holy', Francisco Delicado apostrophizes the saint, 'you who have given relief to the oppressed, refuge to the wandering, and comfort to the sick. O, you incomparable patron, intercede for the salvation of us all'. The caption to the right identifies the female saint: 'The blessed Martha was a virgin, eloquent, beautiful and kind to all; with Sirius as her father and Eucharia as her mother she was an amiable hostess to Christ and the Apostles'. The word 'hospita' off Martha's head means 'hostess' and is the root of the word 'hospital', from Latin 'domus hospitalis'. Originally these 'houses of hospitality' were hostels to pilgrims, but later they were used for accommodating the sick and poor in line with the social work of the monasteries.

'Flumen Rodanus' (bottom right) stands for the river Rhône and 'tarascurus' for a monster in Provençal folklore (la Tarasque). The monster is shown devouring a small child – a symbolism which is probably connected with the 'morbus gallicus,' or the monstrous dragon from France. If this is the allusion, the attitude toward the neighbouring country is the same as that expressed by another Italian, Giorgio Sommariva, in his satirical poem *Enarratio Satyrica* (Venezia, 1496), the first known Italian mention af syphilis. According to Sommariva's argument, 'France, the perfidious enemy of Italy', has attempted to conquer Italy by means of 'a foul disease' (un morbo putridoso), after its military attempt at conquest in 1494–95 proved a failure (see pp.5–7).

* Sommariva's poem is reproduced in Sudhoff, 1912, p.18.

*Discoverie of the Large, Rich, and Bewtiful Empire of Guiana* (1596), and it was, therefore, available in Shakespeare's London. One of the chapters treats 'Of the Guaiacan and of the holy Wood' (Monardes, 1580, fol.10ᵛ) and advances the observation that 'Our Lord God would from whence the euill of the Pox came, from thence should come the remedy for them' (fol.10ᵛ). Having presented this theologico-medical doctrine of specifics ('Providence places the remedy next to the disease'), Monardes-Frampton goes on to describe the pox and the various 'Opinions of this euill':

> 'Some called it the Leprosie, others Swine-Poxe, other[s] Mentegra, others the Deathly Euill, others Elephansia, without certeyne assurance what disease it was. For they were ignorant that it was a newe disease, and they would reduce it to some already known and written of. An nowe we come to our *Guaiacan*, whose name was giuen by the Indians, and of them very well knowne, and so they haue called it and do call it, in all the world, calling it also the woodde of the Indias. Of this woodde many haue written and much, one sorte saying that it was *Ebano*, others that it was a kinde of Boxe, with many other names whereby they haue named it. It is a newe tree and neuer seene in our partes, nor in any other of the discoueries, and as the country is new, so is the tree a new thing also…it is well neere like to blacke, all is very hard as much and more then *Ebano* is.' (fol.11ᵛ)

Monardes-Frampton concludes that *Guaiacan* 'is a maruellous remedie to cure the disease of the Poxe' (fol.12ʳ), and finally gives a description of 'How the water of the woodde is made' (fol.12ʳ) (see Figure 20). The wood is also called 'the holy Wood'(fol.10ᵛ), thus reflecting the Latin name *lignum sanctum* under which it became known in Europe.[*] In an interesting way, however, the author also speaks of the 'euill seede' of 'the euill tree' (fol.11ʳ), thus associating 'The wood of the Indias' (fol.10ᵛ) with 'the Measelles of the Indias' (fol.11ᵛ), as 'the Poxe' is also called.

Attention should finally be drawn to a treatise by the Paracelsian syphilographer Phillipp Hermann (16th century) which was 'put into English by Iohn Hester' and printed in London 1590 under the title *An Excellent Treatise Teaching How to Cure the French Pockes, &c.* It deals with a cure composed of 'drinkes made of *lignum guaiacum*' and admits that 'there hath beene a great abuse committed by diuers' in the preparation and administration of the drug (Hermann, 1590, part 2, ch.1, p.29). It goes on to assert that 'The auncients in times past haue had knowledge of this wood, and haue given it his name…for though in all points it doe not agree with that which they call *Hebena*, yet I saie that it can not be anie other, but a certain kind of the said *Hebena*. The auncients describing the said *Hebena* or *Hebenum*, doe saie, that it dooth not swim, but goeth to the bottome like a stone, and that within it is as blacke as ynke, and therefore some doo saie that this is not that *Hebena*' (p.30). But the descriptions given by Dioscorides, Hermann-Hester points out, do not in all points agree with our own descriptions of the same herbs. 'Even so it is with *Hebena*, for that which groweth in India [America] is of another colour then that which groweth in Grecia, and yet notwithstanding it is a kind of *Hebena*, for it goeth to

---

[*]   A similar conglomeration of names may be found in the works of another Spanish writer on the wonders of the New World, José de Acosta (1539–1600). In speaking of the Antilles and their inhabitants, the author notes that 'They likewise bring wood of an excellent qualitie and colour, as ebony, and others, which serve for buildings and joyners. There is much of that wood which they call *Lignum sanctum*, fit to cure the pox' (Acosta, 1880, vol.1, lib.III, ch.22, p.169).

the bottome, as *Hebenum* doth, and is also of the same vertue, curing the same diseases' (p.30).

In another English translation of a foreign book, *De novo orbe or The Historie of the West Indies* (1612) by the Spanish explorer Peter Martyr (1459–1526), the translator, R. Eden, renders a passage in the original which deals with guaiac. The aborigines in Hispaniola, we are told, possessed 'householde stuffe and instrumentes, workemanly made of a certaine blacke and harde shyning wood, which that excellent learned phisition, Iohn babtist *Elisius*, affirmeth to be Hebene' (Martyr, 1612, p.33).

In Shakespeare's *Hamlet* (1600–1), Monardes-Frampton's *Ebano* (1580), Hermann-Hester's *Hebena* or *Hebenum* (1590) and Martyr-Eden's *Hebene* (1612) reappear in the *Hebona* or *Hebenon* with which King Hamlet is poisoned while 'sleeping in my orchard' (1,5:35). In this passage, the King's poisoner is twice compared to a 'serpent' (1,5:36;39), and the criminal act takes place in the context of a love triangle which is described with a mixture of jealousy and horror by the enraged Ghost. The Queen has submitted to the advances of the King's rival, and it is more than intimated that she is implicated in the crime. The Ghost's tale of the royal *drame à trois* is presented in strongly erotic, not to say venereal, terms, and it centres on such words as 'seduce', 'incest', 'adulter[y]', 'lust', 'shameful lust', 'luxury', 'lewdness', 'sin', 'act', 'will', 'sleeping', 'couch', and 'bed' (1,5:42–83). 'Sleeping within my orchard', the Ghost tells Hamlet,

> Upon my secure hour thy uncle stole,
> With juice of cursed Hebona [Hebenon]* in a vial,
> And in the porches of my ears did pour
> The leperous distilment, whose effect
> Holds such an enmity with blood of man
> That swift as quicksilver it courses through
> The natural gates and alleys of the body,
> And with a sudden vigour it doth posset
> And curd, like eager droppings into milk,
> The thin and wholesome blood. So did it mine;
> And a most instant tetter barked about,
> Most lazar-like, with vile and loathsome crust,
> All my smooth body.
> Thus was I, sleeping, by a brother's hand
> Of life, of crown, of queen, at once dispatched,
> Cut off even in the blossoms of my sin,
> Unhouseled, disappointed, unaneled,
> No reck'ning made, but sent to my account
> With all my imperfections on my head.
> O, horrible! O, horrible! most horrible! (1,5:59–80)

---

* The first edition of Hamlet – the Bad Quarto or pirated edition of 1603 (Q1) – renders the key passage as 'With juice of Hebona In a viall'. The second Quarto of 1604 (Q2) – printed partly from a corrected copy of the bad First Quarto, partly from Shakespeare's foul papers – and all subsequent quartos (Q3, Q4, Q5, and Q6) read 'Hebona', as follows: 'With juyce of cursed Hebona in a viall'. The Folio of 1623 (F1) and all subsequent folios read 'Hebenon'.

THE SYPHILITIC INFECTION IN HAMLET

*The Jew of Malta* (c. 1589) by Christopher Marlowe (1564–1593) refers, like *Hamlet*, to 'The juice of Hebon, and Cocytus breath, and all the poisons of the Stygian pool' (3,4:98–9), thus indicating that there was a common Elizabethan tradition connecting *Hebon*, *Hebona* or *Hebenon* with ebony wood in its 'juicy' or medicinable aspect where the wood could be poisonous. Since there is no evidence that ebony wood itself was ever regarded as poisonous, and since Shakespearean texts have *ebon* and *ebony* elsewhere in its traditional association with blackness (*Venus and Adonis* 1. 948, *2 Henry IV* 5,5:37, *Love's Labour's Lost* 4,3:243–4, *Twelfth Night* 4,2:38), the unique form of the wood in *Hamlet* (1,5:62) suggests associations in Shakespeare to a related, yet different plant. This can only be 'Lignum Guaiacum, commonly called Pockwood' (Hermann, 1590, *To the Reader*), which in Shakespeare's time was closely connected with ebony, as we have demonstrated. The associative patterns of the Ghost's tale further emphasize the venereal implication of the 'Hebona...juice', which is compared to a '*leperous* distilment' running as 'swift as *quicksilver*' and producing effects on the skin which are indistinguishable from the '*tetter*' of a secondary syphilitic eruption (Figure 16).*

Shakespeare's associative pattern bears a curious resemblance to a syphilitic passage in John Lyly's satirical tract *Pappe with a Hatchet* (1589), which Shakespeare is likely to have read as a newcomer to London when the Marprelate controversy was at its height and engaged the pens of the capital's leading literary figures. 'But

---

* The identification of the poison with which King Hamlet is killed has been a bone of contention among Shakespearean scholars for many years. Marshall Montgomery was the first who identified the poison with guaiac (Montgomery, 1920, pp.23–6). Other scholars have attempted to identify the poison with ebony, but for reasons stated above this seems weak on all sides. The case for the yew-tree (*Taxus baccata*) is equally doubtful. Thomas Cooper (1517–94), Shakespeare's contemporary, in his *Thesaurus Linguae* (London, 1578) takes pains to translate *Taxus* twice, rendering it as 'A tree like firre, bearing bearies that are poyson. Also the tree called yew'. *Hebona* or *Hebenon* as synonyms for the yew-tree are nowhere to be found in Elizabethan literature. The closest connection are three references to 'heben' in *The Faerie Queene* (1589–96) by Edmund Spenser (1552?–99), where the word *perhaps* may be interpreted as referring to the yew-tree (Nicholson, 1880–6, pp.21–31. Cf. also Harrison, 1880–6, pp.295–321). However, it is not only philology which is against the yew-theory as meaning *Hebona* or *Hebenon*. Although it is true that the yew was known for a deadly poison – it is even called 'cursed' in Philemon Holland's (1552–1637) translation of Pliny's *Natural History* (1601, I, 463) – Shakespeare only mentions 'yew' four times and none of these connect it with any poisonous qualities. 'My shroud of white, stuck all with yew, O prepare it', sings the clown in *Twelfth Night* (2,4:55), while the witches in *Macbeth* howl: 'Gall of goat, and slips of yew, Slivered in the moon's eclipse' (4,1:27). Shakespeare's associations to 'yew' are the normal gloomy ones because of its use in England as a churchyard tree, hence the 'dismal yew' in *Titus Andronicus* (2,3:107). It is only in the fourth and final reference that there is the possibility of connecting the plant with death-burial *and* poison. 'Thy very beadsmen', Scroope tells the King in *Richard II*, 'learn to bend their bows Of double-fatal yew against thy state' (3,2:116–7). On this background it is unlikely that the yew would be at the back of the poet's mind when he wrote *Hebona* or *Hebenon*; and, in addition, the 'leperous' and 'lazar-*like*' skin effects or 'tetter' of the herbal decoction carry far stronger associations to pockwood than to yew.

Another group of scholars speculate that *Hebenon* might refer to *henbane*, and ingeniously explain that *Hebenon* by metathesis could stand for *henebon*, that is, *henbane*, of which the most common species, *Hyoscyamus niger*, is a narcotic (Bradley, 1920, pp.85–7). Pliny in his *Natural History* (XXV, 17) writes of the henbane plant: 'An oil of its seeds causes mental derangement if it is poured into the ears'. Although this is a close association, the poison poured into the King's ears in *Hamlet* caused death and not insanity as it does in the Pliny reference. Thus the effects ascribed to henbane in Pliny and Elizabethan herbal lore show little correspondence with what Shakespeare describes. Alternative identifications have fixed on hemlock and deadly nightshade (belladonna), but these suggestions rest on an even weaker basis than the identifications of *Hebenon* with the yew and henbane. (For a summary of the above discussion, see Macht, 1918, pp.165–70.)

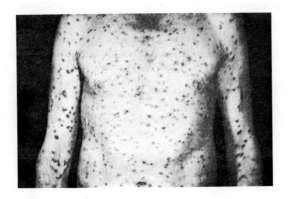

Figure 16. Photo of skin rash of a secondary syphilitic eruption showing macular-papular syphilide on trunk and extremities (Nielsen and Schmidt, 1985, p.83). 'For more than two centuries syphilitic eruptions were classed as pustules or crust', C.C. Dennie observes in *A History of Syphilis*. 'To many observers the manifestations were the primary indications of the new disease. In the 1830s, Jean Louis Alibert proposed that they be given the name of Syphilids, as the lesions are known today' (Dennie, 1962, p.36). Shakespeare's description of the symptoms seems to cover both the roseolar syphilide and the papular syphilide. The former represents the earliest skin lesion of syphilis and usually appears as a generalized and macular rash or 'tetter', erupting four to eight weeks after the primary chancre. The papular syphilide may occur where the roseolar rash was situated or may appear on normal skin. The papules are the commonest and most characteristic of the secondary syphilitic eruptions. They are widely distributed over trunk, arms and legs, and are found on the palms, soles, face and genitals. As the result of endarteritis obliterans and diminution of blood supply, scaling of the surfaces of the papules is common, and crusted lesions are usually seen among the papules of the papular syphilide. When scaling lesions predominate, the rash is called the papulosquamous syphilide. Sometimes the spots are large and plaque-like with considerable waxy scaling on the surface. These may resemble the crusted lesions of psoriasis and have then been referred to as the 'psoriasiform secondary syphilide' (King and Nicol, 1975, p.33).

softe Martins, did your Father die at the Groyne?', Lyly maliciously asks the Puritan extremist Martin Marprelate, in defence of the bishops and the Anglican Church. 'It was well groapt at, for I knewe him sicke of a paine in the groyne. A *pockes* of that religion, (quoth Iulian Grimes to her Father) when al his haires fell off on the sodaine. Well let the old knaue be dead…Martins conscience hath a periwig; therefore to good men he is more sower than wig: a Lemman [whore] will make his conscience *curd* like a *Posset*…with your painted consciences [you] have coloured the religion of diuers, spreading through the *veynes* of the Commonwealth like *poyson*, the doggednes of your deuotions; which entring in like the smooothnes of oyle into the flesh, fretteth in time like *quicksiluer* into the bones' (Lyly, 1902, vol.3, pp.399, 406–7; italics added).

The syphilitic value of Shakespeare's associations to 'quicksilver' in the ghostly tale of *Hamlet* is confirmed not only by its function as an anti-syphilitic in the poet's time but also by the second appearance of the word in the canon. In *2 Henry IV*, 'quicksilver' occurs in a marked syphilitic context, with reference even to the poisoned blood of this infection. 'Sit on my knee, *Doll'*, Falstaff tells his syphilitic prostitute, Doll Tearsheet. 'A rascal bragging slave! The rogue fled from me like *quicksilver.*' 'I'faith', Doll replies, 'and thou followedst him like a church. Thou whoreson little tidy Bartholomew boar-pig, when wilt thou leave fighting a-days, and foining [copulating] a-nights, and begin to patch up thine old body for heaven'

(2,4:223–30). When shortly afterwards Hal arrives at the scene, Falstaff greets him with the words: 'Thou whoreson mad compound of majesty, by this light flesh and corrupt blood [*Leaning his hand upon Doll*], thou art welcome' (2,4:291–3).

The '*corrupt blood*' of Falstaff's syphilized 'light' wench figures as another important associative element in the ghostly tale in *Hamlet*. Here the 'Hebona…juice' is presented as entering the '*blood* of man' and 'cours[ing]' through The natural gates and alleys of the body', that is, flowing through its ducts and veins. The effect of the poison is to 'curd[le]' and coagulate the blood, thus producing a 'tetter' or 'vile and loathsome crust' on the King's 'smooth body'.

This is precisely the way in which the physicians of the 16th century imagined the syphilitic infection to work its poisonous effects on the human body. As early as 1519, Ulrich von Hutten had speculated on 'the secret causes of this disease' (Hutten, 1533, fol.3ᵛ),[*] whose systemic nature baffled the doctors of the age. In the second chapter of *De guaiaci medicina et morbo gallico*, he presents both the astrologers' explanation which 'fetch the cause of this infirmite from the sterres' (fol.3ᵛ), and the physicians' opinion that the disease is due to 'yll and habundant humours…whose sharpnes streking out to the outward partes of the body burneth and dryeth the skynne, and fylleth it ful of scabbes' (fol.4ʳ). He goes on to state his own opinion, shared with a number of others,

'that this infirmite cometh of corrupt, burnt, & enfect blode. And al these thynges were in doubtful disputation, the nature thereof not yet knowen, but now it is knowen, they be also appued. for in myn opinion this sicknes is no other thing but a postumation, & rotting of unpure blode: the whiche after it beginneth to drie, it turneth into swelling & hard knobbes, the which thinge procedeth of the lyuer corrupt.' (fol.4ʳ)

William Clowes repeats these views in the second chapter of *A Briefe and Necessary Treatise* (1596), in which he examines 'The maner of taking this sicknesse' (Clowes, 1596, p.150). He mentions dangerous gateways of the body such as the sexual parts, the mouth, and the anus (omitting the ears!), and proceeds to describe the way in which the poison courses through the veins of the body:

'Any outward part being once infected, the disease immediately entreth into the blood, and so creepeth on like a canker from part to part, untill it commeth to the liuer, where being once entred, it corrupteth the fountaine of blood, and thence sendeth forth the infection by the veines into euery part of the body…the effects thereof (as I gather) are these, it corrupteth the blood, and poisoneth the whole humors of the body, and breedeth in the parts thereof pains and aches, virulent and malignant ulcers, nodes, or knobby hardnes, foule scabs, tetters, and ringwormes both in the hands and feete, and callous ulcers about the priuy parts…Moreouer, venemous pustules and scabs upon the forehead, browes, face, and beard, and in other parts of the body.' (pp.153–4)[**]

---

[*]   Hutten's work is quoted after the English translation by Thomas Paynel (1533).

[**]  'Some doo fall into thys foule disease', says Phillipp Hermann in *An Excellent Treatise Teaching Howe to Cure the French Pockes* (1590), 'through companying with women, where [they] through the secret parts are first infected, then the blood throughout the whole body, & lastlie the sinewes, the flesh and bone' (Hermann, 1590, pp.2–3). Von Hutten's, Shakespeare's and Clowes's ideas of the way in which the syphilitic poison enters through 'The natural gates and alleys of the body' in order to corrupt the blood and 'swift as quicksilver' to reach the entire organism are curiously modern. In the primary stage of syphilis, the infection becomes systemic within a few hours of exposure, the spirochetes passing through the mucous membranes into the

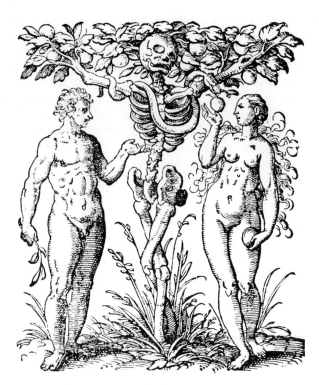

Figure 17. The woodcut of the Fall was executed by the Swiss artist Jobst Amman (1539–91) and forms part of his illustrations for *De conceptu et generatione hominis* (Frankfurt, 1587) by the famous Swiss gynecologist Jacob Rueff (c. 1500–88) (Rueff, 1587, p.1[r]). The picture's symbolism describes the kind of sexual drama which may have influenced the associations in the world's greatest poet when creating his greatest dramatic scene. The serpent with the apple forms part of a skeletal figure which we suggest identified with Claudius. He is described by Hamlet as 'He that hath killed my king and whored my mother' (5,2:64). After the Ghost's revelation that Claudius is 'that incestuous, that adulterate beast…[who] won to his shameful lust The will of my most seeming-virtuous queen' (1,5:42; 45–6), Hamlet's first embittered reaction is: 'O most pernicious woman! O villain, villain, smiling, damned villain!' (1,5:105–6). 'Revenge [my] foul and most unnatural murder', the Ghost roars at Hamlet, 'Murder most foul, as in the best it is; But this most foul, strange, and unnatural' (1,5:25;27–8).

Another 'foul, strange, and unnatural' murder took place in the 16th century when Francois I (1515–47) was venereally poisoned by his mistress, 'la belle Ferronière', without her knowing. Her jealous husband, the famous jurist Ferron, had infected himself with syphilis and passed on the disease to his wife in order to take revenge on his royal rival (Bäumler, 1976, pp.64–5). A similar 'foul play' (1,2:256) in a Bohemian setting could have brought the poet's infection at the hands of a rival who had infected a common love object that had proved unfaithful. Such a triangular drama might explain many peculiar features in *Hamlet*, which according to Ernest Jones reflects 'some overwhelming passion that ended in a betrayal in such circumstances that murderous impulses towards the faithless couple were stirred but could not be admitted to consciousness…His way of responding was to compose a tragedy whose theme was the suffering of a tortured man who could not avenge [in real life] his injured feelings' (Jones, 1949, pp.114, 120). The protagonist, who identifies completely with his father, displays a deep-seated revulsion for Gertrude which is in excess of the facts as they appear. Similarly, Claudius becomes the object of Hamlet's consuming hatred and rivalry, finally to suffer violent death at the Prince's hands. Psychologically, the protagonist's experience with the treacherous couple results in a disillusioned and cynical conception of life, accompanied by a profound misogyny which makes him view all women as prostitutes, even the chaste Ophelia. Without warrant in his sources, Saxo and Belleforest, Shakespeare has finally transformed his play into a poisonous drama which takes place at a literal as well as figurative level, with fatal consequences for all the parties involved (see further pp.229–33).

A final important feature of King Hamlet's poisoning is the associative pattern established by Shakespeare in the third act, where Hamlet stages a re-enactment of the murder in order to prove Claudius's guilt. The poisoner-actor is addressed by Hamlet in this way: 'Begin, *murderer, Pox*, leave thy damnable faces and begin' (Q1 and F1: 3,2:246–7). 'A pox on you' was the favourite Elizabethan curse and it did not apply to the small pox but to the great pox. This same meaning of the word surfaces later in the play, where the gravedigger mentions the 'many *pocky* corses now-a-days that will scarce hold the laying in' (5,1:158–9), the reason being that they are '*rotten* before [they] die' (5,1:157).

## 'CURSED HEBONA' – 'THE WOODDE OF DEATH'

It is true that guaiac was an *anti-lueticum*, and so the action of the 'juice' or decoction in *Hamlet* may seem strange because it acts as a poison producing the same symptoms as the disease for which it was supposed to be a cure. Apart from the poetic freedom allowed an artist in describing a drug and its medical symptoms, there is evidence that Shakespeare's contemporaries regarded guaiac as poisonous and just as danger-ous as quicksilver if administered incorrectly.

In Monardes-Frampton's *Joyfull Newes out of the Newe Founde Worlde* (1580), guaiac is also described as 'the euill tree' (Monardes, 1580, p.41), and in William Bullein's great medical treatise *Bulleins Bulwarke of Defence againste All Sicknes, Sornes and Woundes* (1562), the author terms guaiac 'the woodde of death' if it is used in a faulty manner (Bullein, 1562, *The Booke of Simples*, fol.lxi$^v$). An entire page of Bullein's treatise is devoted to a description of 'what euill[s] haue happened through the abusing of Guaicum emong the imperikes' (fol.lxi$^r$). According to Bullein, the 'wodde was not a litle abused of a great number of ingnorante, murdering, shameles practisioners, whiche haue taken vpon them, to binde sicke men to a law, obseruyng the new diet, onely with *Guaiacum*…Experiens hath learned vs sufficiently, by the deathes of many which haue ben slain in this purgatorie of this folishe Phisicke, ignorantly vsed, or this *Guaicum* rather folishly abused for money' (fol.lxi$^r$).

In his depiction of the guaiac cure, Bullein expressly distinguishes between a correct and a faulty application of the American wood, which in the hands of doctors may turn out to be either the wood of life or the wood of death: 'And now let vs retourne againe vnto our *Guaiacum* or *Lignum vite*, called the woode of life, whiche through couetousnesse, haue been rather made the woode of death, through longe newe diates, to small effecte to many, though fortunate to fewe. *Marcellus* my brother, when your frende *Senior F. Neapolitani* was smitten with the Pox, his heere fell awaie, he could not slepe for boneache, his breath did stincke, Lorde how pale he looked, his muskles consumed, the skabbes appered, vnder whom where deepe hooles grauen with putrified matter, etc. but now his hedde is couered with heere, his skinne cleane, rose coulered in his cheekes, full of strength, he sleapeth verie well, and is in health' (fol.lxi$^v$).

---

bloodstream and, hence, into every organ of the body. When the disease is discovered through the primary lesion – the chancre – it has already infected the lymph glands and thus poisoned the entire organism. Like AIDS, syphilis is a malady of the blood and hard to catch except by the most intimate contact; the only proven routes of contagion of both diseases are blood, sex and childbearing.

In order to understand the dangerous aspects of the American wonder drug, one must examine the entire cure of which it was part. During the 16th century, guaiac was apparently prepared and administered according to several formulae, but certainly one of the earliest, most detailed, and most universally used was that of Ulrich von Hutten. According to the recipe provided by the author in the seventh chapter of his book, the wood was either to be broken into very small pieces, or reduced to sawdust or powder. One pound of the prepared wood was to be mashed with eight pounds of water for a day and a night, and then simmered slowly over an gentle fire in a well-covered vessel filled only two-thirds full. The brew was to be simmered for at least six hours or until it was reduced to one half of the original volume. The chemist was to ensure that the mixture did not boil because the decoction in that case would lose something of its original power. The foam which floated during the cooking was to be skimmed off and used for anointment of the syphilitic sores. The remaining liquid was the medicine proper, to be drunk during the whole treatment in accordance with the greatest fasting possible, by whatever diet.

During the whole *regimen*, the patient had to sit in a continously heated room where every crack was filled, so that he was exposed as little as possible to the noxious influence of the air. The sweating induced by the guaiac had to be supported in every conceivable manner in order to further the chief function of the Holy Wood, which, according to von Hutten, was 'not to breake, or plucke away the bloudde, but by lyttell and lyttell to amende and purify hit (in whiche bloudde being corrupte, resteth al the force and strength of this disease) and to expelle and diuide from the body the hurtefull humours, that are norisshementes of this disease, from some in theyr vrin and sweatynges, and from other som in theyr sieges [stools]. And whan of this disease a man begynneth to waxe whole, than the fyrst operation of Guaiacum is to make a man to sweate, and secondly by the passages of the vrine it purgeth; by whiche meanes it fetcheth out and voydeth marueylous foule fylthynesses'(Hutten, 1533, fol.61ᵛ–62ʳ).*

Von Hutten consoled his readers that the ordeals of the guaiac cure were possible to endure only because of the power inherent in the Holy Wood to preserve life in a feeble body. However, he sternly admonished every patient to abstain entirely from wine and women during the treatment: 'It is playnly knowen, that he shall dye without remedy, that vseth any woman before the xl [fortieth] daye after the cure is begonne, either bycause the body so emptied, is not able to suffer the iniurie of that acte, or elles bycause god wyll not that any man shulde vse such his great benefyte vnpurely' (fol.35ᵛ).

THE DANGERS OF THE GUAIAC CURE

In England the guaiac cure appears to have been well established by the middle of the 16th century since William Bullein (d. 1576), Thomas Gale (1507–87), and John Banister (1540–1610) mention it. Both Bullein and Gale provide detailed

---

* Taken internally, probably the only physiological actions of guaiac are a sense of warmth in the stomach, sweating, and active purging. A well-marked rash, attended with considerable itching, and resembling that of copaiba used in the treatment of gonorrhea, is said sometimes to appear (Munger, 1949, p.208).

recipes for the decoction of the wood and prescriptions as to how the cure is to be carried out in a proper manner, 'as by experiens we se, there is no better remedy, then sweatyng, and the drinkyng of Guiacum, vsyng it in due tyme and order', as William Bullein says of the 'Poxe' (Bullein, 1562, *The Booke of the Use of Sicke Men and Medicenes,* fol.lxviiiv). Thomas Gale also emphasizes that patients, having ingested the medicine, 'must sweate, for in sweating is the chiefest matter that is required in the maner of cure. They muste use all other maner of necessarye thynges, as sleepynge, quietnes, company and a conuenient place, and aboue all thynges to be kept close in all tyme of their cure, lesse that the ayre might enter in and stoppe the powers' (Gale, 1563a, p.84).

John Banister states that mouth ulcers 'if [they] proceed *A morbo venereo*' (Banister, 1575, fol.25ᵛ) are treated by diet, purgation, decoctions of guaiacum and touching the ulcer with sublimated rose water. He also mentions corroding 'Vlcers of the priuie partes' (fol.57ᵛ) which could well be syphilis, chancroid or herpes genitalis, and finally repeats that 'When the Ulcers proceed through the Frenche pockes, a thinne diet must be vsed with the decoction of *Guiacum,* or vse vniuersall [mercurial] vnctions' (fol.62ᵛ).

Once more, however, we hear sceptical voices as to the efficacy of the guaiac cure. During a discussion between two doctors quoted in Thomas Gale's *Certain Workes of Chirurgerie* (1563), one of them mentions the guaiac cure which a certain 'Doctour Cunyngham' is said to have improved upon. But the other doctor is sceptical and says: 'I judge his newe inuented way of curation to be extreme and dangerous to the pacient, for both the fumes, unguents, and strayte order of diet with the wood, are wel knowen to be dangerous, and yet many tymes doeth not that whiche they promise' (p.31).

As with quicksilver, guaiac was thought a very dangerous drug if handled improperly. This may be illustrated by the conditions at *Die Fuggerei* in Augsburg, a hospital founded between 1516 and 1523 by the merchant Jacob Fugger (1459–1525), who prospered by importing guaiac wood from America. *Die Fuggerei* consisted of 52 houses for the poor and diseased, and of these, three were reserved for the treatment with *Guajatzischen Holzes,* this being the reason that the houses were called *Holzhäuser.* The violent purgations and sweatings without drink on an empty stomach made it necessary to examine the patients' general state of health before they were admitted to the 'wood houses' for treatment with guaiac. Professional physicians were appointed for this entrance examination, and the dangers of the guaiac cure were further emphasized by the fact that every patient was required to present a document from a priest stating that he had received the holy sacraments, 'because nobody knows what may happen to him during the cure, in particular through the inunction and fumigation' (*weil niemand weiss, was ihm in der Kur sonderlich ob der schmierb und Rauch mag zusteen*) (Weidenbacher, 1926, p.62) (Fumigation by means of guaiac wood also formed part of the treatment).

The dangers of the new remedy were discussed in detail by one of the great syphilographers of the day, the Frenchman Jacques de Béthencourt (16th century). He is known primarily for his introduction of the term *morbus venereus* for *morbus gallicus,* because he was one of the first to recognize the connection between the disease and the goddess of love, Venus. Two other French syphilographers, it should be noted, were just as eager to exonerate their nation and point out the real culprit. Instead of *morbus gallicus* Jean François Fernel (1497–1558) suggested the term *lues venerea* for syphilis (1548), while Thierry de Héry (1500?–1599) proposed the term *la maladie vénérienne* (1552). In Béthencourt's book *Nova poenitentialis quadragesima* (Paris, 1527), the author portrays a judge summing up a discussion between Mercury and Guaiacum as to the advantages of the two kinds of cure which the two allegorical figures represent:

> 'It is true that Guaiacum suits man's constitution better [than Mercury]. However, the treatment with Guaiacum is inhuman because of the extremely severe way of living which is imposed on the patient…And as the nature of Guaiacum has not been sufficiently examined for us by the ancient medical authors, experiments with it present a danger…For these reasons and considerations, arrived at with a calm mind, I shall conclude: the Mercury cure which is supported by the clearly stated principles of Hippocrates and Galen – our venerable popes of medicine – is to be trusted more than Guaiacum'. (Béthencourt, 1527, sig.Ov^(r-v)–Ovi^r)

Ulrich von Hutten's biographer, David Friedrich Strausz (1808–74), relates how the German knight himself died of tertiary syphilis, in spite of his strenuous use of guaiac water. He also informs us that, while many in Germany believed von Hutten had been poisoned, others actually expressed the view that 'the cause of his early death was due less to the disease and more to the murderous guaiac cure which he had taken' (*die mörderische Guaiak-Cur, die er durchgemacht*) (Strausz, 1895, p.497).

Another witness to the dangers of the guaiac cure is Hutten's contemporary Benvenuto Cellini (1500–71), the noted Italian goldsmith and sculptor. He too was a firm believer in the *aqua guayaci*, and in his autobiography he tells of the way in which he cured himself twice in 1532, using 'all the precautions and abstinence imaginable' and drinking guaiac 'contrary to the advice of the most eminent physicians of Rome' (Cellini, 1771, vol.1, p.230). When his second attack of syphilis proved to be more severe than the first one and was attended with a fever, 'I proposed to take *lignum vitae*, but the physicians opposed it, assuring me that if I meddled with it whilst the fever was upon me, I should die in a week' (p.230). In spite of his medical advisers, Benvenuto Cellini drank 'the decoction of *lignum vitae*' (p.230) and dumbfounded the doctors by recovering. But it is clear that the medical authorities of the day were against him, and that he was running a notable risk.

North of the Alps, the famous Swiss doctor Theophrastus Bombastus von Hohenheim, called Paracelsus (1493–1541), examined the powers of the new remedy in his short treatise *Vom Holz Guiaco gründlicher heylung* (Nuremberg, 1529). Paracelsus was alarmed by what he called 'the greatest disease in the whole world' (*die grösste krankheit der ganzen welt*) (Paracelsus, 1922–33, vol.7, p.11), and he strongly

---

Father and son's joint presentation of King Hamlet's lusty 'crimes' in a month of venery and procreation may explain the peculiar behaviour of the Ghost when appearing to Horatio 'like a guilty thing' (1,1:153), its 'countenance more in sorrow than in anger…very pale' (1,2:231;233). In the same scene, Hamlet instinctively feels that the apparition's reason for coming is not to warn the country of military danger, but to disclose 'some foul play' (1,2:256) of the past, some 'foul crimes' (1,5:12) even: 'My father's spirit in arms! All is not well…Foul deeds will rise, Though all the earth o'erwhelm them, to men's eyes' (1,2:255;257–8).

Figure 18. The woodcut from the title-page of Jean Cheradame's French translation of von Hutten's treatise on the guaiac cure (Paris, c. 1525) shows the author in his bed, well blanketed and wearing a nightcap. On the table is a dish of fruit while a bird-cage is suspended from a beam in the ceiling. Its feathered inhabitant is probably intended to bring a bit of cheer to the depression of the guaiac chamber and also to signal by its death that the room had become too air-

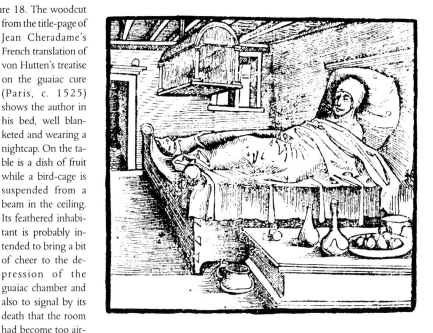

less. In his letter to Willibald Pirckheimer, another syphilitic of the time, von Hutten tells of his staunch friend, Georg von Streitberg, who braved the suffocating heat and stench of Hutten's guaiac chamber, even when he stank most foully (*frequens mihi in hoc valetudinario adfuit, etiam tunc, quum ob morbi foeditatem spurcissime foeterem*), attending to his wants or sitting beside his couch for whole hours at a time, keeping him in good spirits (Burckhard, 1717, p.52). The ordeals of the starved and dried out drinkers of guaiac during their forty days of incarceration were aptly described by Jacques de Béthencourt, earliest of French syphilographers, as 'nova penitentialis quadragesima', a new kind of Lent. The companions of the French king Henry III (*regnebat* 1574–89), for the most part indulgers in the new wood, commonly called the subjection of oneself to a course of guaiac 'suer une diette' (Zimmermann, 1932, p.271). In *William Turners Herball* of 1568, guaiac is called 'Diet woode because they that kepe a Diet for the Frenche poxe or anye other disease hardly curable most commonlye drinke the broth of this woode' (Turner, 1568, p.34).

The guaiac cure's thirty or forty days of severe fasting, heavy sweating and violent purgations are the 'purgatorie' referred to by William Bullein in his description of the abuses of the guaiac cure (p.48). 'Drink every morning a draught of *noli me tangere*', quips another English writer on the pox a generation later, 'and by that means thou shalt be sure to escape the physician's purgatory' ('The Penniles Parliament of Threed-bare Poets' (1608). *The Harleian Miscellany*. London, 1808, vol.1, p.185). A similar 'purgatorie' is probably hinted at by King Hamlet in his ambiguous description of the purgatorial horrors of his 'prison-house' (1,5:14), in which he is 'confined to fast in fires, Till the foul crimes done in my days of nature Are burnt and purged away' (1,5:11–3). This phrasing anticipates the ghostly King's later description of that 'most horrible' (1,5:80) event when he was 'Cut off even in the blossoms of my sin' (5,1:76) and 'sent to my account With all my imperfectionns on my head' (1,5:78–9). Hamlet's description of his uncle's poisoning of his 'sleeping' (1,5:59;74) father seems to move within the same area of venery and guilt. Claudius's real crime is here presented as that of poisoning a man when in the full indulgence of his sensual appetites:

> A [He] took my father grossly, full of bread,
> With all his crimes broad blown, as flush as May;
> And how his audit stands who knows save heaven?
> But in our circumstance and course of thought
> 'Tis heavy with him. (3,3:80–4)

advocated mercurial treatment of the victims of the 'French Disease'. At the same time he warned his colleagues of the toxic effects of 'mercurialism' and advised them to use careful dosage and less toxic mercury preparations. The miracles ascribed to guaiac by von Hutten he vigorously rejected in *Vom Holz Guaiaco gründlicher heylung*, which was the first of a number of studies on syphilis to which Paracelsus dedicated himself. The only miracle Paracelsus conceded to the American wonder drug was the ever continuing and growing revenue which it brought to the coffers of the holders of the guaiac import monopoly, the Fuggers of Augsburg. 'They have brought you a wood', he wrote in 1528 of Charles V and the Fuggers, 'but where is its [medical] virtues?' (*ein holz hant sie euch bracht, wo ist aber der wagen de virtutibus?*) (p.418).

In 1565, in Strasbourg, a disciple of Paracelsus, Michael Schütz (also called Toxites), collected and published the observations of Paracelsus on the subject, and titled the collection *Holtzbüchlein*. This little book begins: 'It is not untrue that the wood I name *Xilohebenum* (also called *sanctum* or *guaiacanum*) is a good and useful herb' (Schütz, 1565, quoted after Montgomery, 1920, p.26). However, Schütz goes on, it is now clear and '*am tag*', 'that the use of that same [medicine] is not properly understood or carried out' and that its use has fallen very much into the hands of quacks and has been subject to misuse and led to imposture, with the result that

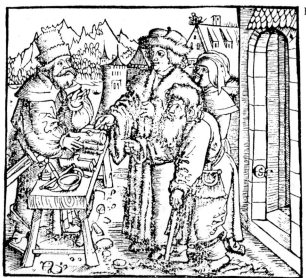

Figure 19. The woodcut adorns the title-page of Thomas Murner's German translation of Ulrich von Hutten's treatise on the guaiac cure, published at Strasbourg 1519. A physician with two patients, one with a staff and a bandaged leg, seems to be bargaining for some of the American wood, sold by a merchant (left) who is ready to weigh the precious wood with his pair of scales. With his short 1529 treatise *Vom Holtz Guaiaco gründlicher heylung*, Paracelsus denounced von Hutten's book and the popular guaiac cure, which he by and large deemed as having no effect on the disease. Paracelsus reiterated these views in the lengthy treatise *Von der Frantzösischen Kranckheit Drei Bücher* (Nuremberg, 1530), in which he attacked the doctors of the day as 'impostors'. Enraged, the Leipzig Medical Faculty sent its dean Heinrich Stromer of Auerbach – founder of 'Auerbach's Cellar' – to Nuremberg, where the Senate of the town subscribed to the doctors' demand for censorship. While Paracelsus fled the city, the Senate issued a decree that prohibited the printing of his planned 'Eight Books on the French Disease' (*Vom Ursprung und Herkommen der Franzosen samt der Recepten Heilung, act Bücher*). The Fuggers and the physicians of Germany had finally won the battle establishing the precedence of guaiac over other cures.

many sick persons have been destroyed (*verderbt*) by this cure (p.26). Schütz in his *Vorrede* points out that many people spoke of quicksilver, or 'Theophrasti medicamenta' as a 'poison with which people were killed', to which he counters that 'I could give many examples from recent years of the way in which the wood Guaiacum through inunction, fumigation and baths has killed many honest people and also grievously ruined many, so that they have lifelong been incapable of work and have considered death more desirable than life' (p.26).

In England, the writer Thomas Nashe (1567–1601) gave expression to similar mixed feelings about guaiac in his *Lenten Stuffe* (1599), where he speaks somewhat contemptuously of the physicians' 'soueraigne *Guiacum*', naming it along with 'their mithridates of fortie seuerall poysons compacted, their bitter *Rubarbe* and torturing *Stibium*' (Nashe, 1910, vol.3, p.176). Still later, another British writer, Patrick Browne, observed of the *lignum vitae* in his book *The Civil and Natural History of Jamaica* (1756): 'The pulp of the berries purges and vomits very violently…The resinous parts of the tree…are esteemed specifics in old venereal taints, chronical rheumatisms, and other disorders arising from the sizyness of the juices; and generally administered in decoctions…but great care must be taken to moderate or temper the native acrimony of these medicines in the beginning of a course, and to prepare the body for the use of them; the neglect of which has been frequently the cause of very dismal consequents in those warm climates, and may probably have the like effects sometimes in colder regions' (Browne, 1756, p.226).

In concluding this section, one may point out that Paracelsus was in many ways ahead of his time. His denunciation of the guaiac cure was not the least of his prophetic observations. Modern medicine has proved that guaiac is wholly without effect on syphilis, and so we may relegate the cure with the Holy Wood to one of the many blind alleys of medical history. Robert S. Munger in his essay on *Guaiacum, the Holy Wood from the New World* (1949) concludes: 'Certainly of all the exotic remedies used through the centuries in the treatment of the greatest of all social diseases, none was more lauded, and at the same time less efficacious than the Holy Wood from the New World' (p.226).

DREAMS OF A 'WONDER DRUG'

On the theory that wherever a disease occurs naturally, there will also be found drugs for its treatment, many new drugs were introduced from the New World for use against syphilis. In addition to guaiac, the chief drugs of this sort were china root, sassafras, and sarsaparilla. Decoctions were usually made from the roots of these plants and drunk in copious quantities. China root, *Smilax sinensis*, was given, as stated by Fracastoro, largely as a sudorific by the Chinese, who 'use it for many diseases, but especially for the French disease. It induces an incredible amount of sweat and is also drying; it is therefore no wonder that it is efficacious for this disease' (Fracastoro, 1930, pp.283–5).

Sarsaparilla, prepared from the root of the South American plant *Smilax ornata*, is not mentioned by Fracastoro, although it was introduced from the West Indies at about the same time as china root was imported from the East in 1535. It quickly became known as a 'blood purifier' and was used until 1914, mainly in old tertiary syphilitic cases with chronic ulcers which did not yield to arsenic, mercury, iodides or bismuth treatment.

Yet another American plant, *Sassafra officinale*, was used in the treatment of the New World disease. 'Sassafras', wrote John Woodall in *The Surgeons Mate* (1617), 'is of a hot and drie temperament in the second degree, commended in taking away obstructions, corroborating the inward parts, helping the asthmatique and Nephretike, clensing the reines from grauell, discussing winde, good for womens diseases, and against any kinde of fluxion, and the *Morbus Gallicus*, or French pox it is a good medicine' (p.98).

A homely plant, saffron (*Crocus sativus*), is mentioned by Shakespeare as an anti-syphilitic in a bawdy context in *All's Well That Ends Well*, where the knavish and lecherous Parolles recommends 'villainous saffron' for all 'unbaked and doughy youth' (4,5:2–3). Such use of the term is also provided by the Dominican friar Thomas Moulton, who in his *Mirrour of Glasse of Health* (1539) gives 'A good drynke for the pox. ca.[pitulum] cxviii. Take salendine and englyshe saffron, the weyght of an halfpenny and a farthyng wort of graynes a quarter of longe pepper, a pany weyght of mase and stale ale, stampe youre herbs and pouder youre suffron and medle them all togither and than drinke it' (capitulum cxviii).

There is no evidence that any of these plant preparations had the slightest effect on syphilis. Yet they themselves produced no harm and, since the disease tends to be self-limiting, they may have given the appearance of producing some benefit.[*]

On top of these sudorifics and purgatives came a plethora of popular medicines for the pox, some of them collected in *A Rich Store-House of Treasury for the Diseased...Now Set Foorth for the Great Benefit and Comfort of the Poorer Sort of People That are Not of Abilitie to Go to the Physitions* (1596). After giving two recipes based on guaiac and quicksilver, the anonymous author 'A.T.' finally presents the common man with 'A good Medecine to kill the great Pocke': 'Take a good quantity of Camphire, and lay it to the place where the pocke is, and it will presently eate it cleane away. Probatum est' (A.T., 1596, fol.62ʳ).

In the forefront of medical speculation and experimentation was the dream of producing the great panacea for all disease – syphilis included. Such visions flourished among the practitioners of a new and revolutionary brand of science known as alchemical or Paracelsian medicine. One of the leading iatrochemists in England was the London distiller and translator John Hester, who, in the final chapter of his Paracelsian treatise *The Key of Philosophie* (1596), disclosed a method 'To make oil of gold' (p.106) and thereby to obtain the great panacea. At the end of a long and complicated process of alchemical distillation and rectification, Hester promised his labouring reader that 'thou shalt finde an oile in the receiuer, the which is not to bee bought for any money: For because it helpeth al diseases in mans bodie, both inwardly and outwardly: although they bee neuer so euill, as the Pestilence, the Poxe, the wolfe, the canker, consumptions, the dropsie, and the leper' (p.110).

---

[*] The Oslo Study of untreated syphilis, which was undertaken by C.P.M. Boek (1845–1917) until 1910 and after that by eminent successors until 1951, demonstrated the high incidence of spontaneous resolution of primary and secondary syphilitic lesions. The Oslo Study confirmed the view that many of the 'cures' attributed to mercury and other specifics could be more justly ascribed to the fluctuating nature of cutaneous luetic infection (Gjestland, 1955, pp.356–64).

Such visions of a 'wonder drug' provided little hope for victims of the hideous disease ravaging Europe as a tragic by-product of the Age of Discovery. The numerous writings on syphilis and the experimental cures waged against it by the physicians of the age inaugurated a revolutionary development in medicine which four hundred years later produced a panacea so great that it could even cure the pox. With the discovery of penicillin, scientists, after their centuries-long battle against 'the serpentine disease', could finally proclaim: 'Sex is here to stay, syphilis not' (Bäumler, 1976, p.13).

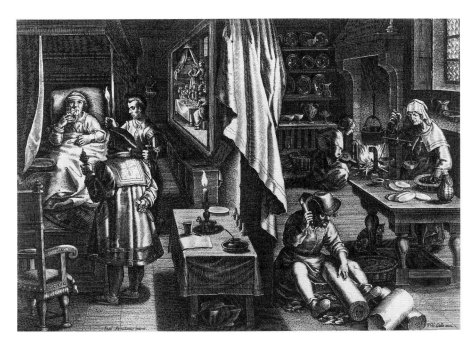

Figure 20. The engraving above shows a sick-room interior in which each of the stages of preparing the guaiac infusion is featured. In the lower right corner a man is seated on the floor, cutting chips from a log of guaiac. A woman standing nearby weighs the wood chips, while in the background a young woman attends the cooking of the pot of guaiac. In the left half of the engraving, the unfortunate syphilitic lies abed, drinking the decoction. An attendant stands ready to refill his cup, while a physician holds before his eyes a small replica of the Holy Tree. The painting on the wall opposite the patient renders the cause of his disease by depicting a brothel. A similar connection between syphilis and brothels is made by William Bullein when introducing guaiac to the English public in his medical treatise *Bulleins Bulwarke of Defence againste All Sicknes, Sornes and Woundes* (1562). Here William Bullein says of 'the wood of life, called *Guaicum*' that 'it might be a meane to make whole, and clense the filthy stinking corrupted boddies, of his [God's] disobedient children, which haue liued in most shamles lust and lechery, among painted stinkyng harlots, for which offence, they be smitten with the plague, called the French Pockes, an euill most noysome to nature, cosin iarman [neighbour] to the incurable Leprosie. This *Guiacum* I say wil not onely make a Pockie body clene, but also is good to clense any of the principall humours, whan thei do abound' (Bullein, 1562, *The Book of Simples*, fol.lx[r]). The caption of the engraving reads: 'Hyacum and lues venerea: the decoction of this tree when it is drunk will assuage the soft members which haue caught the disease'. Engraving by Theodor Galle (1571–1633) after an original design by Jan van der Straet (1523–1605). The engraving is the sixth of a collection of nine plates entitled *Nova reperta* and published in the last quarter of the 16th century in the Netherlands (Brinkman, 1982, pp.37–40).

CONCLUSION

Mercury in the treatment of syphilis came into view almost as early as the disease itself – Arabian medicine having provided a precedent for the use of *Unguentum Saracenicum* in its fight against leprosy and a number of other skin diseases. In England, a recipe for a mercurial ointment against syphilis is found as early as the late 1490s (see pp.58–9), indicating that use of the metal as an anti-syphilitic agent must have spread to the British Isles fairly early. In 1543, Traheron's English translation of Giovanni de Vigo's *Practica copiosa in arte chirurgica* (1514) provided the reading public with the Italian doctor's use of mercurial plasters in the treatment of syphilis. In the second half of the 16th century, the use of mercurial chemotherapy must have been a fairly established feature among English surgeons, for in the 1560s, 70s and 80s a number of leading members of the profession appear to have endorsed the tenet that 'Quicksiluer maye bee conueniently ministred in ointmentes, to heale the Pox' (Bullein, 1562, *The Book of Simples*, fol.lxxiii$^r$). Foremost among the advocates of this procedure were William Bullein (1562), John Banister (1575), William Clowes (1579), and John Read (1588).

English iatrochemists such as John Hester (1594) also encouraged the use of mercurial chemotherapy for the pox, a treatment which was ultimately part of Paracelsian doctrine. The new medicine served the barber-surgeons as a weapon in their criticism of physicians as having become divorced from real, and contemporary, medical experience. Both Continental and English writers commented on the failure of physicians to find effective remedies for the *morbus gallicus* and mercilessly attacked medical practitioners for their extreme caution and for clinging to Galenic doctrines and treatments which had little relevance to the diseases prevalent in Renaissance Europe. Guaiac, an imported wood derivative first made known in English in 1533 in Paynel's translation of von Hutten's treatise on the American wonder drug, rivalled mercury in the treatment of syphilis. Virtually all of the surgeons mentioned above were seen to support the use of the 'Holy Wood' as an effective anti-syphilitic – although critical voices were sometimes heard in the chorus. Since the theory behind the power of mercury to cure disease was basically a theory of humours, mercury was often used in enormous doses, quite against practical medical sense. In the same way, guaiac was regarded in the theory of humours as a sudorific, apt to 'expel and divide from the body the hurtful humours that are nourishments of this disease', as von Hutten explained (see p.48).

In 1546, Fracastoro announced in *De contagione* that guaiac 'of all remedies is that which is in most general use' (Fracastoro, 1930, p.277), but by the last quarter of the 16th century guiacum wood appears to have lost much of its popularity. Although Clowes mentions it, he strictly favours mercury inunctions, and in 1596, the Scottish surgeon Peter Lowe concludes: 'Among the foure wayes to heale this disease, I esteeme this [guaiacum wood] to be the most weake & most uncertaine, the which opinion is confirmed by all those that have written and practiced in this matter' (Lowe, 1596, sig.C3$^r$). Although mercury and guaiac were the two most popular treatments for most of the 16th century, medical writers advocated many other remedies as well including vegetable infusions, sulphur baths, hydrotherapeutic measures, and a variety of dietary and fasting cures.

# 3

# ENGLISH AND THE POX

At the end of the 15th century the Sinister Shepherd invaded England. His appearance marked yet another point in the spread of syphilis by soldiers and sailors from the European continent – a transmission which in the Age of Discovery brought the disease to nearly every part of the globe. In India syphilis was first recognized around 1500, after the arrival of Vasco da Gama, who had left Portugal in 1497. Shortly afterwards it appeared in Canton, China, and by 1512 the disease had reached Kyoto, Japan's capital at that time (Dohi, 1923, pp.36–7, 52). Syphilis spread over the known world with startling speed within a few years of 1493.

## SHADOW ON THE LAND

A number of sources provide evidence that syphilis made its appearance in England and Scotland in the latter half of the 1490s, and that, once more, the disease had followed the front lines and trade routes of soldiers and sailors. This is seen with particular clarity in Scotland, where syphilis was first reported in 1497 in the thriving merchant seaports of Edinburgh, Aberdeen and Glasgow. Similarly, the general spread of the disease in 1497–8 has been traced by scholars to the immigration of Perkin Warbeck, a Flemish Jew, and his men in 1496.[*] Perkin Warbeck claimed to be the Duke of York, the younger of the two princes murdered in the Tower of London in 1483. Warbeck's claim to the English throne was supported by the enemies of Henry VII (*regnebat* 1485–1509), one of whom was the Scottish King James IV (*regnebat* 1488–1513). When Perkin Warbeck arrived in Edinburgh in 1496, he was attended by a motley crowd of 1400 foreign adventurers and mercenaries – an ideal instrument for the dissemination of the new disease.

Three months before Warbeck left Scotland for an abortive raid on England, the town council of Aberdeen issued an order designed to check the spread of syphilis. This order, dated April 21, 1497, is the earliest official record of the disease in Britain. The order does not merely imitate the measures currently in use against plague but recognizes the venereal element in the spread of the disease. It calls for all loose women to desist from their vice and sin of venery and instead to take up

---

[*]    Comrie, vol.1, 1932, pp.199–202 and Morton, 1962, pp.175–6. The early history of syphilis in Scotland has been covered by these scholars.

regular work to support themselves, on pain of being branded with a hot iron on their cheek and banished from the town:

> 'April 21, 1497. The said day, it was statut and ordanit be the alderman and consale for the eschevin [avoidance] of the infirmitey cumm out of Franche and strang partis, that all licht weman be chargit and ordanit to decist fra thair vicis and syne of venerie, and al thair buthis and houssis skalit [emptied], and thai to pas and wirk for thar sustentacioun, vnder the payne of ane key of het yrne one thar chekis, and banysene of the toune.' (Comrie, 1932, vol.1, p.200)

Five months later, on September 22, 1497, the town council of Edinburgh passed 'Ane Grandgore Act' ordering all inhabitants of the town afflicted with syphilis, together with those who professed to cure it, into banishment to the barren little Island of Inchkeith in the Firth of Forth (p.200).[*]

Two of the earliest records of the existence of syphilis in England were brought to light by J.F.D. Shrewsbury in 1970. The original records are in the 1493–4 *Early Chronicles of Shrewsbury* which bear witness that the town of Shrewsbury was affected at that time: 'And about thys tyme began the fowle scabbe and horryble syckness called the freanche pocks' (Shrewsbury, 1970, p.133). Similarly, in 1494, the *Chronicle of Lynn* (Ireland) notes: 'In this yer begane the ffrence pockes' (p.133). Lynn was a seaport, but Shrewsbury had no doubt been infected via Chester and Bristol, where syphilis may have been imported via the wine trade from Bordeaux.[**]

Soldiers may also have been responsible for the transmission of the disease, for Joseph Grünpeck mentions in his *Libellus de mentulagra, alias morbo gallico* (1503) that English soldiers fighting in Italy in 1496 had acquired syphilis (Fuchs, 1843, p.57). On their way home, they would have crossed the Channel and entered the main road to the Continent in Kent. Significantly, the earliest prescription in English for syphilis has come from that area. It is found in a parchment manuscript from the districts around Sandwich, a seaport eleven miles north of Dover. The manuscript contained notes by a certain squire, John Langley, on 'Reseytes of Rents' for various manors around Sandwich, but it also contained 'An Approved Medicine for the French Pox'. Translated into modern language the treatment prescribes:

> 'Take a pound and a half of Barrowese grease, a quarter of a pound of brimstone and as much of turpentine, and half an ounce of quicksilver, and stamp all these in a mortar until the quicksilver be fully amalgamated with the other ingredients and then anoint the patient with it, all his body, and wrap him closely in a sheet, and put him to bed with plenty of clothes over him, so that he may sweat. Serve him in this fashion four or five times, and let him sweat each time four hours. And if his

---

[*] Syphilis in Scotland was recognized under a variety of names such as gor, gore, grandgore, grangore, grantgore, glengor, glengore, glengoir, glengour, the French seikness, the Spanje seiknes, the seiknes of Napillis, pockis, and rognole. The earlier names are probably from the French meaning 'large sore'.

[**] Morton, 1962, p.193 quotes Jeanselme, 1931, p.93 for this information, which in turn derives from Bloch, 1901–11, pp.66–7. Blochs quotes Simon, 1857–60, vol. 2, p.53, while Simon quotes Girtanner's *Abhandlung über die venerische Krankheit*, 1788–9, vol. 1, p.49. Girtanner, without quoting his sources, states: 'In England zeigte sich die krankheit zuerst 1498 zu Bristol. Sie wurde aus Frankreich dahin gebracht, und zwar von Bordeaux, von welchem ort sie auch lange der namen behielt'. The use of the term 'Spanje pockis' by the Scottish poet William Dunbar (1465?–1530?) in his *General Satyre of Scotland* (1507) (Morton, 1962, p.177) may indicate that the populace recognized that the pox had been spread from the ports of Spain with which Scotland was in regular connection. The English physician Andrew Boord who was born about 1480 mentions that 'whan that I was yonge they were named the spanyshe pockes' (Boord, 1547, fol.lxxxxvi[r]).

mouth is sore you must give him honey of roses in a saucer, and take a quantity of lint and roll it up and make the patient hold it between his teeth, so that his mouth keeps open and the water and corruption may run out.' (Cock, 1924, pp.869–70)

Langley's property lay on the main road from France and the Continent, and those living along the route were of necessity in close touch with travellers. Two to six people often slept in a bed; cups were not washed; cleanliness was a virtue not much cultivated, and personal contact, though not always of a sexual nature, was incessant. Life in the camps, on the other hand, was exceedingly promiscuous. With the roads swarming with soldiers, sailors, camp followers, and adventurers, many infected abroad must have brought their disease with them into this, the nearest part of England to the Continent. It is likely that syphilis was well known in this district and that a squire, such as John Langley, would have made a note of 'an approved remedy' to help his dependants, for medicine in those times was largely practised by heads of families.

Another 15th-century document dealing with syphilis is a manuscript of seven folio pages in the Sloane Collection entitled *The tretece of the pokkis: and the cure by the nobull counsell of parris.*[*] This manuscript was discovered by Charles Creighton and published with a commentary by E.L. Zimmermann in 1937 (Zimmermann, 1937, pp.461–82). The manuscript, which Zimmermann dates 'probably not much later than 1500' (p.480), is of interest in that it is the first attempt to present in English a foreign medical treatise on syphilis. The anonymous translator copied his manuscript from the second edition of the Italian physician Gaspare Torella's *Tractatus cum consiliis contra pudendagram seu morbum gallicum* (Rome, 1498). The English scribe penned fragments of only four of the five *consilia* found in Torella's syphilis tract of 1498, and the 'counsels' transcribed cover a variety of vegetable and mineral medicines and a number of purging and sweating regimens for the cure of 'the pokkis'.

The first remedy mentioned is 'A syrop mervelus & expert with weche inumerable hathe been cured', a drink 'of so meche vertu that it heylyth not allonly in this cause butt it preservyth a man allso from lepre yf it be oftyn dronkyn' (pp.461–3). Another remedy provided by the Italian doctor is a 'pill' which not only purges continuously but also without excessive effects. It had been applied to a syphilitic mason, it claimed, and after a few days the man could 'cast stonis and allso walke withowte a staffe' (p.466), the cure being completed with the mason's visit to a hot chamber at the end of a week's treatment: 'The vij day he enterd a stew & there wasshin & swett and delyverd of all maner of spotts or pokkis and soo whole and went to his labur' (p.467). The last of the cases presented by Gaspare Torella deals with 'a bysshopp of tolett [Toledo]' who 'was paynid in tollerably withe puscules & dolorus burnings o the armis shulders nek & leggs or the shynnes as the bones shuld part from the flesh' (p.468). He too was restored by Torella's cures and medicines '& thanked be god he was delyvered of all dolors…& thus with godds grace the pa[tients] shalbe perfetly cured and allso preserved. and thus endythe the cures of this sekenes' (p.471).

---

*   Manuscript Sloane, no. 398, folios 147–53. The British Library.

THE DRAGON'S TEETH

Another early reference to 'the pokkis' is in the book of the *Privy Purse Expenses of Elizabeth of York*, the queen of Henry VII. Under the date of March 15, 1503, an entry informs us that a sum of 40 shillings has been paid on behalf of a certain John Pertriche, 'oon of the sonnes of mad Beale'. The sum appears to have been the amount that the youth cost her majesty for food, clothing and incidental expenses during the preceding year and includes 20 shillings that were 'payed to a surgeon which heled him of the Frenche pox'. The physician's fee was as much as all the other expenses for the year combined (Nicolas, 1830, p.104).

In his *Annals of Henry VII* (dealing with the years 1485–1509), the English chronicler Bernard André (16th century) mentions that the sweating sickness of 1508 was 'followed by a far more detestable malady, to be abhorred as much as leprosy, a wasting pox which still vexes many eminent men' (*et quæ multos adhuc vexat egregios alioquin viros tabifica lues*) (André, 1858, p.126).

In a homiletic work printed in 1509, Bishop John Fisher (1459–1535) gives a similarly dark picture of the situation, viewed this time from the other end of the social scale. In the course of his enumeration of the many diseases inflicted upon man, Fisher refers to God's latest scourge by describing the spectacle of men 'vexed with the frensshe pockes, poore, and nedy, lyenge by the hye wayes stynkinge and almost roten aboue the grounde, hauynge intollerable ache in theyr bones' (Fisher, 1876, p.240).

Yet another tragic picture of poverty and venereal disease is presented by the early Tudor poet Robert Copland (*floruit* 1508–47), who in his poem *The Highway to the Spital-House* (1536) describes the applicants crowding before a London hospital. Already, in 1517–8, the Lord Mayor and his Aldermen had ordered 'that all such poore people as been visited with the great pokkes outwardly apperyng or with other great sores or maladyes tedious, lothsome or abhorrible to be loked vppon & seen to the great anoyaunce of the people, be nat suffred to begge and aske almes in churches & other open places, but that they be sent to thospytalles' (Anderson, 1933, p.417). It is the 'porter' of one of these London hospitals who in Copland's poem points out to him a group of 'Weak men sore wounded by great violence, And sore men eaten with pox and pestilence' (Judges, 1965, p.5). 'And as we talked there gathered at the gate', the poet goes on,

> People as methought of very poor estate,
> With bag and staff, both crooked, lame and blind,
> Scabby and scurvy, pock-eaten flesh and rind,
> Lousy and scald, and peelèd like as apes,
> With scantly a rag for to cover their shapes,
> Breechless, barefooted, all stinking with dirt,
> With thousand of tatters, drabbling to the skirt,
> Boys, girls, and luskish strong knaves,
> Diddering and daddering, leaning on their staves,
> Saying, "Good master, for your mother's blessing,
> Give us a halfpenny towards our lodging!" (p.3)

Robert Fabyan (d. 1513), an English chronicler of the early 16th century, informs us in *The Great Chronicle of London* that in 1506 Henry VII took measures to close the brothels on the Bankside in Southwark, London:

> 'This yere the stewis or comon bordell beyond the watyr ffor what happ or concyderacion the sertaynte I knowe nott, was ffor a seson Inhibyt and closid upp, But It was not long or they were sett opyn agayn, albe It the ffame went that where beffore were occupyed xviij [18] howsys, frrom hens fforth shuld be occupyed but xij [12].' (Fabyan, 1938, p.331)

Although Fabyan proclaims that he did not know 'for what event or consideration' 'the stews or common bordellos' of London were closed up, it is fairly certain that their suppression was connected with the early ravages of 'the pokkis'. Henry VII's regulation of the bordellos was in line with administrative practice abroad, where the closing of the brothels was one of the first prophylactic measures undertaken by authorities to stem the epidemic of syphilis. It is important to notice, however, that the suppression of the stews was not for long, and that according to Fabyan twelve of them were soon reopened.[*]

Furthermore, the women who had been deprived of their occupation by the royal proclamation established themselves in localities on the other side of the Thames. This exodus, which ironically helped to spread syphilis in the growing metropolis, was described in a satirical poem entitled *Cocke Lorelles Bote*, printed in 1509 soon after the accession of Henry VIII:

> There came suche a winde fro wynchester
> That blewe these women ouer the ryuer,
> In wherye, as I wyll you tell.
> Some at saynt Kateryns stroke a grounde,
> And many in holborne were founde;
> Some at saynt Gyles, I trowe,
> Also in aue maria aly, and at westmenster,
> And some in shordyche drewe theder
> With grete lamentacyon. (Rimbault, 1842, p.6)

While the poem stresses such localities as St. Katherine's by the Tower, Holborn, St. Giles's in the Fields, Ave Maria Lane, near the west door of St. Paul's, Westminster, and Shoreditch beyond Bishopsgate, other sources identify, on the fringes of the

---

[*] The Bankside brothels of London were of ancient origin and situated in Southwark under the jurisdiction of the Bishop of Winchester, who had a substantial income collecting rents from these houses of ill fame. Standing in a row along the Surrey side of the Thames, a little above London Bridge, they were wooden erections, each with a stair down to the water, and each with its river front painted with a sign like a tavern. The Elizabethan chronicler and antiquary John Stow (1525?–1605), whose invaluable book *A Survey of London* (1598 and 1603) served as the basis of information for many later commentators and historians, said: 'Next on this banke was sometime the Bordello or stewes, a place so called, of certaine stew houses priuiledged there, for the repair of incontinent men to the like women...These allowed stew houses had signes on the frontes, towardes the Thames, not hanged out, but painted on the walles, as a Boares heade, the Crosse keyes, the Gunne, the Castle, the Crane, the Cardinals Hat, the Bel, the Swanne, &c. I have heard ancient men of good credite report, that these single women were forbidden the rightes of the Church, so long as they continued that sinnefull life, and were excluded from christian buriall, if they were not reconciled before their death. And therefore there was a plot of ground, called the single womans churchyard, appoynted for them, far from the parish church' (Stow, 1908, vol.2, pp.54–5). For a history of these houses of ill fame, see Burford, 1976, pp.115–63.

extramural wards, Lambeth Marsh to the south; Hog Lane and Whitechapel to the east, outside Aldgate; 'Pickt-hatch' near the Charterhouse, beyond Aldersgate, in the north-west; Clerkenwell, especially Turnmill Street, just west of the Charterhouse; and localities in the western liberties such as Leather Lane and White-friars (Burford, 1976, pp.114–5; Chalfont, 1978, pp.142–3, 185–6, 198–9. See also Lupton, 1632, pp.50–5).

Even if *Cocke Lorelles Bote* shows that prostitution cannot have been absent within the City Walls, the sources indicate that the vast majority of brothels were situated in 'the sinfully polluted suburbs', as a later London author called them (Dekker, 1925, p.31).

Among the few allusions to syphilis encountered in English sources at the time of the accession of Henry VIII, a royal proclamation of May 15, 1513 may bear on the subject. Before going to war with France, Henry VIII forbade prostitutes in the train of his army, at the same time as he introduced a new and savage penalty for whores infringing the prohibition. Both measures may be viewed as an attempt to safeguard the efficiency of his forces by protecting them from syphilitic infection. In the proclamation, Henry VIII solemnly ordered that 'no common woman presume to come within the King's host [army], nor nigh the same by the space of three miles, upon pain if any so be taken to be burned upon the right cheek at the first time. And if any be taken with the host, or within three miles of the same, after she or they have be so burned, then she or they to be put into ward of the provost marshal, there to remain in prison as long as shall please the marshal and to have further punition as by him shall be thought convenient' (Larkin and Hughes, 1964–9, vol.1, p.113).[*]

Two years before the royal proclamation, there is a record from Oxford, 1511, when it appears that one of the students there had been infected with syphilis and lost his job as a result of the disease. 'One John Friendship Fellow of Merton College', the antiquary and historian Anthony Wood (1632–95) records, 'was ordered to leave that place because he had the French Pox' (Wood, 1786–90, vol.1, book 1, p.514).

In 1519 a London printer published *William Horman's Vulgaria*, which was perhaps the best-known Latin-English dictionary used in Tudor grammar schools. In the chapter 'De corporis dotibus et cladibus', the book gives useful advice to its young readers about venereal disease: 'The frenche pockes is a perilous and wonderfull sykenes: for it infecteth only with touchynge' (Horman, 1926, p.57).

Such warnings served to fuel an epidemic of anxiety which was not relieved by the opinions of the medical establishment. In Andrew Boord's medical encyclopedia of 1547, *The Breviary of Helthe*, the author asserted that the cause of syphilis 'doth come many wayes, it maye come by lyenge in the shetes or bedde there where a pocky person hath the nyght before lyen in, it maye come with lyenge with a pocky person, it may come by syttynge on a draught or sege [privy] there where as a pocky person did lately syt, it may come by drynkynge oft with a pocky person, but specially it is taken when one pocky person doth synne in lechery the one with another. All the kyndes of the pockes be infectiouse' (Boord, 1547, fol.lxxxxvi<sup>v</sup>).

---

[*] The editors have modernized the text.

Such warnings were given yet another twist by the Scottish surgeon and syphilographer Peter Lowe, who in 1596 informed the public that syphilis might be contracted by 'receiuing the breath of such as are infected, and by sitting on the priuie after them, & sometimes by treading bare-footed on the spettle of those which haue been long corrupted' (see p.20).

## SYPHILIS AND THE CLERGY

One of the most interesting early allusions to syphilis comes from sources related to the English Reformation. The fact that syphilis was used to discredit Romish priests is one of the few indications we have of its existence in that country. 'A pocky priest' was a phrase of the time, and in Simon Fish's *Supplication of Beggars*, which was compiled in 1524 and read to Henry VIII shortly thereafter, the weightiest plea for the dissolution of the monasteries was the scandalous lives of priests, monks, and friars. Wrote Simon Fish: 'These be they that haue made an hundreth thousand ydell hores yn your realme, whiche wolde haue gotten theyre lyuing honestly, yn the swete of theyre faces, had not theyre superfluous rychesse illected theym to vnclene lust and ydelnesse. These be they that corrupt the hole generation of mankind yn your realme; that catche the pokkes of one woman, and bere theym to an other; that be brent wyth one woman, and bere it to an other; that catche the lepry of one woman, and bere it to an other; ye, some of theym shall bost emong his felawes, that he hath medled with an hundreth wymen' (Fish, 1871, p.6).

The characterization of monasteries as reservoirs of venereal infection also appears in a letter from Erasmus who, on a visit to the country in 1516, spoke of 'the great multitude of monasteries in which religious discipline has fallen so low that in comparison with them there is more sobriety and more innocence in a brothel' (Erasmus, 1974–82, vol.4, p.25). Similarly, the author of *The Image of Ypocresye*, an anonymous anti-clerical poem from 1533, talks of the monks' engagement with 'Your closse chambred drabbes, When masse and all is done, The paynes to release' (Furnivall, 1868–72, vol.1, p.194). North of the English border, George Bannatyne (1545–1608) compiled a large collection of Scottish poems (1568) in which he quotes a special word for the clergy:

> 'Sic pryd with prelates so few (s)till preach and pray,
> Sic haut of harlottis with thame bay the nicht and day.' (Bannatyne, 1770, p.42)

Not only were funds for hospitals and parish schools often misappropriated by the Scottish clergy, but in 1549 the provincial council of Edinburgh passed a resolution exhorting prelates and clergy to keep their own illegitimate children 'in thair companie'. Little improvement seems to have been produced, for by 1558–9 legal limits were laid down of how much church property might be purloined for the marriage dowries of bastard daughters (Morton, 1962, p.178). The Archbishop and head of the church in Scotland was John Hamilton of St. Andrews, a man who was visited by Gerolamo Cardano, the Italian physician, regarding the Archbishop's asthma. The prelate also obtained the following advice from the physician in Latin: 'Regarding sexual intercourse: it is certainly not good or beneficial, but when there happens to be a necessity it ought to take place between two sleeps, to wit, after midnight, and it is better to exercise this function three times in six days, e.g. once in every two days rather than twice in one day, and then to wait for ten days' (p.178).

So close did the association of a sexual vice and its attendant disease become with the priesthood that James I (*regnebat* 1603–25), writing long afterward concerning the sentiments of his mother, Mary Stuart, the Queen of Scots (*regnebat* 1542–67), describes her forbidding Archbishop Hamilton 'to use the spittle' in his own baptism, for the reason that she would not have 'a pokie priest to spet in her child's mouth'. These, says King James, were 'her owne words' (Creighton, 1891, p.415; Morton, 1962, p.179).*

In England, Simon Fish's *Supplication of Beggars* was followed by another attack on the clergy which came to herald the Reformation in that country. In 1529 the unpopular Cardinal Thomas Wolsey was charged with having had intentions of killing King Henry VIII by infecting him with his own 'foul and contagious disease of the great pox'. Happily for the Cardinal, he died the following year (possibly of venereal disease) and so managed to escape trial for treason. He did not, however, escape being derided for his syphilitic infection by two malicious poets. In a violent satire against the prelate entitled *Rede me and be nott wrothe* (1528), William Roy has two priest's servants named Watkyn and Jeffraye exchange information about the Cardinal. 'He hath no wyfe, But whoares that be his lovers', says Jeffraye to Watkyn, who wonders: 'Yf he use whoares to occupy, It is grett marvell, certaynly, That he escapeth the Frenche pockes'. To which Jeffraye replies: 'He had the pockes, with out fayle, Wherfore, people on hym did rayle With many obprobrious mockes' (Roy, 1812, p.32).

The second attack came with the poem *Why come ye not to Court* (c. 1523), written by John Skelton (1460?–1529), the King's court poet. 'This Naaman Sirus', Skelton sneered at the 'leprous' Cardinal, who 'Spareth neither maid ne wife' (Skelton, 1964, p.314),

---

*   Mary Stuart was well acquainted with syphilis, for there seems little doubt that her second husband, Darnley, and probably her third, Bothwell, suffered from the disease. R.S. Morton concludes: 'According to the Lords of the Congregation, Darnley, who was 21 years of age and known to be addicted to both alcohol and women, was "poysned". Mary's secretary, Nau, said he had smallpox. Mary herself, however, spoke of him as this "pockish man". When she visited him in Glasgow at the time of his illness she noted, "I thought I should have been killed by his breath: and yet I sat no nearer to him than in a chair by his bed and he lieth on the further side of it". By the time she visited him his rash was fading and he had alopecia. When Darnley finally moved to Kirk O'Fields near Edinburgh to convalesce he had a special bath on Saturday, February 8, 1567. All this rather suggests that he had a salivation of mercury and gives support to a diagnosis of syphilis. Before Mary's visit to Glasgow the royal couple had last met in October, 1566, at Jedburgh. Mary received a letter from him on November 5 at Kelso. The contents of this letter are unknown, but she was heard to cry out that she wished she could die and she was under the care of her physician for some weeks thereafter. Various suggestions regarding the contents of the letter have been found unsatisfactory for one reason or another, but I would suggest that Darnley told Mary he had syphilis and perhaps even accused her of being its source – perhaps this letter is the first recorded use of the contact slip…Two months after Darnley's murder at Kirk O'Fields, Mary married Lord Bothwell. About the end of July she said she was "seven weeks gone with child." At the end of August she miscarried twins and had a fever. This obstetrical accident would be too early in pregnancy to be precipitated by syphilis. After the skirmish at Carberry the following summer, Bothwell, as Great Admiral of Scotland, contrived his escape to Norway where he was imprisoned. He died at the age of 43 in Denmark in April, 1578, after a mental illness which lasted at least 5 years and suggests general paralysis of the insane' (Morton, 1962, p.179).

So fell and so irous,
So full of melancholy,
With a flap afore his eye,
Men ween that he is poxy,
Or else his surgeons they lie…
He is now so overthwart,
And so painéd with panges,
That all his trust hanges
In Balthasar… * that healed Domingo's nose
From the pustuled poxy pose,
Now with his gummes of Araby
Hath promised to heal our cardinal's eye.
Yet some surgéons put a doubt
Lest he will put it clean out,
And make him lame of his nether limbes.
God send him sorrow for his sinnes! (pp.342–3)

## A SYPHILIZED 'MAGNIFICENCE'

Another poetic manifestation of Skelton's hostility to Wolsey is the interlude *Magnificence*, written in the style of the morality plays and expressly warning Henry VIII against 'Largesse and Liberty' (Skelton, 1964, p.210) and evil counsellors. The character 'Magnificence', symbolizing a too liberal prince, is finally beaten down by 'Adversity', who commands a variety of choices. 'Of sorrowful servants I have many scores', the allegorical figure asserts, leprosy, syphilis and gonorrhea appearing to be some of them:

> Some I make lepers and lazars full hoarse;
> And from that they love best some I divorce;
> Some with the marmoll [inflamed sore] to halt I them make;
> And some to cry out of the bone-ache;
> And some I visit with burning of fire. (p.224)

Reduced to the figure of 'Poverty', Magnificence in his misery is reviled by the allegorical figures of 'Counterfeit Countenance', 'Crafty Conveyance' and 'Cloaked Collusion', who 'bequeath him the bone-ache' (p.235) before the trio retires to taverns and brothels of the Bankside in Southwark: **

CL. COL.   But now let us make marry and good cheer!

C. COUNT.   And to the tavern let us draw near.

CR. CON.   And from thence to the halfe street,
            To get us there some freshe meat.

---

\*   Balthasar de Guercis, surgeon to Catherine of Aragon, the King's first wife.
\**  A number of medical historians have assumed that Henry VIII acquired syphilis as a young man, transmitted it to several of his wives, and died with gummatous ulcers upon his legs and general paralysis of the insane. This diagnosis would account for the many miscarriages and still-born children of his Queens, for his 'sorre legges' in the latter half of his life, and for his marked and tragic change in character. However, the syphilitic diagnosis has been contested by other medical historians, recently by J.F.D. Shrewsbury (1952, pp.141–85) and N.R. Barrett (1973, pp.216–33).

CL. COL.     Why, is there any store of rawe mutton
                 [prostitutes]?

C. COUNT.   Yea, in faith, or else thou art too great a glutton!

CR. CON.    But they say it is a queasy meat;
                 It will strike a man mischievously in a heat.

CL. COL.     In fay, man, some ribs of the mutton be so rank
                 That they will fire one ungraciously in the flank.

C. COUNT.   Yea, and when ye come out of the shop,
                 Ye shall be clappéd with a collop,
                 That will make you to halt and to hop.

CR. CON.    Some be rested there that they think on it forty days,
                 For there be whores there at all assays.

CL. COL.     For the passion of God, let us go thither! (Skelton, 1964, p.235).

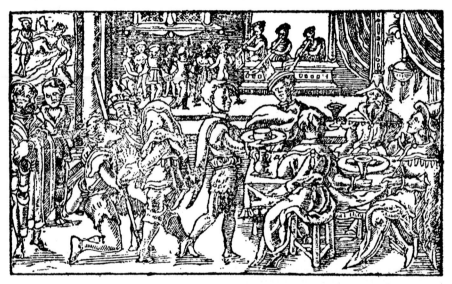

Figure 21. The woodcut adorns the title-page of an interlude called *Jack Juggler* (third edition, c. 1565–70).[*]
Interludes, which succeeded morality plays in the evolution of Elizabethan drama, also relied on an
edifying plot enacted by allegorical figures. Wanton Youth led astray by Pride, Sloth and Lechery was
a popular theme, and is reflected in the woodcut's rendering of the biblical story of the Prodigal Son.
This was the general subject of a group of interludes written about 1540–75, chief of which are the
anonymous *Misogonus* (c. 1560) and Georg Gascoigne's (1525?–77) 'tragicall comedie', the *Glasse of
Government* (1575). On the woodcut, the repentant son is received by his father (foreground left) having
wasted his wealth and health in taverns and brothels (background and foreground right).

In the morality plays and interludes of the 16th century, references to syphilis are rare. One is found
in *Hyckescorner* (1513–16) where Pity remarks that 'Courtyers go gaye and take lytell wages, And
many with harlottes at the taverne hauntes…On themselves they have no pyte [pity]. God punyssheth

---

ENGLISH BOOKS ON SYPHILIS IN THE 16TH CENTURY

In 1533 the first book on syphilis appeared in the English language. Its translator was Thomas Paynel, a canon of Merton Abbey, who had previously translated the *Regimen Salernitanum*, a popular health guide of the times. Going one day into the city to see about a new edition of this work, Paynel was asked by his printer if he would like to translate a book on the French pox 'wryten by that great clerke of Almayne, Ulrich Hutten knyght' (Hutten, 1533, *The Preface*). 'How nedefull and howe beneficiall to the common welth were it', said the printer, 'For almoste into euerye parte of this realme, this mooste foule and peynfull disease is crepte, and many soore infected therwith' (*Ibid.*). The English edition of Hutten's work was published under the title *De Morbo Gallico* (1533), and it soon became a best-seller. Two more editions followed rapidly in 1536, followed by three more in 1539, and a seventh edition in 1540. Apparently there was a great demand for the book and its medical information.

The second book on syphilis to appear in the English language was Bartholomew Traheron's translation in 1543 of Giovanni de Vigo's famous *Practica copiosa in arte chirurgica* (Rome, 1514) (see pp.9–10). The book summed up all the surgical learning of its time, and in its fifth chapter, entitled *De morbo gallico* de Vigo, gives one of the

---

full sore with grete sekenesse, As pockes, pestylence, purple[s] and axes' (Manly, 1897, vol.1, p.406). Another reference is found in *Misogonus* (c. 1560) where a quack called Cacurgus asserts that 'I have all things that grows in the Indian land. I can cure the ague, the measles and the French pock, The tetter, the morphew, the bile, blain, and weal' (Farmer, 1906, p.218).

A third reference is found in *Nice Wanton* (1547–53) where Iniquity tempts a 'fayre wenche' called Dalilah to whoredom and gaming. After a long interval, according to the stage directions, Dalilah 'commeth in ragged, her face hid or disfigured, halting on a staffe', and displaying a panoply of the symptoms of tertiary syphilis:

> Alas, wretched wretche that I am!
> Most miserable caitife that euer was borne!
> Full of payne and sorow, croked and lame,
> Stuft with diseases, in this world forlorne!
>
> My senowes be shronken, my flesh eaten with pocks,
> My bones ful of ache[s] and great payne;
> My head is bald, that bare yelowe lockes;
> Croked I crepe to the earth agayne;
>
> Mine eie-sight is dimme; my hands tremble and shake…
> Where I was fayre and amiable of face,
> Now am I foule and horrible to se:
> Al this I haue deserued for lacke of grace,
> Iustly for my sinnes God doth plague me. (Manley, 1897, vol.1, pp.468–9)

At the end of the play, Worldly Shame informs the audience that Dalilah, 'The fayre wenche…Is dead of the pockes, taken at the stewes' (p.576), while Ismael, her brother, has been hanged as a thief. 'Thief brother, syster whore, Two graffes of an yll tree' (p.468) thus suffer the fate of all wayward youth: death by hanging and by the pox.

best clinical descriptions of syphilis in the 16th century. He stresses the contagiousness of the disease, its origin from sexual intercourse with an infected person, and its rapid dissemination throughout the body. He describes the primary lesion, the secondary eruptions, the eye lesions and the ulcerations of the nose, and the formation of gummata. He believes that cauterization of the initial sore is an effective treatment, an idea which persisted for centuries. He also believes in the value of purgation and blood-letting, just as he shares the belief of other syphilographers of his age that certain foods should be eaten and others restricted in the diet. A great many drugs, potions, brews, wines and the flesh of different animals are advocated by de Vigo in the treatment of syphilis. He does not seem to have been acquainted with the extract of the Holy Wood but he refers to the specific action of mercury, both upon the lesions and upon the pains so common in the disease. De Vigo's mercurial plasters eventually came into wide use and renown in the medical field, where they still bear his name in the pharmacopoeia.

Traheron published his English translation of de Vigo's *Practica* under the title *The Most Excellent Workes of Chirurgerye, Made and Set Forth by Master John Vigon* (1543). 'I can not telle whether anye man hath receyued the true knowleage, and spirite of Christ, that pitieth not the greate sickenesses, and diseases, wherin we are wrapped on euerye syde', Traheron states in his dedication of the book to the Rev. Richard Tracy. 'For this cause', he goes on, 'I haue thought it not vnprofitable (let some busie speakers, rather than doers bable what they lyste) to bestowe some labour, and tyme, in translatyng this booke, whiche conteynethe so manye goodly remedies, for the diseases that communelye, and iustelye happen vnto vs' (Vigo, 1543, *An Epystole*). In conformity with the learning of his time, Traheron thus gives expression to his belief that diseases are God's punishment for man's disobedience. He expressly includes syphilis in his catalogue of divine plagues:

'God the myghtie gouerner of all thynges, longetyme sythens, hath witnessed, by his excellent prophet Moses, that for the transgression of hys holy lawes, he wolde plage the people with sondrye, and greuouse diseases. Howbeit our blindenes hath ben so great, that in the multitude of moste fylthye, and shameful botches, sores, and other pitious maladies we haue not perceaued, how horrible a thynge synne is, and howe present vengeaunce the dyspisyng, and neglectyng of goddes dredfull commaundementes, bryngeth vppon vs, no not when we haue be burnte wyth fyery carbuncles, nor when our fleshe hath bene toren from the bones, and eaten vp wyth lothsome cankers, nor when we haue ben myserably tormented, wyth that moste fylthy, pestiferous, and abominable dysease the Frenche or spanyshe pockes.' (*Ibid.*)

In spite of man's pride, wickedness and 'corrupte byrthe', Traheron still manages to sustain his belief in the 'vnmeasurable mercye' of his Maker, 'whych in the myddest of our abomination, and deseruyng of al extreme tormentes, hath euer remembred hys natural goodnesse, both gyuynge vertues to herbes, stones, trees, and metalles, wherewyth our euels myghte be eased, and also styrryng vp men to note suche thynges, and to practyse them vpon our paynfull griefes' (*Ibid.*).

Such a divinely inspired man was 'Johanne Vigo', whom Traheron praises for his 'synguler wytte, longe experience, and diligent studye' (*Ibid.*).

'I thynke that nothyng canne better testifie and prooue the connynge of this man', Traheron concludes his preface, 'than that he continued so long, with so great prayse, practysynge at rome, in suche a multitude of pockye curtisanes, neyther priestes, bysshoppes, nor cardinalles excepted as it playnlye appeareth in his booke. For where suche carions ben, the best Aegles wyll resorte.' (*Ibid.*)

Giovanni de Vigo's reputation as one of the eagles of Renaissance medicine was due to the fact that his *Practica copiosa* was virtually the only book before the works of Ambroise Paré (1510–90) to deal with the two new features of Renaissance surgery: the treatment of syphilitic wounds and of gunshot wounds. De Vigo taught that gunshot wounds were poisoned burns and consequently should be treated with cautery and the use of boiling oil. It was not until Paré that physicians realized that gunshot wounds were not 'poisonous', and therefore were to be healed by soothing applications rather than boiling oil. De Vigo's cauterization of syphilitic wounds was more correct in its assessment of the poisonous nature of the wound, but his pseudo-Hippocratic tenet that 'diseases not curable by iron are curable by fire' proved as harmful to those with wounds from syphilis as it did to those with wounds from firearms.

The most drastic treatment of syphilis of the time, de Vigo's 'surgical intervention' was carried out by the numerous surgeons and barbers of the century. The patient was tied down to a table and the chancre cut with a knife to the base of the prepuce. Afterwards the surgical wound was cauterized with a hot iron. Incisions and cauterizations were also made on chancres appearing elsewhere on the skin, in the language of the time called carbonadoes. Here, as in other fields, consultation of barbers and surgeons required a good health. 'I have now been for over five weeks in the surgeons' hands', wrote Erasmus to his friend John Fisher on October 23, 1518, adding that, in his opinion, these people were 'the most dangerous kind of men' (Erasmus, 1968, p.63).

## A 'BREVIARY OF HELTHE' AND A 'BULWARKE OF DEFENCE'

The third medical book in England to mention syphilis was Andrew Boord's *Breviary of Helthe* (1547). Boord (1490?–1549) wrote not only for his peers but for popular appeal, and his *Breviary of Helthe* is the first printed medical book to be written by a physician in English. Syphilis is described in Boord's medical encyclopaedia under the entries *mala frantizoz* and *morbus gallicus*, where Boord provides the reader with the following information:

'*Mala frantizoz* is the araby worde. In latyn it is named *Morbus gallicus* or *Variole maiores*. In englyshe it is named one of the first kyndes of the french pockes the which be skabbes and pimples lyke to leprosyte, wherfore for this matter or sicknes loke in the capytle named *Morbus gallicus*...*Morbus gallicus* or *Variole maiores* be the latyn wordes. And some do name it *Mentagra*, but for *Mentagra* loke in *Lichen*. In englyshe *Morbus gallicus* is named the french pockes, whan that I was yonge they were named the spanyshe pockes the which be of many kyndes of the pockes, some be moyst, some be waterashe, some be drye, and some be skoruie, some be lyke skabbes, some be lyke ring wormes, some be fistuled, some be festered, some be cankarus, some be lyke wennes, some be lyke biles, some be lyke knobbes or knurres [burres], and some be vlcerous hauynge a lytle drye skabbe in the midle of the vlcerous skabbe, some hath ache in the ioyntes and no signe of the pockes and yet it may be the pockes. And there is the smal pockes, loke for it in the capytle named *Variole maiores.*' (Boord, 1547, fol.lxxxvii$^r$, fol.lxxxxvi$^{r-v}$)

William Bullein's *Bulwarke of Defence* (1562) is a fourth medical book in English to mention syphilis, which is first described in a cursory manner in the author's introduction of the guaiac cure (see p.49). Later in the book, the disease receives a somewhat broader treatment when it is described by the allegorical figure, Sickness. 'Many men, women, and children now a daies', he says, 'be greuously vexed with a shamefull disease, called the Frenche Pockes, paines in their iointes, no reste, palenesse of culler, fallyng of here, baldnes of hedde and berde, lamenes of limmes, skabbes, filthe, etc.' (Bullein, 1562, *The Booke of Compoundes*, fol.xlvii$^r$). 'In soche cases what is to bee doen', Sickness goes on to ask, 'I praie you tell me gentle Health, for this sicknesse waxeth common, but yet it would faine bee called, but onely a Feuer' (fol.xlvii$^r$). To which Health answers:

> 'Many men haue written moche of this Poxe, after sondry sortes, and diuers waies, and haue killed not a fewe with long diattes, but I will speake that, whiche I do knowe, proued and seen, to haue helped very many. Yet would I not, that any should fishe for this disease, or be to bolde when he is bitten, to thinke hereby to be helped: but rather eschue the cause of this infirmitie, and filthy, rotten, burning of harlottes, etc. As to flie from the Pestilence, or from a wilde fire, for what is more to bee abhorred, then a pockie, filthie, stinkyng carcas. But if through blinde ignoraunce, sodain chaunce, etc. any haue gotten it: then doe thus to be deliuered from it.' (fol.xlvii$^{r-v}$)

Bullein here acquaints the reader with the guaiac cure and with the wondrous properties of the American wonder drug, which he later recommends be combined with

> 'moiste bathe of herbes, or parfumes with Masticke, Stirax oile, etc. Whiche haue vertue to clense skabbes, iche, pox, I say the poxe, as by experiens we se, there is no better remedy, then sweatyng, and the drinkyng of Guiacum, vsyng it in due tyme and order.' (Bullein, 1562, *The Booke of the Use of Sicke Men and Medicenes*, fol.lxviii$^v$)

Bullein finally has a short but interesting note which indicates that syphilis was continuing to spread among the population and that it was a matter of grave concern. While referring to the wounds of a young man who fell into a deep coalpit at Newcastle, Bullein says that he was

> 'healed by an auncient practisour called Mighel, a Frencheman, whiche also is cunnynge to helpe his owne countrey disease, that now is to commonly knowen here in Englande, the more to be lamented: But yet dayly increased, whereof I entinde to speake in the place of the Poxe.' (Bullein, 1562, *The Booke of Simples*, fol.ii–iii)

In A *Dialogue against the Fever Pestilence* (1564), Bullein has one more reference to the pox with the soliloquy of Roger, the servant, who wonders about his future prospects after his master has caught the plague. 'Alas, what shall I doe, poore knaue?' he asks himself. 'I could goe to London, and lurke in some baudie Lane. I knowe an olde stale hore of myne in London; she is married to, an hoddie pecke, John A Noddes…This quene will pick his purse for my sake. She can make false Dice; Hir first housebande was prentise with James Elles, and of hym learned to plaie at the shorte knife and the horn Thimble. But these Dogge trickes will bryng one to the Poxe, the Gallous, or to the Deuill' (Bullein, 1888, p.122). In mentioning this retributive trio, Bullein's perceptive servant shows his awareness of the fate of all wayward youth, so brilliantly described in the interlude *Nice Wanton* (see p.67).

Another contemporary reference to the wide prevalence of the pox appears in *A Diall for All Agues* (1566) by the surgeon John Jones (*floruit* 1579). Here the author makes a cursory reference to 'the Neapolitanes, or rather the besegers of Naples, with the pockes (spred sence [then] to far abrode, through al the parts of Europe, no kyngdome that I haue bene in free, the more pity)' (Jones, 1566, cap.8: *Of the pestilentiall feuer, or plage, or boche,* n.p.).

Three years earlier another well-known Elizabethan surgeon, Thomas Gale, had published his *Certaine Workes of Chirurgerie* (1563) in which he introduces himself 'to the Frindly readers' and reminds them of the value of right 'Chirurgirie' and proper research,

> 'for that ther spring new infirmities in our dayes vnknowen to them before our time. What say you to *Chamæleontiasis*, vulgarly named *morbus gallicus*? Who euer haue written of the nature cause, and accidentes of it? Which is the occasion that so many miserablye haue dyed, and daily perishe of it: and those that haue receiued helth, haue bene so small a numbre.' (Gale, 1563b, first folio)

THE POX AT ST. BARTHOLOMEW'S HOSPITAL

The picture presented by the authors and sources quoted above provides little support for the view that syphilis had declined after its first appearance in epidemic proportions in Britain. Actually, a number of other sources provide cumulative evidence that syphilis was a growing threat to the population and that it consumed an increasing amount of medical resources.

According to John Howes, a grocer and collector of hospital rents, England during the reigns of Henry VIII and Edward VI had spawned a wretched brood of 'poore lame ydell & maysterles men dispersed into dyvers parts of this Realme, but chiefeley about this Cittie of London' (Howes, 1904, p.4). The diseased condition of this group of the population also appears with Howes's statement that, in the last years of Edward VI, 'the streates & lanes in London began to swarme with beggers & roges...the nomber of the poore did so encrease of all sorts, that the churches, streates and lanes Were fylled daylye with a number of Loathsome Lazars botches and sores so that St. Bartholomewes hospitall Was not able to receyve the tenthe parte of those that then were to be provided for' (pp.6–7). In the 1550s, these dermatological symptoms could better be referred to syphilis than to leprosy, a fact which is supported by the admission of these patients to St. Bartholomew's Hospital, a centre for the treatment of syphilitics.

An interesting insight into the prevalence of syphilis in mid-century London is provided by the records of this Hospital, which were examined by Margaret Pelling (Pelling, 1986, pp.82–112). During a twelve month period in 1547–8, the Hospital's surgeons received gratuities for healing 87 patients. Of these, 21 had suffered from syphilis, or about a quarter of those admitted. The Hospital's administrators showed a significant tendency to record cases of pox rather than other diseases –

perhaps an indication of the swelling number of this group of patients. In the 1550s, the poor suffering from syphilis were segregated in a special ward of the Hospital (the Dorter) and provided with nurses, clothing, and mattresses which only these patients were permitted to use. A hot house or sweating ward was also instituted at this time. At one point twenty extra mattresses were urgently needed to prevent cross-infection among the hospitalized (p.97).

The growing number of syphilitic patients is also indicated by the fact that the Hospital's administrators allowed rebates to tenants who accommodated such patients on premises belonging to the Hospital. One house where people were 'laid of the pox' was in Golden Lane, which ran north from Holborn Bridge. So customary did this practice become that worried property owners sometimes introduced a clause into their leases which prohibited letting 'to any butchers or any that shall lay any of the pox, etc.' (p.97).

The syphilitic poor were also placed in St. Thomas's Hospital and in the lazarhouses of St. Bartholomew's and Christ's Hospital. In this respect, Bartholomew's administrators were fortunate in being able to take advantage of the decline of one disease as another appeared on the scene. Toward the middle of the 15th century, leprosy was rapidly declining in Europe, and this was particularly so in England (Newman, 1895, pp.1–150).* When syphilis replaced it as a common scourge at the end of the same century, the almost empty lazarhouses could be used to accommodate the growing number of syphilitic patients.

England had as many as 500 lazarhouses, but unfortunately most of them were converted into barns or business premises with the dissolution of the monasteries during the reign of Henry VIII. St. Bartholomew's Hospital, however, was allowed by its charter of 1547 to keep five or six of these lazars, locks, or 'outhouses' as they were also called. The lazars ranged from Mile End in the east to Hammersmith in the west, from Southwark in the south to Finchley in the north. In spite of the urgent need for these houses, the cost of running them proved too great, so that the number of lazars in use gradually fell. In 1621, only two were left: the 'Lock' for men in Kent Street, Southwark, and the 'Spital' in Kingsland for women. The term 'Lock' then became associated with syphilis, while 'lazar' became a common epithet applied to people infected with the foul disease (see pp.257–9). The inmates of London's lazarhouses were properly described by William Harvey in 1633 as the incurable, the infectious, and the scandalous (Pelling, 1986, p.126).

Anxiety about health in an age of infectious diseases such as plague, syphilis and smallpox prompted a spectacular development in medical science and practice. The best known examples of this development in Tudor times are the grant of the first charter to the College of Physicians of London in 1518; the introduction of the ecclesiastical licensing system in 1514; the amalgamation of the Barbers' and the Surgeons' Companies in 1540, and the foundation or reconstitution of the five royal hospitals in the 1540s: St. Bartholomew's, Christ's, St. Thomas's, Bridewell, and Bethlehem (the madhouse known as Bedlam). Possibly the most notable development was the emergence of Paracelsian medicine and chemotherapy in the later

---

*    Houses listed in the Appendix.

decades of the 16th century – followed by the founding of the Apothecaries' Society in 1617 (Webster, 1979, pp.165–235, 301–34).

During the 16th century, medical services became a major item of consumption for all classes of the population, with physicians and barber-surgeons administering to the needs of the upper and middle classes, while unlicensed practitioners, empirics and quacks took care of the lower classes and the poor.

### THE BARBER-SURGEONS' COMPANY 1540

By 1540, it appears that the pox had become so widespread that it affected the organization of medicine in London. In that year, the barbers and surgeons were incorporated into the Barber-Surgeons' Company by a royal Act which forbade common barbers, or persons merely shaving, to meddle with surgery, except to draw teeth,

> 'forasmuche as suche personnes usyng the mistery or facultie of surgery, often tymes medle and take into their cures, and houses, such [sykke] and diseasid personnes as ben infected with the pestilence, great pockes, and such other contaagious infirmities, & other feates thereunto bilonging, which is very perillous for infecting the Kinges people resorting to their shoppes and houses, there being washed and shaven.' (Vicary, 1888, p.206)

In the ensuing article, the Act of 1540 stipulated 'that no manner of person...presume to keepe any Shop or Barbery or shauing within the City of London, except he be a Freeman of the same Corporation and Company' (Vicary, 1888, p.207; see also Young, 1890, pp.78–81, 586–90).

Pelling, who has studied the barber-surgeons of Tudor England, is probably right in viewing the Act of 1540 as reflecting the barber-surgeons' attempt to establish their ascendancy with respect to all venereal disease (Pelling, 1986, p.196). Apparently, the venereal plague had assumed such proportions by the middle of the century that a monopoly on treatment guaranteed a rich financial harvest. In this respect, it seems that the barber-surgeons' initiative met with a certain success, for the medical and literary sources of the hundred years following the enactment of this Act feature the barber-surgeon as the practitioner to be consulted by a patient suffering from the pox.

An example may be given from the parish record books kept by the clerks of St Botolph without Aldgate, London, from 1583 through 1599. An entry under February 2, 1599, records the burial of

> 'Jhon Akenyead a tapster late dwelling at the signe of the greyhownd in southwarke who for some desase was to be cured by one Mr Foster A chiurgion and did lye at [was lodged at] the house of Ellen wryght a widow dwelling in a garden howse neare hogg lane in the precinct near whyt chaple barres where he dyed and was Buried the second day of februarie Anno 1599 yeares xxv. he was no parishioner with us. – de Morbo gallico.' (Forbes, 1971, p.92)

A tapster from Southwark would be at special risk of infection since the district teemed with brothels and alehouses, both of which were disseminating centres of syphilis. The fact that such districts were a source of substantial income for the barber-surgeons may be gleaned from John Earle's *Microcosmographie* of 1633.

Describing 'A Surgeon', the author says that 'Hee had beene long since undone, if the charity of the Stewes had not relieved him, from whom he ha's his Tribute as duely as the Pope, or a wind-fall sometimes from a Taverne, if a quart Pot hit right' (Earle, 1633, '49. A Surgeon').

In Marston's *The Dutch Courtesan* (1605), the association between brothels, barber-surgeons and syphilis comes easily to Cocledemoy, a knavish citizen, who greets a barber-surgeon's apprentice with these bawdy innuendoes:

COCLEDEMOY    What, a barber-surgeon, my delicate boy?

HOLIFERNES    Yes, sir, an apprentice to surgery.

COCLEDEMOY    'Tis my fine boy. To what bawdy house doth your master belong? What's thy name?

HOLIFERNES    Holifernes Reinscure.

COCLEDEMOY    Reinscure? Good Master Holifernes, I desire your further acquaintance — nay, pray ye be covered, my fine boy; kill thy itch and heal thy scabs. Is thy master rotten? (2,1:162–70)

Cocledemoy resumes his jibes at the surgical profession during his quarrel with Mary Faugh, whom he calls a 'bawd' (1,2:13) and a 'pandress, supportress of barber-surgeons and enhanceress of lotium and diet drink!' (1,2:23–4). Significantly, John Taylor's description of 'A Whore' from 1630 points her out not only as a source of syphilitic infection but also as a source of great income for the surgeons:

> Thus may shee liue, (much honour'd for her crimes)
> And haue the Pox some twelue or 13 times,
> And shee may be so bountifull agen,
> To sell those Pox to three or fourescore men:
> And thus the Surgeons may get more by farre,
> By Whores and Peace, then by the sword and warre.
> And thus a Whore (if men consider of it)
> Is an increasing gainfull piece of profit. (Taylor, 1630, p.111, 'A Whore')

There is also evidence that many physicians regarded the treatment administered by the barber-surgeons as worse than the disease they professed to cure. Thus John Cotta, a famous London doctor, in 1612 launched a violent attack on the barber-surgeons, saying of them that

> 'if they kill, a dead man telleth no tales: or if by chance they saue one life, that shall be a perpetuall flag to call more fooles to the same adventure. This is commonly seene in the vulgar custome of curing the French disease by Barbers and Surgeons, who precipitate commonly euery one alike, and confusedly without respect or order thrust all through the purgatorie of their sweatings, bleeding, vomiting, vnctions, plaisters, and the like.' (Cotta, 1612, p.38)

## THE QUACKS' CHARTER 1542–3

Pelling supports her interpretation of the venereal background of the incorporation of the barbers and surgeons in 1540 by drawing attention to the somewhat puzzling Act of 1542–3, the so-called Quacks' Charter. Here the licensed surgeons of London were condemned for 'mynding oonelie theyre owne lucres, and nothing the profite or ease of the diseased' (Vicary, 1888, p.208). Caring for money only, the licensed surgeons were presented by the Act as people who had 'sued, troubled, and vexed, divers honest persones, aswell men as women, whome God hathe endued with the knowledge of the nature, kinde, and operacion, of certeyne herbes, rotes and waters, and the using and mynistering of them to suche as been pained with customable diseases' (p.208). These ailments were specified as 'any outwarde sore…wounde, appostemacions…scaldinges, burninges, sore mouthes, the stone, strangurye, saucelin and morfew [scurvy and scaly eruptions], and suche other lyke dis-eases'(pp.208–9).[*] The majority of the cutaneous conditions listed could easily be references to syphilis, just as 'strangury', or prostatitis, was a not uncommon side effect of gonorrhea. Moreover, 'scaldings' and 'burnings' were popular terms for such 'customable diseases' as syphilis and gonorrhea (see pp.258–68).

The royal Act of 1542–3 concluded that since most surgeons were in fact quite ignorant and often caused their patients more harm than good,

> 'it shalbe lefull [lawful] to everye persone, being the Kinges Subject, having knowledge and experience of the nature of herbes, rotes, and waters, or of the operacion of the same, by speculacion or practyse, within any parte of the Realme of Englande, or within any other the Kinges Domynions, to practyse…without sute, vexacion, trouble, penaltie, or losse of theyre goodes.' (Vicary, 1888, p.209)

In this way, the Quacks' Charter opened the way for competition between common practitioners and the barber-surgeons, and if Pelling is right in her interpretation of the venereal disease implications of this Act too, it may reflect an official attitude that all available measures be used to halt the venereal plague and that treatment should be available to all classes (Pelling, 1986, p.97).

The skeleton of such an official health policy may be further discerned in an important act which was passed in the last year of Henry VIII's reign.

## PROCLAMATION OF HENRY VIII AGAINST THE STEWS 1546

In *A Chronicle of England during the Reign of the Tudors from A.D. 1485 to 1559*, the historian Charles Wriothesley (d. 1561) writes under the heading for the year 1546: 'The yeare, at Easter, the stewes was putt downe by the Kinges proclamation made there with a trumpett and an harold at armes' (Wriothesley, 1875, p.163). At about the same time (1542), it appears that the stews at Chester were also suppressed (see p.99). Henry VIII's 'proclamation to avoyd the abhominable place called the *Stewes*' was addressed to the Mayor and Sheriffs of London, and it read as follows:

> 'The King's Most Excellent Majesty, considering how by toleration of such dissolute and miserable persons as, putting away the fear of Almighty God and shame of the world, have been suffered to dwell besides London and elsewhere in common, open places called the stews, and there without punishment or correction exercise their abominable and detestable sin, there hath of late increased and grown such enormities as not only provoke instantly the anger and wrath of Almighty God, but also engender such corruption among the people as tendeth to the intolerable annoyance of the commonwealth, and where not only the youth is provoked,

---

[*]  In contemporary dermatological literature, morfew, morphea, morphew and similar words always seem to refer to a scaly eruption, perhaps a symptom of scurvy (see Copeman and Copeman, 1969, pp.307–8).

enticed, and allowed to execute the fleshly lusts, but also, by such assemblies of evil-disposed persons haunted and accustomed, is daily devised and conspired how to spoil and rob the true laboring and well-disposed men, for these considerations hath by advice of his council thought requisite utterly to extinct such abominable license and clearly to take away all occasion of the same: wherefore his majesty straightly chargeth and commandeth that all such persons as have accustomed most abominably to abuse their bodies contrary to God's law and honesty, in any such common place called the stews now about the city of London, do, before the Feast of Easter next coming, depart from those common places and resort incontinently to their natural countries with their bags and baggages, upon pain of imprisonment and further to be punished at the King's majesty's will and pleasure.

Furthermore his majesty straightly chargeth and commandeth that all such house-holders as under the name of bawds have kept the notable and marked houses and known hostelries for the said evil-disposed persons; that is to say, such householders as do inhabit the houses whited and painted with signs on the front for a token of the said houses, shall avoid with bag and baggage before the Feast of Easter next coming upon pain of like punishment at the King's majesty's will and pleasure.

Furthermore the King's majesty straightly chargeth and commandeth that all such as dwell upon the banks called the stews near London, and have at any time before this proclamation sold any manner victuals to such as have resorted to their houses, do before the said Feast of Easter cease and leave off their victualing and forbear to retain any guest or stranger into their house either to eat and drink or lodge, after the Feast of Easter next coming, until they have presented themselves before the King's majesty's council and there bound themselves with surety in recognizance not to suffer any such misorder in their house, or lodge any serving man, prentice, or woman unmarried, other than their hired servants, upon the pain before specified.

The King's most excellent majesty also chargeth and commandeth that no owner or mean tenant of any such whited house or houses, where the said lewd persons have had resort and used their most detestable life, do from the said Feast of Easter presume to let any of the houses, heretofore abused with said mischiefs in the streets called the stews aforesaid, to any person or persons before the same owner or mean tenant intending to make lease as afore so present the name or names of such as should hire the same to the King's majesty's council, and that before them the lessee hath put in bond and surety not to suffer any of the said houses to be abused as hath been in times past with the said abomination, upon like pain as before is mentioned.

Finally, to the intent all resort should be eschewed to the said place, the King's majesty straightly chargeth and commandeth that from the Feast of Easter next ensuing there shall no bear-baiting be used in that row or in any place on that side the bridge called London Bridge, whereby the accustomed assemblies may be in that place thoroughly abolished and extinct, upon like pain as well to them that keep the bears and dogs which have been used in that purpose as to all such as will resort to see the same.' (Larkin and Hughes, 1964–9, vol.1, pp.365–6. Westminster, 13 April, 1546, 37 Henry VIII)*

In this important document, the 'dissolute and miserable' agents of prostitution are described as having engendered by their 'abominable and detestable sin' not only dangerous 'enormities' in the Commonwealth but also a 'corruption' of the same along with the spread of theft and crime. In order to wipe out these spiritual and

---

*    The editors have modernized the text.

physical evils, the Act of 1546 banishes all bawds from their brothel-houses and all whores to their home parishes. Lessees as well as their tenants are to enter bonds for the observance of this order and see to it that neither prostitution nor victualling take place in their houses.

In a final effort to strangle the serpent of whoredom, the royal proclamation cracks down on the 'bears and dogs' of the Bankside in the pious hope that the banishment of another popular entertainment will discourage resort to the area. Bear-baiting and bull-baiting went hand in hand with gaming and wenching, haunting of taverns and alehouses, and watching of theatre performances. These were all studies to be pursued at the 'Beares Colledge', as the red-light district of Southwark was popularly called (Jonson, 1925–52, vol.8, p.87, Epigramme 133), and according to a variety of sources from Tudor and Stuart England, the education was formidable in all subjects.

## THE KING'S TRUMPET BLOWN IN VAIN

As it turned out, King Henry's herald had blown his trumpet in vain, for during the reign of Henry's son Edward VI (*regnebat* 1547–53), whoredom seems to have flourished stronger than ever and to have spread to a much wider area of the capital. 'You have put down the stews...Ye have but changed the place, and not taken the whoredome away', Archbishop Hugh Latimer (1485?–1555) told the King and his Lords in one of his interminable sermons, delivered in 1549 (Latimer, 1844, pp.133–4).

> 'There is more open whoredom, more stewed whoredom than ever was be-fore...God is dishonoured by whoredom in this city of London; yea, the Bank, when it stood, was never so common! If it be true that is told, it is marvel that it [London] doth not sink, and that the earth gapeth not and swalloweth it up. It is wonderful that the city of London doth suffer such whoredom unpunished.' (pp.134, 196)

According to Latimer, conditions in the country as a whole did not seem to differ greatly from those in the capital. 'Lechery is used throughout England, and such lechery as is used in none other places of the world', he told the King in the last of his court sermons, delivered in the Lent of 1550. 'And yet it is made a matter of sport, a matter of nothing; a laughing matter, and a trifle' (pp.257–8).[*]

Latimer finished his sermon on the subject by demanding the death penalty for adultery, stating his conviction that such a measure 'might be a remedy for all this matter. There would not be then so much adultery, whoredom, and lechery in England as there is' (p.244).

After the boy-king's death at the age of fifteen, Edward VI was succeeded by his half-sister Mary Tudor (*regnebat* 1553–58), who married Philip II of Spain and made a bloody attempt to reintroduce Catholicism in England. The change of the system might have furthered a more liberal official attitude toward prostitution, since Roman Catholic countries displayed a greater toleration of this institution than Calvinist and Lutheran countries. Actually there are signs that clergymen of the old

---

[*]  cf. Thomas Becon's similar statement in Becon, 1843, p.41 and Becon, 1844, p.643.

guard appear to have scented morning-air, for in his *Description of England*, written in 1577–87, the chronicler William Harrison (1534–93) says of the year 1545:

> 'The Stewes & publike bordell houses about London & in other places in England, are abolished & so continue vntill the time of Quene Mary; in whose daies, some of the Clergy made labour to haue them restored againe; & were very likely to haue obteined their sute if she had liued a while longer; soche trees, soche frute: "for the stewes," saith one of them in a sermon made at Paules cross, "are so necessary in a common welth, as a iaxe [lavatory] in a mannes house": his name I spare, sith it shall suffice that it beginneth with the same letter that papa dothe.' (Harrison, 1877, pp.li–lii)

Since Harrison wrote in the 1570s and 1580s, the pope alluded to must be Gregory XIII (1572–85), and so the bishop who preached from St. Paul's Cross was very likely Stephen Gardiner (1483?–1555), the Bishop of Winchester. Gardiner had been rusticated during Edward VI's reign, but under 'Bloody Mary' he was restored to power and was even appointed Lord Chancellor. His 'shameles whordom' came under attack in 1542 by the Puritan preacher Henry Brinklow, who openly accused him of keeping other men's wives, and suggested that 'If all the bysshops of Ingland were hanged which kepe harlots and whorys, we shuld haue fewer pompos bysshops than we haue' (Brinklow, 1874, p.64).

Another sidelight on the clergy during Mary's reign is provided by the scandalous life of one of the most prominent clergymen in the land, Dr. Hugh Weston (1505?–58). In 1553 Weston was installed as Dean of Westminster but, according to a contemporary source, he was also known to have been 'sore bytten wyth a Wynchester gose' and to have been much practised in the art of passing his infection on to others (see pp.258–60). 'Winchester goose' was an Elizabethan slang expression for either a syphilitic prostitute from Southwark or a person infected with the pox (see pp.214–9). The Dean's promiscuous habits became so outrageous that he had to be removed from office in August 1557 by Cardinal Pole.

A third source testifying to the liberal winds blowing during the reign of Queen Mary is the former prostitute Anus in Thomas Randolph's (1605–35) play *Hey for Honesty, Down with Knavery* (1651). 'Ah, Turnbull Grove! shall I nevermore be beholding to thy charitable shades?', she wistfully reminisces.

> 'Ah! 'twas a good world when the nunneries stood. O, their charitable thoughts that took so much compassion on poor women, to found such zealous bawdy-houses! Had not [Thomas] Cromwell been an eunuch, he had never persuaded the destruction of such places set up for such uses. 'Twas a good world, too, in the days of Queen Mary' (4,3:461). (Randolph, 1875, vol.2, p.461)

Any prospects of a return to the system of licensed prostitution in force prior to the Act of 1546 were cut short by the death of Mary in 1558. She was followed by her half-sister Elizabeth I (*regnebat* 1558–1603), who repealed the Marian legislation which had reconciled England with the Pope and introduced a new Act of Supremacy that concluded the reformation of the Church begun by her father. Her long, conservative reign made no legislation against prostitution as such but entrenched the tradition against legalized prostitution and licensed brothels which her father had adopted by his closing of the stews of Southwark in 1546.

Whether or not the royal cure might have proven worse than the ailment was a question raised by the clergyman and popular author Thomas Fuller (1608–61). Writing on the subject of 'The Harlot' in his sprawling work *The Holy and the Profane State* (1642), Fuller concluded his observations on prostitution by saying of the harlot that

'*She dieth commonly of a lothsome disease.* I mean that disease, unknown to Antiquity, created within some hundreds of years, which took the name from Naples. When hell invented new degrees in sinne, it was time for heaven to invent new punishments. Yet is this new disease now grown so common and ordinary, as if they meant to put divine Justice to a second task to find out a newer. And now it is high time for our Harlot, being grown lothsome to her self, to runne out of her self by repentance. Some conceive that when King Henry the eight destroyed the publick Stews in this Land (which till his time stood on the banks side on Southwark next the Bear-garden, beasts and beastly women being very fit neighbours) he rather scattered then quenched the fire of lust in this kingdome, and by turning the flame out of the chimney where it had a vent, more endangered the burning of the Commonwealth. But they are deceived: for whilest the Laws of the Land tolerated open uncleannesse, God might justly have made the whole State do penance for whoredom; whereas now that sinne though committed, yet not permitted, and though (God knows) it be too generall, it is still but personall.' (Fuller, 1938, vol.2, p.360)[*]

---

[*] Fuller in 1655 amplified his views on the subject in his *Church History of Britain from the Birth of Jesus Christ until the Year MDCXLVIII*, in which he advances his 'Argument[s] *pro* and *con* about Stewes':

1. Mans infirmity herein since his Naturall corruption is grown so generall, it is needfull to connive at such Houses, as a kinde of remedy to prevent worse incontinency with Married women, the whole land being the cleaner for the publick Sincks or Sewer of Stewes.

1. It is absurd to say, and belibelleth Divine Providence, That any thing is really Needfull that is not Lawfull. Such pretended necessity created by bad men must be annihilated by good Laws. Let Marriage run in its proper channel, being permitted to all persons; and then no need of such noysome sinks which may well be dammed up. The malady cannot be accounted a remedy: For whilest Matrimony is appointed and blessed by God to cool the heat of Lust, Whoredome doth double the drought thereof.

2. As Moses permitted Divorcement to the Jewes, Stewes may be connived at on the same accompt for the hardnesse of mens hearts.

2. Christians ought not so much to listen to Moses his permission, as to Christ his reprehension thereof. Besides some faults had a cover for them in the twi-light of the Law, which have none in the sun-shine of the Gospel.

3. Strange women were no strangers in Israel it self under their best Kings; two of that trade publickly known, pleaded before King Solomon. These were publickly repaired unto and known by the attire of an Harlot.

3. Christians must conform themselves to the necessary members and commendable ornaments of the Jewish Commonwealth, but not to the wennes and ulcers thereof.

4. Many great Families were preserved thereby, whose younger Brethren abstaining from Marriage, did not cumber the same with numerosity of Children.

4. Where Harlots have preserved one house, they have destroyed an hundred. Besides, we must not doe Evil, that Good may come thereof. Nor can many Children be accompted evils to men, which are blessings from God.

5. Such Stewes are Fashionable in forreigne Nations; yea, in Rome it self.

5. Let the Paramount Whore tolerate Whores, which as a branch of Popery was now banished England; more honour it is for us to go before forraign Nations in Reformation, than to follow them in their Corruptions.

6. The suppressing of Stewes would not make men more chaste, but more close: not more sincerely honest, but secretly wanton. In all populous places, male-incontinency will meet with a female counterpart, and so reciprocally.

6. This undeniable truth is sadly granted. Perchance there may now be moe Englishfolk Adulterers, but England was then a Adultresse, so long as Stewes were openly licensed. It was a Nationall sin, when publickly permitted; which now is but personall, though too generally committed (Fuller, 1655, pp.240–1).

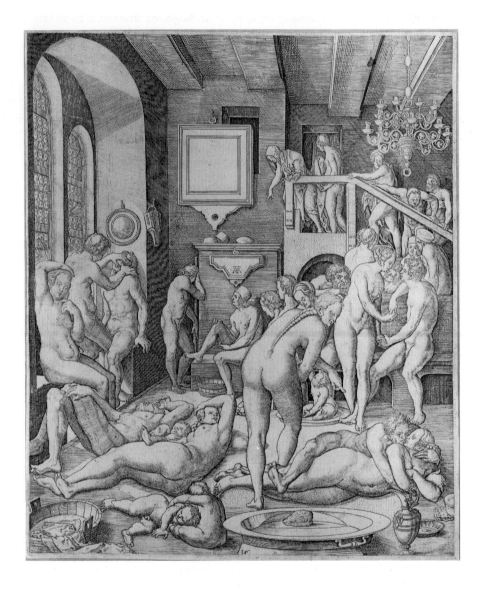

Figure 22. Engraving of a 16th-century bath house and brothel by Virgil Solis (1514–62), Den kongelige
Kobberstiksamling, Copenhagen. Camden makes a common mistake in his derivation of the word 'stew'
for brothel. There were, for many years, ponds or stews on the South bank of the Thames, in which
fish were kept, and these small bodies of water are clearly visible in some maps of the 16th and 17th
centuries. However, the stew–brothel relationship is a legacy of the Roman conquest when the
association between steam-baths and bawdy houses was common. During the Renaissance, this was
further reinforced by the practice of sweating as a cure for syphilis. In Shakespeare's *Measure for Measure*
(1604–5), the Constable refers to the bawd of the play, Mistress Overdone, as 'a bad woman; whose
house, sir, was, as they say, plucked down in the suburbs; and now she professes a hot-house; which I
think is a very ill house too' (2,1:63–6).

The connection between bath establishments and brothels in Shakespeare's time is confirmed by one of Ben Jonson's humorous epigrams, *On the New Hot-House* (1616), in which it says:

> Where lately harbour'd many a famous whore,
> A purging bill, now fix'd vpon the dore,
> Tells you it is a hot-house: So it ma',
> And still be a whore-house. Th'are Synonima. (Jonson, 1925–52, vol.8, p.29)

In 1633 the aldermen of London received an order to see that the bath establishments in different parts of the town were not visited by prostitutes, and that the baths specially reserved for women were not frequented by young men, vagabonds and people of ill-fame (see pp.125–6). So great was the revulsion against bagnios and stews that when, in 1649, the well-known physician and abortionist Peter Chamberlen (1601–83) petitioned Parliament for permission to open bath establishments all over England and published a brochure on the subject, his request was rejected by the Puritans now in power on the grounds of morality (*Biographisches Lexicon der hervorragenden Ärzte aller Zeiten und Völker.* Vienna and Leipzig, 1884, vol.1, p.695).

---

Fuller's conclusion that the King was justified, that the situation has been remedied, and that sin is now considered to be personal, rather than openly tolerated by the State, presents a sanguine view of the situation which was shared by another famous writer and historian of the previous generation, William Camden (1551–1623). Working on his monumental study *Britain, or a Chorographicall Description of the Most Flourishing Kingdomes England, Scotland, and Ireland*, which was published in Latin in 1586, Camden, at the time of writing (1583), supports the royal action to abolish brothels and speaks of them in the past tense:

> 'The Bishops house of Winchester [in Southwark was] built by William Giffard Bishop, for his Successours, about the yeare of our Lord 1107. From which along the *Tamis* banke there runneth Westward a continued raunge of dwelling houses: where within our fathers remembrance was the *Bordello* or *Lupanarie*, for so the Latines terme those little roomes or secret chambers of harlots wherein they filthily prostituted their bodies to sale, because they after the manner of ravening she-wolves catch hold of silly wretched men and plucke them into their holes. But these were prohibited by King Henry the Eighth, at which time England was growne to excessive lasciviousnesse and riot; which in other Nations are continued for gaine, under a specious shew of helping mans infirmity: Neither, of these Strumpets and brothel-houses, doe I thinke that this place in our tongue tooke the name *Stewes*, but of those *Ponds* or *Stewes*, which are heere to feed Pikes and Tenches fat, and to scowre them from the strong and muddy fennish taste.' (Camden, 1610, p.434)

Despite the statements of Fuller and Camden, there is evidence that the efforts of Henry VIII to rid Southwark of licensed brothels only encouraged the development of unlicensed ones. As early as 1550, only four years after the royal proclamation, the Puritan preacher Robert Crowley (1518?–88) said:

> The bawdes of the stues
> be turned all out;
> But some think they inhabit
> al England through out.

> In taverns and tiplyng houses
> many myght be founde,
> If officers would make serch
> but as they are bounde. (Crowley, 1872, pp.13–4)

Crowley here discloses a problem that was also revealed by other critics of the time such as the Puritan preachers and social and moral reformers like William Clowes, Thomas Nashe, Samuel Rowlands and Thomas Dekker (see pp.106–21). 'London, what are thy Suburbes but licensed Stewes?' was their common cry, 'Can it be so many brothel-houses of salary sensuality and six-penny whoredome (the next doore to the Magistrates) should be sette vp and maintained, if brybes dyd not bestirre them?' (Nashe, 1910, p.148). Thomas Nashe, of course, did not mean that the State had once again taken over the regulation of prostitution, but rather that public apathy, general promiscuity, and private interest had permitted the presence of a social institution which everybody knew to be a centre for the dissemination of venereal disease. This position was supported more than a quarter of a century later by John Taylor, the 'Water Poet' (1580–1653), who wrote in 1630:

> The Stewes in *England* bore a beastly sway,
> Till the eight *Henry* banish'd them away:
> And since those common *whores* were quite put downe,
> A damned crue of priuate *whores* are growne,
> So that the diuell will be doing still,
> Either with publique or with priuate ill. (Taylor, 1630, p.110, 'A Whore')

## CONCLUSION

The sources quoted above show that sailors and soldiers were the prime transmitters of syphilis to the British Isles, thus reiterating a pattern already experienced on the Continent. Another source of infection appears to be the clergy, whose members were unmarried and therefore tempted to promiscuous sexuality, a situation also paralleled in conditions in pre-Reformation Europe. The sources also show a spreading of syphilis during the early years of the 16th century, a development which led to the closure of the brothels in 1506 on the Bankside in London. Ironically, this measure forced Bankside prostitutes to move to other parts of the city so that syphilis was spread to the suburbs of London as well.

In rural areas the new disease also appears to have spread on the wings of prostitution, promiscuity, and alcoholism, so that in 1533 a local source states that 'almost into every part of this realm, this most foul and painful disease is crept, and many sore infected therewith' (p.67). Another early source describes syphilis as 'a wasting pox which still vexes many eminent men' (p.60), indicating that in England, as on the Continent, syphilis knew no social distinctions and raged equally among the nobility and the lower classes of society.

Sources further indicate that syphilis absorbed an increasing amount of medical resources and that a large number of admissions to hospitals and lazarhouses were syphilitic patients. The incorporation of the Barber-Surgeons' Company in 1540 has been interpreted as an attempt on the part of barber-surgeons to monopolize the treatment of syphilis and to capitalize on a disease which, according to Pelling, had by 1600 achieved such prominence that it shared with scurvy the distinction of being a regular factor affecting prognosis and the rate of healing of conditions in general (Pelling, 1986, p.98). Sources pertaining to the decades after 1540 clearly indicate that it was the barber-surgeons and not the physicians that were most heavily involved in the treatment of syphilitic patients, and that this clientele was a source of great income for them.

The Quacks' Charter of 1542–3, apparently another reaction to the rapid spread of syphilis, seems to reflect an official attitude that all available measures should be used to halt the venereal plague and that treatment should be offered to all classes. A sign that official health policy focused on the spread of syphilis may also be seen in the proclamation of Henry VIII against the stews in 1546, which put an end to licensed prostitution. The closure and prohibition of public brothels appears to have sparked a debate on licensed versus unlicensed prostitution, obviously prompted by the realization that 'private whores' represented a greater potential for the dissemination of venereal disease than 'public whores'.

According to the preachers and moralists of the time, 'whoredom' does not seem to have diminished after 1546, when a number of clergymen and Puritan preachers advocated the death penalty for adultery in order to stop the moral, social and physical corruption following in the wake of widespread promiscuity.

# 4

# AN AGE OF UPHEAVAL

Then as now there are four factors to consider in the epidemiology of syphilis: (1) the reservoir of infection; (2) the infecting organism; (3) the susceptible host; and (4) the means of transmission. While the spirochete *Treponema pallidum* is the infecting organism, the infected man or woman its host, and the means of transmission sexual intercourse in well over 90 per cent of the cases, the reservoir of infection, or the source of syphilis that keeps it alive, is prostitution. The men and women who confine their sexual relations strictly to one mate do not infect anyone but themselves and are unimportant factors in the persistence of syphilis, because their syphilis dies with them. It is the sexually promiscuous, whether men or women, who perpetuate syphilis; and among these the greatest source of the spread is prostitution, whether clandestine or public.

## THE SOCIODEMOGRAPHY OF SEXUALLY TRANSMITTED DISEASES

Throughout history prostitution has been most common in settings characterized by poverty, a high degree of transiency, social disintegration, and a double standard of sexual behaviour (Holmes, 1990, p.31). Tudor England became a classic example of such a setting because of sweeping changes which took place at the time in almost all areas of culture and society. Profoundly affecting every class and individual, this transformation of the English nation during the 16th century presented a number of critical features, of which the most important were: (1) widening of the gap between the propertied classes and the proletariat due to economic expansion in foreign trade and domestic agriculture and manufacturing; (2) growing poverty among the wage earners of town and village as a result of land shortage, labour surplus, rising prices, cheap money, and declining wages; (3) large scale migration in the wake of booming population, growing unemployment and radical changes in the medieval system of land tenure and communal farming; (4) social disintegration in the expanding cities, above all London, as a result of overcrowding, unemployment, poverty and crime; (5) growing promiscuity in the wake of economic prosperity, social inequality, increasing consumption and the rise of an entertainment industry.

The spiritual and physical disruption of the medieval, fossilized church and the establishment of a new state religion during the same period introduced an element of religious and ideological confusion which intensified the sense of living in an age of transition and revaluation of all traditional norms. These trends and their dynamic interplay created an almost ideal environment for the Sinister Shepherd to graze his sheep.

## ECONOMIC AND SOCIAL UPHEAVALS OF THE 16TH CENTURY

From the early 16th century onward there was a great upsurge of interest in England in the problems of poverty and vagrancy. This growth of interest was fired by an increase in the number of vagrants. Contemporary records abound with complaints about the 'huge nomber of Beggers and Vacaboundes [that] doe breede here in Englande' (Harrison, 1877, p.216) – 'this rascall rablement raung[ing] about the countrey' (Viles and Furnivall, 1880, p.21) and compounded of 'all theeues and caterpillers in the commonwealth' (Harrison, 1877, p.217). Some of these accounts doubtless exaggerate, but it seems certain that the number of vagrants and of the poor generally did grow. Unemployment, poverty and vagrancy were the social evils of Elizabethan society, and they were caused by economic, agricultural, demographic and social changes which made themselves felt from the early 16th century onward.

If Tudor poverty and vagrancy had any one starting point, it may have been the disruptions caused by the Wars of the Roses (1455–85) in which Henry VII finally succeeded in curbing the overmighty nobility and in abolishing its private armies. The immediate result was to drive out of employment many professional soldiers as well as servants of noble households. Vagrants who were former soldiers and servants became progressively more numerous as the century progressed, if only for the obvious reason that England's history of ever increasing warfare abroad with France and Spain led ultimately to ever greater numbers of demobilised soldiers and sailors flooding the labour market.

The dissolution of the monasteries by Henry VIII may have added new numbers to this ever-growing army of vagrants. Monks and nuns who had to rely solely on their pensions were in a critical financial situation – one which was made worse when the legal status of itinerant friars, proctors and pardoners was no longer recognized during the Reformation, and the mendicants became vagrants in the eyes of the law. Those who suffered most from the closing of the monasteries were domestic servants such as gardeners, butlers, cooks and launderers, who had found it difficult to obtain alternative employment, and the unknown number of poor who had come to rely on the monasteries for their charity.

Another larger social group was forced to take to the road by changes in agriculture and the form of landholding which took place at the beginning of the Tudor era. One such change was a direct result of the Black Death, which claimed an enormous number of lives at the end of the Middle Ages. Since the raising of sheep required fewer workers than other forms of husbandry, the English wool industry had flourished increasingly up to the early 1500s. The boom in the cloth trade with the Netherlands during the early and middle years of the century added a further impetus. As a result of this development, many landlords took to enclosing common lands for sheep pasture and forcing tenants out of their small holdings.

In the first part of Thomas More's *Utopia* (1516), Raphael Hythloday argues that men are being punished and even executed for crimes to which they have been driven by hunger and need. A primary social evil, Hythloday suggests, is the practice of enclosing common land in order to raise sheep, thus depriving the working man of his traditional right to graze his animals. 'Your sheep', he exclaims,

> 'that were wont to be so meek and tame, and so small eaters, now, as I hear say, be become so great devourers and so wild, that they eat up, and swallow down the very men themselves. They consume, destroy, and devour whole fields, houses and cities. For look in what part of the realm doth grow the finest and therefore the dearest wool, there noblemen and gentlemen, yea and certain abbots...leave no ground for tillage. They enclose all into pastures; they throw down houses; they pluck down towns, and leave nothing standing, but only the church to be made a sheep-house.' (More, 1962, p.26)

The unemployment resulting from enclosure had the deplorable consequences of furthering drunkenness, gaming, stealing and prostitution, evils which could only by redressed by 'restoring husbandry and tillage' (p.28). Concluded More's mouth-piece:

> 'Now bawds, queans, whores, harlots, strumpets, brothel-houses, stews; and yet another stews, wine-taverns, ale-houses, and tippling houses, with so many naughty, lewd, and unlawful games, as dice, cards, tables, tennis, bowls, quoits, do not all these send the haunters of them straight a-stealing, when their money is gone? Cast out these pernicious abominations; make a law that they which plucked down farms and towns of husbandry shall re-edify them, or else yield and uprender the possession thereof to such as will go to the cost of building them anew.' (p.28)

## POVERTY AND PROSTITUTION

The social evils of the enclosure movement as More described them were compounded by the fact that England during the 16th century was caught up in a vast European spiral of rising prices, declining real wages, and devalued currency. Between 1500 and 1540, prices in England doubled, and they doubled again in the next generation. In 1450 the cost of wheat had been what it was in 1300; by 1550 it had tripled.

Another critical development was the erosion of the purchasing power of the currency by more than two-thirds during the middle of the century. Rising costs emanating from the general price rise and the devaluation of the currency caused landlords to seek compensation for inflationary pressures. Even those tenants who were protected by the customary and common laws faced the renewal of their leases at much less favourable rents, while peasant farmers who held their tenure either by copy (a document recorded in the manor court) or by unwritten custom were evicted. As the medieval system of land tenure and communal farming broke down, more and more farm workers became dependent on wages as their sole form of income, and progressively fewer were guaranteed employment on their fathers' farms.

According to the social critic Robert Crowley, enclosure and eviction were responsible for the undermining of the 'commonweal', and in a tract entitled

*Information and Petition against the Oppressors of the Poor of This Realm* (1549) he analyzed the features of the rural crisis. Crowley saw a primary difficulty in the attitude of landlords who squeezed every penny out of their lands and tenants so that the poorest among them could get no property or income of their own. Leasemongering which piled rent upon rent on each piece of property, and the inflationary valuation caused by land surveyors drove men of modest means out of the land market. In consequence, the children of the poor came to a bad end, and boys quite capable of following the liberal arts – 'whereof the realme hath great lacke' (Crowley, 1872, p.166) – had to resign themselves to menial work in support of their impoverished parents. Girls suffered in other ways, striking out into a bleak path where prostitution lay at the end of the road. 'What modeste, chaste, and womanly virgins haue, for lacke of dourie, ben compelled, either to passe ouer the days of theyr youth in vngrate seruitude, or else to marye to perpetuall miserable pouertie', Crowley asked eloquently in his tract.

> 'What immodeste and wanton gyrles haue hereby ben made sisters of the Banck (the stumbling stock of all frayle youth) and finaly, moste miserable creatures, lyeinge and dieynge in the stretes ful of all plages and penurie! What vniuersall destruction chaunceth to this noble realme by this outragious and vnsaciable desyr of the surueiers of landes!' (p.166)

Local riots and disturbances against rising rents and the encroachment of fenced pastures increased in the 1530s and 1540s as landlords enlarged the size of their flocks until ruminants outnumbered human beings three to one. Although inflation temporarily injected new life into the economy, it affected the growing number of people who had to rely solely on wages adversely. During the period 1500 to 1640, despite a threefold increase in monetary terms, real wages dropped by as much as 50 per cent. Wage workers found themselves in real difficulties, and their plight was made worse by the fact that few of them had alternative sources of income. Many of these people – perhaps one-third in the cities, one-fifth in the rural districts – were on, or just below, the poverty line, and a similar number were barely above it. Not surprisingly, food riots were far from uncommon in a century where bad harvests were relatively common and disastrous ones not infrequent. On the average, there was a harvest failure every four years during the 16th century (Pound, 1971, pp.15–16, 80–1).

Inflation and the wool trade thus combined with the enclosure movement and changes in the medieval system of land tenure to create economic and social upheaval in which land surplus, labour shortage, low rents, and high wages were replaced by land shortage, labour surplus, high rents, and declining wages.

The steady rise in population was perhaps the most critical feature of all in this upheaval, and it increased in intensity as the century progressed. As England slowly began to recover from the demographic catastrophe of the Black Death, the population, which in 1400 may have dropped as low as 2.5 million, was back up to about 3 million by 1550, and half a century later was over 4 million. By 1650 the population explosion in England itself hit 5.2 million, while the total for Britain (including Scotland, Ireland, and Wales) reached 7.7 million.[*]

William Lambarde (1536–1601), a historian and justice of the peace, commented on 'the dearth of all things' and 'the overgrown number of us' (Read, 1962, p.182).[**] 'The number of our people is multiplied', he complained, 'it is both demonstrable to the eye and evident in reason' (p.182).[***] The topographer and historian William Harrison (1534–93) presented a similar picture in his *Description of England* (1577–87), while also recording the opinion of the Malthusians of his day: 'Some also doe grudge at the great increase of people in these daies, thinking a necessarie brood of cattell farre better than a superfluous augmentation of mankind' (Harrison, 1877, p.215).

The cumulative impact of all these forces created a situation which Elizabethan society could do nothing to control, even if it had been able to identify it with greater certainty. The result was a large-scale migration of individuals, of impoverished and unemployed men and women, of vagrants and beggars in search of food, charity or work – a *Völkerwanderung* which served to disseminate such highly contagious diseases as bubonic plague, smallpox, syphilis and gonorrhea.

## VAGRANTS AND VAGRANCY IN ELIZABETHAN ENGLAND

New types of infection are always dangerous, and travel and communication are their best friends. One of the sources of the spread of syphilis among the rural and urban population in England may be studied in two pioneering accounts of vagrancy written in the 1560s, John Awdeley's *Fraternitye of Vacabondes* (1561) and Thomas Harman's *Caveat for Common Cursetors* (1567). These books describe in detail the subculture that was formed by individuals forced on the road, including the patterns of unsocial behaviour, organized criminal activity, and gross promiscuity to which the culture became adapted.

At the top of the pecking order of vagabonds were the 'upright men' who not only had the right to help themselves to a share of any other vagrant's possessions, but also the right to intercourse with anyone's woman. 'An Vpright man', explains Awdeley,

> 'is of so much authority, that meeting with any of his profession, he may cal them to accompt, & commaund a share or snap vnto him selfe, of al that they haue gained by their trade in one moneth. And if he doo them wrong, they haue no remedy agaynst hym, no though he beate them, as he vseth commonly to do. He may also commaund any of their women, which they cal Doxies, to serue his turne.' (Viles and Furnivall, 1880, p.4)

Next in the hierarchy of vagabonds were the 'curtals', who according to Awdeley 'vseth commonly to go with a short cloke, like to grey Friers, & his woman with

---

[*]   See E.A. Wrigley and R.S. Schofield: *The Population History of England, 1541–1871*. London, 1981, pp.208–10. The two authors of this classic study conclude: 'From 1541 to 1656 the population grew from 2.7 million to 5.2 million, almost doubling in 115 years, an increase equivalent to an average growth rate of 0.56 per cent per annum…The economy was clearly incapable of making effective use of the additional labour coming onto the market and real wages suffered a drastic fall' (Wrigley and Schofield, 1981, pp.210, 411).

[**]  See also Hurstfield and Smith, 1972, p.47.

[***] cf. also p.47.

him in like liuery, which he calleth his Altham if she be hys wyfe, & if she be his harlot, she is called hys Doxy' (p.4). Other categories included the ruffler, the prigman, the palliard, the swigman, the tinkard, the rogue, and so forth. Harman is more expansive on the subject of 'doxies' than Awdeley, who dismisses them curtly as 'their women' (p.4). 'These Doxes', says Harman,

> 'be broken and spoyled of their maydenhead by the vpright men, and then they haue their name of Doxes, and not afore. And afterwarde she is commen and indifferent for any that wyll vse her, as *homo* is a commen name to all men. Such as be fayre and some what handsome, kepe company with the walkinge Mortes, and are redye alwayes for the vpright men, and are cheifely mayntayned by them, for others shalbe spoyled for their sakes: the other, inferior, sort wyll resorte to noble mens places, and gentlemens houses, standing at the gate, eyther lurkinge on the backesyde about backe houses, eyther in hedge rowes, or some other thycket, expectinge their praye, which is for the vncomely company of some curteous gest, of whome they be refreshed with meate and some money, where eschaunge is made, ware for ware: this bread and meate they vse to carrye in their greate hosen; so that these beastlye bryberinge breeches serue manye tymes for bawdye purposes.' (pp.73–4)

The promiscuous activities of these 'doxies' roaming the countryside and disseminating venereal diseases to all levels of the population were known also to Thomas Dekker. Writing a generation later, he observed in *The Belman of London* (1608) that

> 'These *Doxyes* will for good victuals or a small peice of money, prostitute there bodies to seruingmen if they can get into any conuenient corner about their maisters houses, & to ploughmen in barnes, haylofts or stables: they are common pick-pockets, familiars (with the baser sorts of cut-purses,) and oftentimes secret murtherers of those infants which are begotten of their bodies.' (Dekker, 1884–6, vol.3, p.107)[*]

Harman further informs us that before a woman is deflowered by an upright man, she is called a 'dell', described by the author as

> 'a yonge wenche, able for generation, and not yet knowen or broken by the vpright man. These go abroade yong, eyther by the death of their parentes, and no bodye to looke vnto them, or els by some sharpe mystres that they serue, do runne away out of seruice; eyther she is naturally borne one, and then she is a wyld Dell: these are broken verye yonge; when they haue béene lyen with all by the vpright man, then they be Doxes, and no Dels. These wylde dels, beinge traded vp with their monstrous mothers, must of necessytie be as euill, or worsse, then their parents, for neither we gather grapes from gréene bryars, neither fygs from Thystels. But such buds, such blosoms, such euyll sede sowen, wel worsse beinge growen.' (Viles and Furnivall, 1880, p.75)

Other varieties of female vagrants included 'autem morts', whom Harman describes as women married in church, 'for Autem in their Language is a Churche; so she is a wyfe maried at the Church, and they be as chaste as a Cowe I haue, that goeth to Bull euery moone, with what Bull she careth not' (p.67). Another variety was the so-called 'walking morts' who were not married, although they often pretended to

---

[*]   Dekker's source for his observations on vagrancy in the *The Belman of London* and *Lanthorne and Candlelight* is generally felt to be Harmann's *Caveat* so that Dekker may be characterized as a secondary source in this area.

be so by presenting themselves as widows with needy children or as wives left alone by husbands on active service (p.67).

Harman records a conversation with one of these 'walking morts' whom he interviewed in the summer of 1566 in his house at Crayford near Dartford in Kent. Harman was a country magistrate, but ill health prevented him from taking an active part in the affairs of the county, and so he turned his disability to account by keeping close observation on the travellers upon the neighbouring highroad. The 'walking mort' told Harman that a year ago she had travelled into East Kent by the sea-coast while expecting yet another child by an unknown father. Gathering oysters and mussels on the beach, she happened to fall into a deep hole where she would have been drowned by the oncoming tide if she had not been rescued by a man whom she recognized as a farmer 'of some welth' and with 'a very honest woman to his wyfe' (p.69). However, the farmer's price for saving the woman was her promise to have intercourse with him in his barn at 9 o'clock the same evening. The indignant woman disclosed the plan to the farmer's wife who had 'donne me so much good' (p.69), as she informed Harman, and the two women agreed that the 'walking mort' should call out 'fye, for shame, fye' when the farmer was about to embrace her in the hay. At the sound of the watchword, the farmer's wife promised her to 'bée harde by you wyth helpe' (p.70), and

> 'So my dame lefte me settinge by a good fyre with meate and drynke; and wyth the oysters I broughte with me, I hadde great cheere: shée wente strayght and repaired vnto her gossypes dwelling there by; and, as I dyd after vnderstande, she made her mone to them, what a naughtye, lewed, lecherous husbande shée hadde, and howe that she coulde not haue hys companye for harlotes, and that she was in feare to take some fylthy dyseaase of hym, he was so commen a man, hauinge lytle respecte whome he hadde to do with all; "and," quoth she, "nowe here is one at my house, a poore woman that goeth aboute the countrey that he woulde haue hadde to doe withall."' (p.70)

After deliberation, the farmer's wife and her female neighbours decided to teach the adulterous husband a lesson he would not forget for a long time, and so they agreed on a plan which, as the wife explained to the woman, was devised as 'some remedy to make my husband a good man, that I may lyue in some suerty without disease, and that hée may saue his soule that God so derelye bought' (p.70). At the appointed hour, the 'walking mort' turned up in the barn, and as she gave the watchword, the women came out of their hiding to give the naked farmer a sound beating 'that the bloud braste plentifullye oute in most places' (p.73).

After the chastisement, the women told the farmer 'that he shoulde from that tyme forth knowe his wyfe from other mens, and that this punishment was but a flebyting in respect of that which should followe, yf he amended not his manners' (p.73). Apparently the Falstaffian story had a happy end, for the 'walking mort' told Harman that 'I here a very good reporte of hym now, that he loueth his wyfe well, and vseth hym selfe verye honestlye; and was not this a good acte? nowe, howe saye you?' To which Harman gave the woman his reply of acknowledgement: 'It was pretely handeled' (p.73).

### 'ROTTEN', OR SYPHILIZED, VAGRANT WHORES

The last two classes of female vagrants commonly met with on the English roads were the so-called 'bawdy baskets' and 'demanders for glimmer'. As her name implied, the 'bawdy basket' offered more for sale than the laces, pins, needles and ribbons which she carried in her basket. 'And as they walke by the waye, they often gaine some money wyth their instrument, by such as they sodaynely mete withall. The vpright men haue good acquayntance with these, and will helpe and relieue them when they want. Thus they trade their lyues in lewed lothsome lechery' (Viles and Furnivall, 1880, p.65).

The 'demander for glimmer', finally, was a woman who travelled from place to place with false documents certifying that she had lost all her goods through fire, 'for glymmar, in their language, is fyre' (p.61). Harman observes that these women, like all female vagrants, are 'easlye perswaded to lykinge lechery' (p.62) and that an average demander 'would wekely be worth vi. or seuen shyllinges with her begging and bycherye' (p.61).

At the lowest level of the wandering proletariat of prostitutes was the younger generation, the children of vagrants, who were called 'kinchin coes' if they were boys, and 'kinchin morts' if they were girls. Harman shows no sympathy with these children born into a life of vagrancy, for he observes that 'A Kynchen Co is a young boye, traden vp to suche peuishe purposes as you haue harde of other young ympes before, that when he groweth vnto yeres, he is better to hang then to drawe forth' (p.76). As to the 'kinchin mort', Harman informs the reader that she 'is a lytle Gyrle: the Mortes their mothers carries them at their backes in their slates, whiche is their shetes, and bryngs them vp sauagely, tyll they growe to be rype, and soone rype, soone rotten' (p.76).

Harman's last reference is to the medlar, 'a fruit rotten before it is ripe', and therefore an Elizabethan slang expression for a prostitute. 'He that marries a whore looks like a fellow bound all his lifetime to a medlar-tree', says Ward in Middleton's *Women Beware Women* (1657), 'and that's good stuff; 'tis no sooner ripe but it looks rotten, and so do some queans at nineteen. A pox on't!' (4,3:98–102). Significantly, 'rotten' was a common Elizabethan euphemism for a person infected with the pox. The *locus classicus* is the graveyard scene in Shakespeare's *Hamlet* (1600–1) where the Prince asks the grave-digger: 'How long will a man lie i'th' earth ere he *rot?*' To which the sexton replies: 'Faith, if a be not *rotten* before a die – as we have many *pocky* corses nowadays that will scarce hold the laying in – a will last you some eight year or nine year' (5,1:158–61). 'She is Rotten, and ready for an Hospital', says the Emperor Valentinian of a 'holy Whore' in Fletcher's *The Tragedy of Valentinian* (1610–14) (4,1:55).

'De hot Neapolitan pox rot him' (2,2:44–5), curses the prostitute heroine Franceschina in Marston's *The Dutch Courtesan* (1605), while another bawd in Dekker's *The Honest Whore* (1630) tells a customer that 'We have meats of all sorts of dressing; we have stewed meat for your Frenchmen, pretty light picking meat for your Italian, and that which is rotten roasted, for *Don Spaniardo*'. To which the customer replies: 'A pox on't' (3,3:12–5). In similar fashion, Sordido in Middleton's *Women Beware Women* (1657) says of an indiscriminate man-about-town: 'He may

The above groups of persons were the people specifically mentioned by William Clowes as disseminating agents of syphilis, both in the capital and in the country – the *Lues Venerea* following in the wake of 'the licentious and beastly disorder of a great number of rogues and vagabondes: The filthye lyfe of many lewd and idell persons, both men and women, about the citye of *London*, and the great number of lewd alehowses, which are the very nests and harbourers of such filthy creatures' (Clowes, 1579, fol. Bi$^v$). The last connection is an interesting one which had surfaced in the citizens' complaints in 1527 to the City's authorities that London's 'innumerable typelyng and ale houses aswell in sellars [cellars], dark lanes as in other places' were characterized by 'moche evill rule…as welle by nyghte as by daye, playing at dyse, cardes & vnlaufulle games with kepyng of bawdry & horedome and lodgyng of vacaboundes' (Anderson, 1933, pp.75–6).

The connection between alehouses, vagrancy and the spread of syphilis we shall study more closely in the next section.

## ALEHOUSES AND PROSTITUTION

During the 16th century the number of alehouses exploded all over England as a result of swelling population, rising unemployment, increasing migration, the beginnings of urbanization, spreading poverty, growing alcoholism, and better brewing methods. Ale was a beverage brewed of fermented malt and water, and in the Middle Ages it was a popular drink which many people brewed at home. With the rising standard of living in the 16th century and the development of better brewing technology, the demand grew for stronger and more palatable beverages. The revolution in drinking taste, which was largely complete by the 16th century, saw a change in England from the consumption of poor quality, spiced ale to hopped beer which was stronger, more tasty, and easier to make on a commercial basis. Beer was not only more economical to brew, but could also be stored longer than ale without deteriorating, and the ensuing price differential between the two beverages was highly influential in promoting demand for the new product at a time when real wages were declining (Clark, 1983, p.97).

However, factors of price and taste were not the only ones involved, for equally important in the history of public drinking was fashion. In 1547 Andrew Boorde in his *Dyetary* admonished his countrymen that 'water is not holsome sole by it selfe for an Englysshe man' (Boorde, 1870, p.252), and his countrymen took his advice to heart. Writing in the 1570s, Reginald Scot asserted that beer was rapidly gaining ground in Kent because the 'most part of our countrymen do abhor and abandon ale as a loathsome drink' (Clark, 1983, p.97). Another reason for the proliferation of beer was growing competition among alehouse-keepers to provide the cheapest and strongest tipple. In 1612 the constables of Calne in Wiltshire contended that the alehouse-keepers all vied to brew the strongest ale, while in the next decade a draft parliamentary bill declared that it was 'now the common practice for everyone to strive to exceed [each] other in the strength of their beer' (p.99).

The English alehouse of Elizabethan and Stuart England should more properly be called a beerhouse, since it was the change from ale to beer that brought the decline in domestic brewing for home consumption and the consequent rise in the number of alehouses. In his classic study on *The English Alehouse: A Social History 1200–1830* (1983), Peter Clark concludes that there may have been as many as 24,000 alehouse-keepers in England by the time of the government survey of 1577, including a substantial number of unlicensed owners. Assuming a population of about 3.4 million, this would make for one alehouse to every 142 inhabitants. By the time of the government survey in the 1630s, the number of licensed alehouses had grown to about 32–35,000, with possibly another 15–20,000 unlicensed premises. With a population of about 4.9 million by the 1630s, there may have been one alehouse for every 89–104 inhabitants – a significantly higher ratio than in 1577 (pp.43–4). In the towns the alehouses were spread evenly throughout the community, while in the country they clustered along the main trading routes, in the woodland areas, and in all but the smallest villages.

While the landlord of the inn or tavern looked after the upper and middling classes of society, it was the alehouse-keeper who ministered to the needs of the lower orders of society – small farmers, craftsmen, artisans, labourers, apprentices, servants, vagrants and the indigent. The alehouse-keeper came from the same social background, and from the data collected by Peter Clark it seems likely that at least some of the growing number of alehouse-keepers which so worried the authorities were recruited from the large force of near destitute subsistence migrants that besieged the villages and towns of Elizabethan and Stuart England (p.78).

The establishment of an alehouse was not an insuperable difficulty, for it could often be the back kitchen of a mean dwelling, standing in some obscure back street and run frequently without a licence. Beer could be bought on credit from the prosperous class of brewers, and the only capital investment was for a few benches and tables for the customers. Furthermore, the alehouse-keeper might supplement his income by letting out a room or a barn to vagrants for a penny a night.

Running an alehouse was a family business and the keeper's wife was the one who welcomed the guests, served them liquor and kept them happy with smiles, kisses and, as ballads frequently rehearsed, sometimes more intimate favours. Larger alehouses might have one or two servants, and the girls employed in the tippling dens were generally expected to amuse the customers. In Jacobean Anglesey, for instance, it was said that 'most of our alehouses have a punk besides, for if the good hostess be not so well shaped as she may serve the turn in her own person, she must have a maid to fill pots that shall be fitting' (p.84).

Writing in 1617, Barnabe Rich claimed that a man at an alehouse might have 'his pot of ale, his pipe of tobacco and his pocksy whore and all for his 3d' (Rich, 1617, p.16).[*]

The profits of prostitution were probably split between the girl and the alehouse-keeper, but the money might also stay in the family. One Essex tippler had his eldest son run a gaming table, while the daughter of the house served as a bawd (Clark, 1983, p.84). At Mother Bowden's alehouse in Chelmsford, 'the harlot her daughter' offered her services to customers at a price, while her mother sold 'ale or beer without licence', according to the statement of the justices of the peace (Emmison,

---

[*]  Quoted by Clark, 1983, p.149.

1970, p.26). Of the 12 unlicensed victuallers presented before them at Chelmsford in 1567, three or four were further charged with keeping brothels.[*]

It is small wonder that many alehouse-keepers had a bad reputation and that they were often accused of keeping a 'lewd and disordered house'. In Philip Massinger's play *A New Way to Pay Old Debts* (1633), an alehouse-keeper named Tim Tapwell describes how he 'with a little stocke, Some forty pounds or so, bought a small cottage, Humbled my selfe to marriage with my [wife] *Froth* here; Gaue entertainment'. To which a prodigal named Welborne replies: 'Yes, to whores, and canters, Clubbers by night'. 'True', answers Tapwell, 'but they brought in profit' (1,1:59–63) (Massinger, 1976, vol.2, p.301). Similarly, in Thomas Lodge and Robert Greene's didactic play *A Looking Glasse for London and England* (1598), the Clown muses that

> 'seeing I haue prouided the Ale, who is the puruaior for the wenches? For, masters, take this cup of me, a cup of Ale without a wench, why, alasse, tis like an egge without salt, or a red herring without mustard.'

To which the First Ruffian answers: 'Lead vs to the Ale, weele haue wenches inough I warrant thee' (1,3:262–7) (Greene, 1905, vol.1, p.153).

Before receiving their licence, alehouse-keepers were frequently required by the justices of the peace not to harbour rogues and vagabonds, not to allow bastard births on their premises, not to serve meat in Lent, and not to allow prostitution (Emmison, 1970, p.203). These regulations, of course, were far more often breached than observed, and William Clowes seems to have had his reasons for denouncing 'the great number of lewd alehowses' as disseminating centres of syphilis.

Writing in 1612, the 'High-Constable' who gave Dekker his information for *O per se O* attributed the vast increase in wenching to 'the almost infinite numbers of tipling houses'. In a book posthumously published in 1638, Thomas Dekker reported that in London

> 'A whole street is in some place, but a continued *Ale-house:* Not a shoppe to be seen between a Red *Lattice*, and a Red *Lattice*, no workers, but all drinkers: not a Tradesman at his occupation, for every Tradesman keepes (in that place) an *Ale-house*. It is an easier life, a lazier life, a Trade more gainefull.' (Dekker, 1638, sig. K3ᵛ)

In the same book, Dekker devotes a whole chapter (XVI) to 'The abuses of Ale-houses', comparing the tippling dens to 'an Epidemicall disease, a generall calimity, an Impostume as wide as a Kingdome…Roam[ing] like *Tettars* over the body of the Commonweale' (sig. K3ʳ). These medical metaphors clearly indicate that Dekker was well aware of the connection between alehouses, prostitution and the dissemination of syphilis.


## 'LEWD ALEHOWSES'

The large number of teenagers and young adults at the alehouse, many of whom were servants, apprentices, or migrant labourers, was another major force in the epidemiology of venereal diseases. For this group of young people, the alehouse functioned as a hotel and social club where one could meet people of one's own

---

[*]    P. Clark: 'The Alehouse and the Alternative Society', in Pennington and Thomas, 1978, p.59.

age without supervision from parents or masters and where a variety of sexual liaisons might be conducted, ranging from courtship through casual fornication to prostitution. With a growing proportion of the population in their late teens and twenties and a rising age at marriage – 28–29 years for men and 26–27 years for women (Wrigley and Schofield, 1981, p.423) – there was inevitable pressure for illegitimate sexuality.

A final reason for the proliferation of alehouse prostitution was the sexual imbalance in larger towns during the 16th and 17th centuries, where the demographic picture was characterized by a substantial surplus of women (Clark and Slack, 1976, pp.87–8).* Many of these females were poor, recent immigrants and desperate for work, and service in an alehouse as a maid or a whore – or more often both – was an obvious way of keeping starvation from the door. These women and their employers appear in the description given by William Clowes of

> 'the great number of lewd alehowses, which are the very nests and habourers of such filthy creatures: By meanes of which disordered persons some other of better disposition are many tymes infected, and many more lyke to be.' (see page 108)

In 1540 the town leaders at Chester promulgated an order which throws an interesting light on the conditions described above. 'Whereas *all* the taverns and alehouses of this city, be used to be kept by *young women* otherwise than is used in any other place of this realme', the burghers indignantly observed,

> 'whereat all strangers greatly marvel and think it inconvenient, whereby great slander and dishonest report of this city hath and doth run abroad; in avoiding whereof, as also to eschew such great occasions of wantonness, brawls, frays, and other inconveniences as thereby doth and may arise among youth and light disposed persons, as also damages to their masters, owners of the taverns and alehouses: Ordered, that after the 9th of June next, there shall be no tavern or alehouse kept in the said city by any woman between *fourteen* and *forty* years of age, under pain of forty pounds forfeiture for him or her that keepeth any such servant'. (Hemmingway, 1831, vol.1, p.147)**

Two years later, in 1542, the mayor of the town, William Beswicke, broke with the problem of prostitution in general by issuing an ordinance for the suppression of all stews and brothel houses in the city of Chester (p.146). Four years later the monarch of the country followed in his wake (see pp.75–7).

## WINE, WENCHES AND VENEREAL DISEASES

As demonstrated above, the alehouse played an important part in meeting the social and sexual needs of the lower ranks of English society at a time of major transition. In exploring this function, one should distinguish the alehouse very clearly from the tavern and the inn, which were altogether more respectable establishments. The inn was usually placed in the town's main thoroughfare and was a large spacious building, with a wine license, stabling, and guest rooms where men and women of standing would often meet. Roughly speaking, the principal difference between a

---

*   In London, however, the picture was different due to the large number of apprentices working there; see p.147.
**  Cf. Clark, 1983, p 79

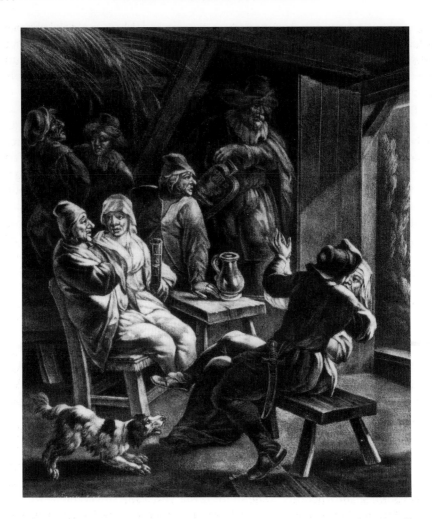

Figure 23. A country alehouse painted by Robert Robinson c. 1680, with traditional music and sexual promiscuity. A primary reason for the growth of alehouse prostitution was high demand, not least from the large number of tramping labourers on the road and away from home. To this transient population as well as to the impoverished villagers and townspeople of the period, the alehouse took on the various functions of a hotel, a social club, an information bureau, a playhouse, a receiving centre for stolen goods, and a brothel.

> So many ale-sellers
> In bawdy holes and cellars,
> Of young folks ill-counsellors,
> Saw I never,

the poet-laureate John Skelton (1460?–1529) complained in the early Tudor period (Skelton, 1964, p.136). In his Rabelaisian poem *The Tunning of Elinour Rumming*, he described the boisterous alehouse of Elinour Rumming in Surrey, which was packed out with a motley crew of 'wenches' and 'housewives' – 'A sort of foul drabbes All scurvy with scabbes' (pp.115–6). In London and other growing towns, the alehouses and tippling dens provided temporary accommodation for the rapid flow of newcomers, enjoying here a variety of popular entertainments such as gaming, cockfighting, dancing, wenching, and the sweet oblivion of drunkenness.

tavern and an inn seems to have been that a tavern also sold wines but did not take in lodgers. The tavern's clientele was comprised of merchants, gentry and other affluent folk, and Thomas Dekker shrewdly urged any man that 'desires to bee a man of good reckoning in the Cittie...[to] take his continuall diet at a Tauerne' (Dekker, 1884–6, vol.2, p.255).

Taverns, like inns, were places for business to be done, investments to be arranged, lawyers and physicians to be consulted, and social gatherings to be held. In London, for instance, the Mermaid Tavern in Bread Street, Cheapside, was renowned for its club of poets, actors, aristocrats and lawyers, who met on the first Friday of every month for drink and talk. The club had been founded by Raleigh, and it included such noteworthy personages as Shakespeare, Jonson, Beaumont, Fletcher, Webster and Donne. Most famous of the taverns of London was the Boar's Head Tavern in Eastcheap, where Sir John Falstaff is supposed to have taken his ease and drunk his deep potations of sack. Here the fat knight also played 'Saturn and Venus...in conjunction' (*2 Henry IV*, 2,4:261) with a young prostitute called Doll Tearsheet, who later died 'i' th' spital Of malady of France' (*Henry V*, 5,1:85–6).

Then, as now, drunkenness and wenching went together, and the higher establishments of social intercourse did not differ in this respect from the lower ones. 'Wines, indeed, *and* girls are good', sings the roaring chorus in John Lyly's aristocratic play *Alexander and Campaspe* (1584), 'But braue victuals feast the bloud. For wenches, wine and lusty cheere Ioue would leape downe to surfet heere' (1,2:109–12). These Falstaffian lines suggest the link between taverns and inns, drunkenness and prostitution – a connection also confirmed by other sources which shows that these establishments were not above offering sexual services to their customers. Waiters and bartenders appear to have operated, then as now, as intermediate links between guests and prostitutes. 'The next places that are fild, after the Playhouses bee emptied, are (or ought to be) tauernes', Dekker observes in *The Guls Hornbooke* (1609), adding that 'if you loue the company of all the drawers, neuer sup without your Cockatrice: for, hauing her there, you shall be sure of most officious attendance' (Dekker, 1884–6, vol.2, pp.254, 258).

'In Taverns there's good wine, and excellent wenches', the Captain muses in Fletcher's *A Wife for a Moneth* (1624) (5,1:66), while Middleton's Father Hubburd asserts that 'luxurious plots are always begun in taverns, to be ended in vaulting-houses' (Middleton, 1885–6, vol.8, p.79). 'At thrifty mother Walker's', he continues his tale, 'we found a whole nest of pinching bachelors, crowded together upon forms and benches, in that most worshipful three-halfpenny ordinary, where presently they were boarded with hot monsieur Mutton-and-porridge (a Frenchman by his blowing)' (p.80). 'Drink hard Gentlemen', the Third Physician tells Thomas, Hylas and Sam in Fletcher's *Monsieur Thomas* (1619), 'And get unwholesome drabs: 'tis ten to one then We shall hear further from ye' (3,1:130).

Other contemporary authors emphasize the dangers of contracting venereal diseases in such establishments of consumption and entertainment. In his *Mirour for Magestrates of Cyties* (1584), George Whetstone (1544?–87) warns the young gentlemen of the Inns of Court against 'Dice, Wine and Lecherie' (Whetstone, 1584, sig.27ʳ) and also against the go-betweens that operate in taverns and inns:

Figure 24. The satirical woodcut from *The Roxburghe Ballads* (vol.1, p.159) illustrates a popular song called *The Industrious Smith* and shows a company of drunken gentlemen smoking, quarrelling and vomiting. The woodcut may serve as an illustration of Barnabe Rich's image of the 'common Drunkard, the very dregges of double Beere, and strong Ale: amongst men a Beast, and amongst Beasts a very Swyne' (Rich, 1616, p.34). The guests are being served by a waitress (left), who may also be the hostess of the inn or tavern. Not all such ladies were as virtuous as the beautiful hostess of 'The George Inn' in *Willobie His Avisa* (1594), whom several gentlemen

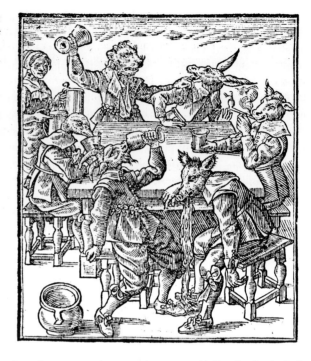

and noblemen in vain attempted to seduce – among them a young man named 'H.[enry] W.[riothesley]', third Earl of Southampton, whose encouraging friend appears to be yet another lecher, identified by the text with 'the old player' 'W.[illiam] S.[hakespeare]' (Willoby, 1966, pp.115–6).

In John Earle's *Microcosmographie* from 1633, the author tells us that a handsome hostess 'Is the fairer commendation of an Inne, above the faire Signe, or faire Lodgings: She is the Loadstone that attracts men of Iron, Gallants and Roarers...Her Lipps are your welcome, and your entertainement her company, which is put into the reckoning too, and is the dearest parcell in it: No Citizens wife is demurer than she at the first greeting, nor drawes in her mouth with a chaster simper, but you may be more familiar without distaste, and shee do's not startle at Bawdry' (Earle, 1633, sig. N2$^{\text{r-v}}$. '72.A handsome Hostesse').

For all the social differences between inns, taverns and alehouses, it appears that the three establishments had one feature in common. 'Drunkenness', complained Barnabe Rich in 1617, 'is now a continuall company-keeper in euery Tauerne, in euery Inne, and in euery Alehouse' (Rich, 1617, p.23). He added that 'there is no hope to keepe out whoredom, where drunkennesse her gentleman usher hath free and quiet passage to leade the way' (Rich, 1616, p.35). Then as now, alcohol and venereal diseases have been inseparable bedfellows.

'The man that is inticed to be a Dicer, of his owne accorde wil be a Horemaster: But (say you) if he haue no acquaintance, the banishment of the Stewes wyl kepe hym chast. But say as the Prouerbe is. *Monie will hyre a guide to go to the Deuile*; And (*certes*) as dailie gheasts at ordinarie Tabls, a man shal fynde neate Bawdes, that onely lyue vppon the brocage of loue, fellowes that wyl procure acquaintaunce for a dumbe man. These be no bashful *Besoigniers*, but such as glory in their facultie. Their common talke shal be Ribaldry, and matter of their profession. To conclude, he that hath aduantage, slily bloweth a meeting of faire women into my yong maisters eares: His company needeth not to be desired. Incontinent desire maketh him wood of their societie. Gods blood, lets goe, straight he cryeth, and with more haste, then good speede, they go to some blind brothel-house wher (peraduenture) for a Pottle or two of wyne, the imbracement of a paynted Harlot, and the French Pockes for a reckoning, the *Punie* payeth fortie shillings.' (Whetstone, 1584, sig.26ᵛ)

In similar fashion, Thomas Dekker warns young gentlemen against squandering their money and health in taverns and inns: 'The Ignorant prodigall drownes all the Acres of his Auncestors in the bottom of a wine-seller, or buries them al in the belly of a Harlot' (Dekker, 1884–5, vol.4, p.35). Not for nothing did Sir John Harington, the godson of Elizabeth I, call attention to

> 'The chiefest of all our sensual pleasures, I meane, that which some call the sweet sinne of letcherie, though God knowes, it hath much sowre sawce to it; for which notwithstanding, many hazard both their fame, their fortune, their friends, yea their soules; which makes them so oft breake the sixth commaundment.' (Harington, 1962, p.84)

CONCLUSION

The sources quoted in this chapter on the social, economic and demographic developments in England during the 16th century bear out the connection between poverty and prostitution. With about one third of the population in the cities living on, or just below, the poverty level, and a similar number barely above it, conditions were favourable for prostitution and for the concomitant dissemination of syphilis and other venereal diseases. The spread of these diseases was also furthered by the massive migration of impoverished villagers and townspeople during the period, and by the proliferation of alehouses, which became centres of alcoholism, prostitution, and venereal disease.

Peter Clark's statistics amplify the sinister implications of this retributive trio. Clark concludes that by the time of the government survey in the 1630s, there may have been one alehouse for every 100 inhabitants – a significantly higher ratio than in 1577. If William Clowes is also right in viewing 'lewd alehowses' as sources of syphilitic infection, one potential brothel for every 100 inhabitants represents an alarming figure. Of course not all alehouses were 'lewd' establishments, but sources show that alehouses, like the theatres, were favourite haunts of prostitutes. The explosion of the number of alehouses during this period may thus be viewed as furthering infection from syphilis on a grand scale, especially since these establishments were stopping places for a large transient part of the population. In addition, alehouses were centres for the consumption of alcohol, a primary effect of which is the temporary breaking down of moral resistance and a willingness to take chances which the individual would not take in a sober condition. We may assume that William Clowes had good reasons for denouncing 'the great number of lewd alehowses' as disseminating centres of syphilis. By 1606, yet another critic of England's social mores, Thomas Dekker, called drunkenness and lechery the 'two plagues that now run ouer all the Kingdome' (Dekker, 1884–6, vol.4, p.13).

# 5

# CHRONICLERS OF SYPHILIS AND PROSTITUTION

Throughout history prostitution has been most common in settings characterized by poverty, a high degree of transiency, and social disintegration (Holmes, 1990, p.31). All these factors converged in the capital of England, which during the 16th century became a centre of prostitution and a hatching station of venereal disease on a grand scale. During the reign of the Tudors, London was the fastest growing area in the world, and at the turn of the century it had become the world's greatest metropolis. From a city of perhaps 50–60,000 souls around 1500 it had become one of 120,000 in 1530, 200,000 in 1600 and 375,000 in 1650 (Beier and Finlay, 1986, p.48).

'She is the great Bee-hive of Christendom', the hack author Donald Lupton (d. 1676) stated in 1632 (p.1), when London had consolidated its lead in overseas and domestic trade and established itself as the economic centre of Western Europe. Half a century earlier John Lyly in *Euphues and his England* (1580) had presented the Elizabethan view of the English capital:

> '*London* [is] a place both for the beautie of buyldinge, infinite riches, varietie of all things, that excelleth all the Cities in the world: insomuch that it maye be called the Store-house and Marte of all *Europe.*' (Lyly, 1902, vol.2, p.191)

The Thames with its swans and multitude of vessels was the thoroughfare of London and the link that connected it with the farthest corners of the earth. The river, asserted Lupton, is 'the glory and wealth of the City, the high way to the Sea, the bringer in of wealth and Strangers' (Lupton, 1632, p.22). 'Sweet Thames! run softly till I end my song', Edmund Spenser (1552–99) had written in his *Prothalamion*, but his view contrasted sharply with a foreign ambassador's judgement that the city stank and was the filthiest in the world. 'Its Italian name, *Londra*', Orazio Busino commented, 'should be changed into *Lorda*, or filthy, which would be well merited by the black, offensive mud which is peculiar to its streets, and furnishes the mob with a formidable missile whenever anything occurs to call forth their disapprobation' (Harrison, 1878, p.52). Except for its two or three main thoroughfares, London was a network of narrow, badly paved lanes, half darkened by the overhanging fronts of the houses, and rendered extremely insanitary by the citizens' habit of depositing all their garbage in front of their doors.

While this method of garbage disposal furthered the spread of rats and bubonic plague, the overcrowding of the City and the sprawling slum quarters of its suburbs helped to spread contagious diseases of all kinds. As early as 1545, massive metropolitan growth provoked desperate complaints of a multitude of

> 'small chambers, cotages and lodgynges for sturdy beggers, harlottes, ydle and vnthryftye persones, whereby beggerye, vagabuncy, vnthryftynes, theefte, pokkes, pestylence, infeccions, diseases & infirmytyes do ensue & daylly growe to the defacynge of the beaultie of the said cit[y].' (Anderson, 1933, p.206)

Half a century later, John Manningham, a student of law, heard Sir William Periam (1534–1604) plead 'in the Chequer', that there were about 30,000 'idle persons and maisterles men' in the City, 'the very scumme of England, and the sinke of iniquitie' (Manningham, 1976, p.113). Precisely who composed the 'idle' and 'unthrifty' persons in the sources quoted above is a matter for debate: some were unemployed, some unemployable, while others belonged to the bottom of society such as rogues and vagabonds and their 'doxies'. The great majority of the 'maisterles' men were unskilled labourers engaged in all sorts of jobs, from work on the wharves and docks to porters carrying all kinds of goods and articles from place to place. The social group of 'maisterles', 'idle' and 'unthrifty' persons was one that lived at a subsistence level and hence was referred to the overcrowded slum quarters of suburban London. Here they were exposed to all kinds of infections such as tuberculosis, smallpox, syphilis and bubonic plague, and the authorities' way of preventing further infection was sensibly enough to effect slum-clearance.[*]

Such measures were explicitly undertaken in 1603 after one of the fiercest outbreaks of bubonic plague in London. A royal proclamation of September 16, 1603, called for demolition of the worst slum quarters of the capital after stating that

> 'the great confluence and accesse of excessive numbers of idle, indigent, dissolute and dangerous persons, and the pestering of many of them in small and strait roomes and habitations in the Citie of London, and in and about the Suburbes of the same, have bene one of the chiefest occasions of the great Plague and mortality.' (Larkin and Hughes, 1973–83, vol.1, p.47)

Many of these slum buildings may be taken to have harboured brothels, just as their clearance may be connected with the events of 1603–4, when the inhabitants of London encountered a mortal threat from the 'twin plague' of bubonic and syphilitic infection (see pp.217–9).

An echo of this dual epidemic and the governmental reaction to it may be perceived in Shakespeare's *Measure for Measure* (1604–5), in which a short scene alludes to the authorities' call for demolitions in the suburban slums of London – thinly disguised as those of the Austrian capital (cf. p.114).

'You have not heard of the proclamation, have you?', Pompey asks the bawd Mistress Overdone, who is ignorant of the news:

MIS. O. What proclamation, man?

POM. All houses [of ill fame] in the suburbs of Vienna must be plucked down.

MIS. O. And what shall become of those in the city?

---

[*] See the relevant proclamations in Larkin and Hughes 1964–9, vol.3, pp.245–8 and Larkin and Hughes, 1973 83, vol.1, pp.47–8.

POM.    They shall stand for seed: they had gone down too, but that a wise burgher put in for them.

MIS. O.    But shall all our houses of resort in the suburbs be pulled down?

POM.    To the ground, mistress.

MIS. O.    Why, here's a change indeed in the commonwealth! What shall become of me?

POM.    Come: fear not you: good counsellors lack no clients: though you change your place, you need not change your trade: I'll be your tapster still; courage, there will be pity taken on you; you that have worn your eyes almost out in the service, you will be considered. (1,2:85–103)

Efforts to control vagrancy, migration and overcrowding were as common and as futile as the regular battles to suppress begging, alehouses and prostitution. Hundreds of newcomers streamed into the capital each day, pouring in on carts and boats and, more commonly, on their feet: villagers from the countryside in search of work and a new life; vagrants and paupers from towns and countryside in hope of casual work or charity; vagabonds and rogues from everywhere in search of a livelihood or a criminal career.

Since London was both the dynamic centre of worldwide trade and finance and the governmental, legal and political centre of England, the capital also attracted immigrants of a higher social status and a better financial background: merchants and traders from England and abroad in search of business and profit; religious and political refugees from the Continent in hope of safer spheres of activity; courtiers and officials from manors and towns in pursuit of power and royal favour.

Bustling with energy and activity, London displayed a *joie de vivre* that was aptly represented by its pleasure-loving inhabitants, who, like Shakespeare's merchants of Venice, put on their 'boldest suit of mirth' (*M. of V.* 2,2:193) for an evening of merriment. It is a reflection of that outlook that earned London its checkered reputation as a hedonist's heaven and, not coincidentally, as the world capital of the sex trade. Evidence of this is provided by a number of sources, chief of which are the treatises of William Clowes and the pamphlets of Robert Greene, Thomas Nashe, Samuel Rowlands, and Thomas Dekker.

## WILLIAM CLOWES'S TEARS OVER ENGLAND AND LONDON

William Clowes can justly be called the first English venereologist. Born in Warwickshire in about 1540, he learned surgery as an apprentice of George Keble, a London surgeon and, in 1569, was admitted to the Barber-Surgeons' Company. He practised both as an army and naval surgeon and in 1575 was appointed one of the surgeons of St. Bartholomew's Hospital and later surgeon to Christ's Hospital. He was also surgeon to Queen Elizabeth and James I. From 1588 and until his death in 1604 he served on the court of the Barber-Surgeons' Company, at the same time as he established himself as the leading English writer on surgery.

His work in venereology resulted in the publication in 1579 of *A Short and Profitable Treatise Touching the Cure of the Disease Called Morbus Gallicus by Unctions*, which afterward ran to several editions. The book was influenced by Traheron's

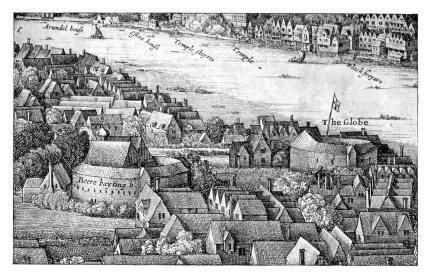

Figure 25. A prominent theme of modern venereology is the influence of dynamically changing demographic and sociocultural forces on the spread of sexually transmitted diseases. In this respect Tudor and Stuart London provides a classic example with its dynamic growth, international trade, rapid immigration, heterogeneous transient population, congested living-quarters, unhygienic conditions, appalling poverty, and freewheeling sexual habits.

The engraving (above) from Wenceslas Hollar's (1607–77) *Long View of London*, (1647, Antwerp), shows a section of one of Europe's biggest sea-ports, famous for its entertainments and forming part of the borough of Southwark, which, according to John Stow's *Survey of London* (1598), 'consisteth of diuers streetes, wayes, and winding lanes, all full of buildings, inhabited' (Stow, 1908, p.52). Here were most of the bull- and bearbaiting rings, most of the theatres, and a large number of brothels, alehouses and taverns in which Londoners, tourists and sailors from all over the world entertained themselves. Known as 'stews', the suburban brothels offered day-and-night visitors the pleasure of a female companion at the price of sixpence, the same as the most costly theatre ticket.

Most of London's prostitutes were fugitives from rural poverty and overpopulation, and with the population explosion of the 16th and 17th centuries supplies were never wanting for the 'flesh trade' of the booming city. London's prostitutes and their customers ran a considerable risk of contracting venereal disease, for, according to William Clowes, the hospitals of London were filled with 'an infinite multitude' of victims of 'the pocks'. The Gargantuan proportions of syphilis in Elizabethan London appears with Clowes's statement from his own practice at St. Bartholomew's 'that among every twentye diseased persons that are taken in, fiftene of them have the pocks'.

Alfred Fournier (1832–1914), one of the leading French authorities on syphilis, gathered together his collection of 50,000 case records built up over decades of practice and estimated that 15 per cent of Parisians were infected with syphilis in the latter half of the 19th century. This figure immediately drew fire from some quarters as being far too high, but Fournier was joined by others who produced similar figures. Henry-Camille-Chrysostôme Leloir said that 13 per cent of Parisians had syphilis. Alfred Blaschko estimated that 10 to 12 per cent of the adult population of Germany had syphilis; Albert Neisser believed it was closer to 15 per cent. In the United States, estimates ranged from 5 to 18 per cent. In Britain one estimate reckoned that between 10 and 20 per cent of the London population were infected with syphilis in the late 19th century (Butler, 1936, p.108. See also Cassel, 1987, p.17). In Tudor and Stuart London, the various demographic, residential, social, economic, and medical trends may well have merged to form a similar incidence, if not higher.

translation of Giovanni de Vigo's *Practica* (see pp.67–9) and by the Spanish physician Juan Almenar's treatise *Libellus de Morbo Gallico* (Venice, 1502). Clowes had translated the latter work and incorporated it into his own 1588 work on surgery, *A Prooved Practice for All Young Chirurgians*.

In the manner of his time, Clowes opened his book with a preface addressed 'To the right worshipfull the Maisters & Gouernors of the Barbars and Chirurgions with all the rest of that Societye in London' (Clowes, 1579, sig.Aii[r]). After this introduction of his treatise to his colleagues in London, Clowes went on to address his circle of lay readers, reminding them of the moral, political, medical and prophylactic aims of his work. At the same time, he gave a number of startling facts and figures of the prevalence of syphilis in Queen Elizabeth's England and Shakespeare's London:

> 'This I will say that the disease it selfe was neuer in mine opinion more ryfe among the *Indians, Neapolitans,* or in *Fraunce,* or *Spayne,* then it is at this day in the realme of *England*: I pray God quickly deliuer vs from it, and to remoue from vs that filthy sinne that breedeth it, that nurseth it, that disperseth it, and that (after the best kinde of cure vsed) by gods iust iudgment agayne reneweth it. It is wonderfull to consider how huge multitudes there be of such as be infected with it, and that dayly increase, to the great daunger of the common wealth, and the stayne of the whole nation: the cause whereof I see none so great as the licentious and beastly disorder of a great number of rogues and vagabondes: The filthye lyfe of many lewd and idell persons, both men and women, about the citye of *London,* and the great number of lewd alehowses, which are the very nests and harbourers of such filthy creatures: By meanes of which disordered persons some other of better disposition are many tymes infected, and many more lyke to be, except there be some speedy remedy prouided for the same. I may speake boldely, because I speake truely: and yet I speake it with very griefe of hart. In the Hospitall of Saint Bartholomew in London, there hath bene cured of this disease by me, and 3 other[s], within this fyue yeares, to the number of one thowsand and more. I speake nothing of Saint Thomas Hospital and other howses about this Citye, wherin an infinite multitude are dayly in cure. So that vndoubtedly vnlesse the Lord be mercyfull vnto vs, and that the magistrates doe with great seueritye seeke correction and punishment of that filthy vice, and except the people of this land doe speedily repent their most ungodly life and leaue this odious sinne, it cannot be but the whole land will shortly be poysoned with this most noysome sickenes.

> The worshipfull masters of the hospitall can witnes that I speake the truth: as also, I with my brethren can testifie with them, with what griefe of minde they are dayly enforced to take in a number of vyle creatures that otherwise would infect many, seeking with lyke care to restrayne this greeuous sinne. And yet the nomber still increaseth. For it hapneth in the howse of Saint Bartholomew very seldome but that among every twentye diseased persons that are taken in, fiftene of them have the pocks: and therefore how carefully it ought to be looked vnto let euery man judge, who hath care of his owne health, or of the safegard of his countrye.' (Clowes, 1579, sig.Bi[v]–ii[v])[*]

---

[*]   In a later edition of 1585, Clowes dropped his estimate slightly to conclude that over his full '9 or 10' years with the Hospital, 'amongst euery twentie so diseased…ten of them were infected with *Lues Venerea*' (fol.2). Clowes's figures may be compared with the incidence of syphilis among admissions to 19th century hospitals in Tunis (121 per 1000 over 20 years) and South America (485 out of 972 admissions in one year) (See Hirsch, 1885, vol.2, pp.79 and 83).

## 'MORBUS GALLICUS' BECOMING A 'MORBUS ANGLICUS'

William Clowes's data regarding the prevalence of syphilis in the England of Elizabeth I and Shakespeare's time are startling. It is true that Clowes was a physician and that his view from the hospital ward and consulting room may have prejudiced his assessment of the situation. Yet other contemporary witnesses seem to agree with Clowes although they were ordinary citizens of the same country. One of these witnesses was Robert Greene (1560?–92), whose keen observations of contemporary life were reflected in his plays, romances and numerous pamphlets. Famous among these were his so-called 'conny-catching' pamphlets in which he described the underworld of Elizabethan England. In *A Disputation between a Hee and a Shee Conny-Catcher* (1592), a London whore named Nan discusses with a petty thief named Lawrence which of them presents the greatest danger to the commonwealth. Describing the contents of his pamphlet, Greene says:

> 'In this Dialogue, louing Country-men shall you finde what preiudice ensues by haunting of whore-houses, what dangers grows by dallying with common harlottes, what inconuenience followes the inordinate pleasures of vnchast Libertines, (not onely by their consuming of their wealth, and impouerishment of their goods and landes, but to the great indangering of their health). For in conuersing with them, they aime not simply at the losse of goods, and blemish of their good names, but they fish for diseases, sicknesse, sores incurable, vlcers bursting out of the ioyntes, and sault rhumes, which by the humour of that villanie, lepte from *Naples* into *Fraunce* and from *Fraunce* into the bowels of *Englande*: which makes many crye out in their bones, whilest goodman Surgion laughs in his purse: a thing to be feared as deadly while men liue, as hell is to be dreaded after death, for it not only infecteth the bodie, consumeth the soule, and waste[th] wealth and worship, but ingraues a perpetuall shame in the forehead of the partie so abused.' (Greene, 1881–6, vol.10, pp.197–8)

From the symptoms enumerated and the geographical origin of the disease, it is clear that Greene is describing syphilis and its general spread among the population through prostitution. 'O Lawrence', says the whore Nan to her petty thief,

> 'enter into your owne thoughts, and thinke what the faire wordes of a wanton will do, what the smiles of a strumpet will driue a man to act, into what ieopardie a man will thrust himselfe for her that he loues, although for his sweete villanie, he be brought to loathsome leprosie: tush *Lawrence*, they say the Poxe came from *Naples*, some from *Spaine*, some from *France*, but whersoeuer it first grew, it is so surely now rooted in *England*, that by S (*Syth*) it may better be called *A Morbus Anglicus* then *Gallicus*, and I hope you will graunt, all these Frenche fauours grewe from whoores.' (p.232)

Greene's discussion between a thief and a whore as to 'whether of them are most pre-iuditiall to the Common-wealth' (p.197) is answered by Nan in an unambiguous way: 'Tush *Lawrence*, what enormities proceedes more in the Common-wealth then from whooredome?' (p.234).

Writing at the end of the same decade, Ben Jonson in *Every Man Out of His Humour* (1599) has this to say of the *morbus gallicus*:

PUNTARVOLO    What, the French poxe?

CARLO            The French poxe! Our poxe. S'bloud we haue 'hem in as good forme
BUFFONE        as they, man (4,3:77). (Jonson, 1925–52, vol.3, p.538)[*]

Reminiscing about his youth, the lecherous Sir Bounteous Progress in Middleton's
*A Mad World, My Masters* (1608) observes: 'Ay, ay, in those days that was a queasy
time; our age is better hardened now, and put oftener in the fire; we are tried what
we are. Tut, the pox is as natural now as an ague in the springtime; we seldom take
physic without it' (4,2:21–5).

A generation later, in 1642, the royal chaplain and popular author Thomas Fuller
(1608–61) observed that 'When hell invented new degrees in sinne, it was time for
heaven to invent new punishments'. One of these was the pox, whose relationship
to God and his countrymen Fuller formulated in this manner: 'Yet is this new disease
now grown so common and ordinary, as if they meant to put divine Justice to a
second task to find out a newer' (Fuller, 1938, vol.2, p.360).

Some years before, another clergyman and famous author, John Donne (1571–
1631), had asked himself the questions: 'Why dye none for love now? Because
woemen are become easyer? Or because these later times have provided mankind
of more new meanes for the destroying themselves and one another: Poxe[,]
Gunpowder, young marriages and Controversyes in Religion?' (Donne, 1980, p.26).

To all appearances, syphilis had spread to a considerable proportion of the
population during the 16th century, so that Dekker in 1605 was able to describe
the pox as a disease that was 'as catching as the plague, though not all so general'
(*Westward Hoe*, 4,1:83–4).

## CLOWES'S STRATEGIES FOR BEHAVIOURAL CHANGE IN THE POPULATION

Despite the importance of behavioural change in the prevention of most sexually
transmitted infections, efforts directed at behavioural change have, throughout
history, proved extremely difficult. Clowes's approach to the problem is interesting
in that his treatise begins with careful delineation of behaviours that need intervention and their respective target groups. In these opening paragraphs, Clowes reveals
a streak of Puritanism which shows in his attitude to syphilis as the 'foul disease'
and in his indignation at people of easy virtue. His focus of attack is emphatically
prostitution and its practitioners, referred to as the 'filthy creatures' of a 'great
number of lewd alehowses', or brothels. The second target group is the sexually
promiscuous and their habits, which he refers to as the 'ungodly life' and 'odious
sin' of 'the people of this land', their fornication threatening 'the whole land' with
poisoning.

In his epistle 'To the frendly Reader', Clowes is still more explicit in his
denunciation of prostitution and debauchery, 'wish[ing] all men generally, and those
which be infected especially to lothe, detest, hate, and abhorre that stinking sinne,
that is the originall cause of this infection, and to pray earnestly to God the heauenly
phisition for his gracious assistance, to the perfect amendement of lyfe, the most
safest, and surest way to remoue it' (1579, sig.Aiii[rv]ff).

---

[*]    See also vol.9, p.464n.

In line with the cultural milieu of his time, Clowes's attempts at formulating a policy for individual behavioural change are based in part on considerations of health, and in part on doctrines of theology. This attitude is an ever present undercurrent in the literature of the time and surfaces in the numerous sermons and homilies of the age, urging fear of personal ruin and eternal damnation as the prime reasons for positive health behaviour. 'Although the lips of an harlot are to the foolish a dropping honeycomb, and her neck softer than oil', the Protestant divine Thomas Becon (1512–67) told his parishioners during the reign of Elizabeth I,

> 'yet at the last is she as bitter as wormwood, and as sharp as a sword. Her feet go down unto death, and her steps haste them into hell: and he that accompanieth himself with an whore, shall go down unto hell, but he that goeth away from her shall be saved: yea, he that maintaineth an whore shall come unto beggary in this world, and after this life shall have his part in the lake that burneth with fire and brimstone.' (Becon, 1844b, p.58)

'Is not whoredom an enemy to the pleasant flower of youth', Becon asked in another of his attacks on promiscuity, 'and bringeth it not grey hairs and old age before the time? What gift of nature (although it were never so precious) is not corrupted with whoredom? Come not the French pox, with other divers diseases, of whoredom?' (Becon, 1844a, p.647).

Like other clergymen on their pulpits, Thomas Becon was particularly emphatic when addressing the youth of the parish. Speaking 'Of the Office and Duty of Young Men Unmarried', Becon stated that 'it is the duty of young men also to keep their bodies unpolluted, undefiled, unspotted, free and utterly estranged from all whoredom and uncleanness, that they may come with pure bodies unto the holy state of honourable wedlock' (p.367).*

Humanist authors such as John Lyly also joined in the campaign for effecting positive behavioural change, advancing not only God and health as arguments but also theories of longevity based on rational Galenic medicine. 'I haue heard wise Clearkes say', observes a beautiful woman in *Euphues and His England* (1580), 'that *Galen* being asked what dyet he vsed that he lyued so long, aunswered: I haue dronke no wine, I haue touched no woman, I haue kept my selfe warme' (1902, vol.2, p.55).

While endorsing moral behaviour as the best way to combat syphilitic infection, Clowes also suggests 'correction and punishment' 'with great severity' of those who make prostitution their trade, and thereby formulates a policy of intervention at the community level. In his epistle to the reader, Clowes is particularly emphatic on this point, 'wish[ing] all magistrates, as the second surgions appoynted by god, euen in the loue of righteousnes, & the Zeale of Gods glory, to haue a watchfull eye, to finde

---

* Such sermons formed part of the campaign waged unremittingly by the Church and parochial authorities against bastardy and to a lesser extent against pre-marital pregnancy. This campaign was carried out through the medium of the ecclesiastical courts which exercised vigilance over the morals of the rank and file of the parish. The courts were empowered to exercise jurisdiction over the entire range of behaviour that lay outside the actual limits of the civil and criminal law, and the object of their prosecutions, it was laid down, was that all who behaved 'wantonly, wickedly, or unchastlie, or unseemly are by the law cannons and constitutions customs and government of the Church of England to be censured and afterwards corrected and punished by the Ecclesiastical Judge to the end that others of them by their punishment and correction may be terrified and affrighted from committing the like offence and scandal and live godly righteous virtuous and chaste lives in all godliness and honesty' (Chambers, 1972, p.43). (See further pp.264–8)

out the offenders in this filthy sinne, and to execute vpon them such seuere punishment, as may terrifie the wicked wretches of the world, from that abhominable wickednes' (1579a)

Clowes also hints at the implementation of prophylactic measures to contain the spread of syphilis by isolating infected persons in hospitals – doctors 'seek[ing] with like care to restrain this grievous sin'. The last and most important aspect of Clowes's treatise is its medical one: the curative measures proposed by the author once the disease has been contracted. In his introductory epistle, Clowes informs the reader of his intention to 'set downe a profitable treatise with sufficient instruction, for the cure of the residew of the sicknes, in the which I haue had sum reasonable experience, and no small practise for many yeares' (1579a). As we have seen above, Clowes advises treatment by mercury while prescribing a variety of dietary and fasting cures (see pp.34–7). In the 1596 edition of his treatise, he widens his armamentarium to include a number of unctions and decoctions made of guaiac and various herbs, roots, berries and flowers.

In summing up the numerous aspects of William Clowes's *Short and Profitable Treatise* (1579), one should emphasize its desperate sense of urgency, its insistent, almost Puritanical, appeal to the individual and to society to take action against the

> '*Lues Venerea*, that is the pestilent infection of filthy lust…A sicknes very lothsome, odious, troublesome, and daungerous…which at this day not onely infecteth Naples, and Fraunce, from whence at the first it tooke his name, But increasing yet daylye, spreadeth it selfe throughout all England and ouerfloweth as I thinke the whole world.' (1579a)

Clowes takes his leave of the reader by admonishing him with these portentous words:

> 'Let me craue thy frendly acceptation of this my harty good will and faythfull zeale to my country, and countrymen, whome I see in these dayes exceedingly afflicted with this noysome and perilous sicknes, vnto whome, notwithstanding, I dare promise no helpe at all: No not by the best and most soueraygne medicens in the whole world except they be at defiance with sinne, and haue wholy bent themselues to walke in the obedience of Gods holy lawes.' (1579a)

## GEORGE WHETSTONE'S 'A MIRROR FOR MAGISTRATES'

Five years after the publication of Clowes's treatise, another citizen of London attempted to call attention to one of the major evils of the time. His name was George Whetstone (1544?–87), and his Bohemian way of life made him a good observer of the problems he wanted to describe. Whetstone was related to a wealthy family, and after an unsuccessful career at court he seems to have haunted gambling houses and brothels and dissipated his patrimony by reckless living. He charged others with having cheated him, and for three years plunged into ruinous litigation, after which he entered the army to fight in Holland against Spain and, finally, to sail with Humphrey Gilbert for the North-West Passage in 1578–9. With a certain success he also tried his hand as a hack-writer and dramatist, and in these fields devoted much energy to denunciation of the depravity of London.

In 1584 Whetstone held up a 'mirror' to its magistrates in the hope that they would see their own problems reflected in another sprawling metropolis of history. Whetstone called his treatise 'A mirour for magestrates of cyties. Representing the ordinances of…Alexander…Severus to suppresse and chastise the notorious vices noorished in Rome by the superfluous number of Dicing-houses, Tauarns, and common Stewes' (1584). To this section Whetstone added a final chapter entitled 'A Touchstone for the time contaynyng many…mischiefes, bred in London by the infection of some of thease sanctuaries of iniquitie'. Not to miss the targets of his campaign, Whetstone dedicated his work to the Mayor of London and his Aldermen and to 'the Gentlemen of the Innnes of Court' (see further p.152).

Like Clowes, Whetstone advocates behavioural change against the scourge of alcoholism and venereal disease, and his treatise is a serious call for moral re-arma-ment, accompanied by radical measures to stop 'this daungerous infection', as he terms the above evils (Whetstone, 1584, fol.3$^r$). Using Alexander Severus as his mouthpiece, Whetstone cites the first oration of the Roman emperor to his senators, according to which 'these daungerous infyrmities in a Commonwealth must be cured as the skilfull Surgion doth a festred sore'.

'Their causes must bee searched and their nourishing humors purged, and then amendment followeth', the good emperor sums up the problem, concluding that

> 'The cause of this inordinate lust, this excessive drunkennesse, this outragious prodigalitye, & to be short, this hel of iniquity among the Romanes, is euill education: of long time there hath bin no man ready to instruct them in vertues, nor willing to reprehend their vices, the nourishment of these euils are the Tauerns, Dicing places, and brothell houses, of whiche Rome hath great store, & and they greater store of guestes: so that to rid the publique weale of this daungerous infection, is fyrste and cheefelye to instruct the youth in good maners, and next to abate the number of these superfluous howses, or at the least, daylie to ouer-see their dooings.' (fol.3$^r$)

Whetstone proceeds to enumerate the 'Lawes, Pains, and Penalties, set downe by Alexander Severus, to punish Offenders against the Weale-publique' (fol.15$^r$), and records with satisfaction that the emperor closed down all taverns, dicing-houses and stews 'of evyll fame: saying: That, if the Owners could not liue, but vpon the vndoynge of others, it were reason, they should starue, by the necessytie of their idle bryngyng vp' (fol.15$^r$). The reformist emperor is presented as introducing even social sanctions to stop the wave of debauchery and dissipation, commanding 'that no Gentleman, *Romayne*, should resorte to any of these Houses, vppon paine, to lose the name of Gentleman' (fol.15$^r$).

In his prefatory Epistle to *A Mirour for Magestrates of Cyties*, Whetstone is quite explicit on the contemporary relevance of Alexander Severus's methods to stamp out vice and corruption. Deploring the growth of vice in London and the prolifera-tion of brothels, taverns and gambling houses, Whetstone declares that the laws are no more than 'written threatninges'; even proclamations have no force against 'brainsick iades' who need a sharper whip. There is need for 'visible Lightes in obscure Corners' (fol.A3$^v$) – informers who could discover the true state of affairs and report abuses to the authorities. Whetstone recapitulates the story of Alexander Severus's wanderings about Rome in disguise to investigate transgressions and mete out stern justice to offenders, drawing a specific parallel with the English scene by comparing Severus's two imperial Censors with Henry VII's agents Empson and Dudley.

In the 1580s, the example of Alexander Severus was eagerly seized on by English reformers demanding stricter measures against the wave of promiscuity and whoredom. The reforming campaign was conducted largely by Puritan extremists who used the opportunity to vent their ideas of an ideal government as opposed to that of the Elizabethan establishment. Writers such as Philip Stubbes and Thomas Lupton called for a theocratic commonwealth which would put an end to the laxity of a society in which fines or standing in a white sheet were considered sufficient punishment for whoredom (Stubbes, 1877–9, p.99). Strict measures, including the death penalty, were urged against prostitution, adultery, incest, and fornication, and if such drastic measures could not be adopted, branding was suggested as an alternative punishment, so that 'honest and chaste Christians might be discerned from the adulterous Children of Satan' (p.99) (see p.18).

George Whetstone's lesson from remote antiquity was later remembered by Sir Thomas Middleton when he became Lord Mayor of London in 1613. During that year he sent spies to find out lewd houses, and even visited some of them himself in disguise, just as he caught as many bawds as he could and had them carted, whipped and banished. He also made a list of all alehouses and victualling houses in the City for purposes of regulation, and finally set all beggars to work, which, he says, was worse than death to them.[*]

Whetstone's tale of the Disguised Ruler was later put to dramatic use by Shakespeare in *Measure for Measure* (1604–5), a play in which Vincentio, the Duke of Vienna, disguises himself as a friar called Ludovico in order to stage a final exposure of vice and whoredom in the Austrian capital – a transparent symbol of London:

> DUKE   My business in this state
> Made me a looker-on here in Vienna,
> Where I have seen corruption boil and bubble
> Till it o'errun the stew: laws for all faults,
> But faults so countenanced that the strong statutes
> Stand like the forfeits in a barber's shop,
> As much in mock as mark. (5,1:314–9)

## THOMAS NASHE'S TEARS OVER LONDON

William Clowes's, George Whetstone's and the Puritans' tears over England and its capital, and their concomitant despair at the impotence of the authorities to enforce the laws of the country were followed by another interesting lamentation in 1593 from the journalistic quarter. Its author was Thomas Nashe (1567?–1601), and the title of his strange report and jeremiad was *Christs Teares over Jerusalem* (1593).

Nashe had made his literary debut with *The Anatomie of Absurditie* (1589), an acrid review of recent literature, and for the rest of his short and turbulent life engaged in pamphleteering, playwriting, novel writing, and violent controversies

---

[*]   *Remembrancia* (1878), iii, 159. The letter is dated July 8, 1614. Quoted by Aydelotte, 1967, p.74.

with the Puritans, whom he hated. The London plague of 1593 brought Nashe face to face with death and seems to have sparked an existential crisis governed by the realization that 'This world uncertain is; Fond [foolish] are life's lustful joys; Death proves them all but toys; None from his darts can fly; I am sick, I must die. Lord, have mercy on us!' ('A Litany in Time of Plague').

On September 8, 1593, the author obtained a license for publishing his series of repentant reflections on the sins of himself and his London neighbours. *Christs Teares over Jerusalem* is a florid religious meditation in which Nashe warns his countrymen during one of the worst plagues to strike England that unless the populace reforms, London will suffer the fate of Jerusalem. '*London*, thou art the seeded Garden of sinne, the Sea that sucks in all the scummy chanels of the Realme' (1910, vol.2, p.158), Nashe opens his sermon of castigation, and proceeds to examine all the 'vices' of the Elizabethan metropolis such as pride, ambition, avarice, vainglory, atheism, discontent, contention, disdain, gorgeous attire, and delicacy. Nashe's fictitious visitor to London concludes his circular tour by studying the sex trade of the booming capital and the promiscuous habits of its pleasure-loving inhabitants:

'To my iourneys end I haste, & discend to the second continent of Delicacie, which is Lust or Luxury. In complayning of it, I am afrayd I shall defile good words, and too-long detayne my Readers. It is a sinne that nowe serueth in *London* in steade of an afternoones recreation. It is a trade that heeretofore thriued in hugger-mugger, but of late dayes walketh openly by day light, like a substantiall graue Merchant. Of hys name or profession hee is not ashamed: at the first beeing askt of it, he will confesse it. Into the hart of the Citty is vncleannesse crept. Great Patrons it hath gotte: almost none are punisht for it that haue a good purse. Euery queane vaunts herselfe of some or other man of Nobility.

*London*, what are thy Suburbes but licensed Stewes? Can it be so many brothel-houses of salary sensuality & sixepenny whoredome (the next doore to the Magistrates) should be sette vp and maintained, if brybes dyd not bestirre them? I accuse none, but certainly iustice somewhere is corrupted. Whole Hospitals of tenne times a day dishonested strumpets haue we cloystred together. Night and day the entrance vnto them is as free as to a Tauerne. Not one of them but hath a hundred retayners. Prentises and poore Seruaunts they encourage to robbe theyr Maisters. Gentlemens purses and pockets they will diue into and picke, euen whiles they are dallying with them.

No Smithfield ruffianly Swashbuckler will come of with such harshe hell-raking othes as they. Euery one of them is a Gentlewoman, and eyther the wife of two husbands, or a bedde-wedded Bride before shee was tenne yeeres old. The speech-shunning sores and sight-ircking botches of theyr vnsatiate intemperance, they will vnblushingly lay foorth and iestingly brag of, where euer they haunt.' (p.148)

In a later passage, Nashe returns to the syphilitic lesions of the infected prostitutes, whose early and tragic end he also describes in vivid terms: 'Ere they come to forty, you shall see them worne to the bare bone. At twenty their liuely colour is lost, theyr faces are sodden & perboyld with French surfets [syphilitic sores]' (pp.149–50). In the middle of his brimstone sermon, Nashe admonishes these women to leave their trade for both physical and moral reasons: 'Make not your bodies stincking dungeons for diseases to dwell in: imprison not your soules in a sinck' (p.154).

Nashe's indignation at the bodily and spiritual debasement of women through prostitution is matched by his shock at his fellow-citizens' promiscuous habits. 'I see reuelling, dauncing, and banquetting till midnight', he details his report, 'I see a number of wiues cockolding their husbandes, vnder pretence of going to their next neighbours labour' (p.151). Economic reflections merge with moral considerations in the manner of the Puritan preachers of the time and have Nashe grumbling at the illegal fortunes made by the city's traders in the flesh. 'Prouident Iustices, to whom these abuses redresse appertaineth', he admonishes the authorities,

> 'take a little paines to visite these houses of hospitality by night, and you shall see what Courtes of good fellowship they keepe. Hoyse vppe Baudes in the Subsidie booke, for the plentie they liue in is princelie. A great office is not so gainefull as the principalship of a Colledge of Curtizans. No Merchant in ritches may compare with those Merchants of maiden-head, if theyr female Inmates were not so fleeting & vncertaine.' (p.151)

In concluding his chapter on 'Lust & Luxury', Nashe lines up with Clowes, Whetstone and the Puritans in making an urgent appeal to the authorities to take severe measures against prostitution: 'I woulde those that shoulde reforme it woulde take but halfe the paynes in supplanting it that I haue done in disclosing it' (p.153). If the abolition of prostitution is too much to ask of the authorities, Nashe finds that the very least they could do is to introduce some kind of regulation of it. This proposal is obviously meant as a prophylactic measure, a way of containing crime, corruption and venereal disease, which Nashe describes so eloquently in his treatise: '*A thousande partes better were it to haue publique Stewes, then to let them keepe priuate Stewes as they doe*' (p.153, italics added).

## SAMUEL ROWLANDS'S TEARS OVER LONDON

Yet another testimony of the flourishing of prostitution in Elizabethan London is provided by a pamphlet published around the turn of the century by the author Samuel Rowlands (1570?–1630?). Between 1598 and 1628, Rowlands wrote a voluminous number of satirical tracts in prose and verse, but he also composed a number of fervently religious poems and two pious tracts entitled *A Sacred Memorie of the Miracles Wrought by...Jesus Christ* (1618) and *Heaven's Glory* (1628).

In *Greenes Ghost Haunting Conie-Catchers* (1602), Rowlands sets out to expose the social and moral evils of the metropolis in the manner of Robert Greene's coney-catching pamphlets. In 'The Epistle Dedicatorie' he promises the reader to reveal 'what grosse villanies are now practised in the bright Sunneshine' (Rowlands, 1880, vol.1, p.4), expressly including in his panorama of vices that of prostitution. 'In this Treatise (louing countrimen) you shall see what...inconuenience may come by following flattering strumpets' (p.4), he begins his satirical attack. He concludes this with an appeal to the authorities to establish strict surveillance and harsh punishment of the practitioners of prostitution in order to stop the venereal plague with its physical and moral corruption of the population:

'I know not, I, what should be the cause why so innumerable harlots and Curtizans abide about London, but because that good lawes are not looked vnto: is there not one appointed for the apprehending of such hell-moths, that eat a man out of bodie & soule? And yet there be more notorious strumpets & their mates about the Citie and the suburbs, then euer were before the [Provost] Marshall was appointed: idle mates I meane, that vnder the habit of a Gentleman or seruing man, think themselues free from the whip, although they can giue no honest account of their life. I could wish, and so it is to be wished of euery honest subiect, that *Amasis* lawe were receiued, who ordained that euerie man at the yeares end should giue an account to the Magistrate how hee liued, and he that did not so, or could not make an account of an honest life to be put to death as a fellon, without fauor or pardon: What then should become of a number of our vpstart gallants, that liue only by the sweate of other mens browes, and are the decay of the forwardest Gentlemen and best wits? Then should we haue fewer conicatching strumpets, who are the verie causes of all the plagues that happen to this flourishing common wealth. They are the destruction of so manie Gentlemen in England. By them many Lordships come to ruine.' (pp.4–5)

'Would it please the honorable and worshipfull of the land to take order for the cutting off of these cosoners, and consuming cankers of this common wealth', Samuel Rowlands concludes his indignant preface, 'they should not only cause a blessing to be powred on this flourishing state, but haue the prayers of euery good subiect for their prosperous healths and welfare' (p.5).

Another famous satirist of the time, Richard Brathwaite (1588?–1673), carried on Rowlands's line of thought by viewing prostitution as a subversive political force, whose 'pollutions' affected the state in almost all areas of life. 'A purple Strumpet', he asserted in *A Strappado for the Divell* (1615), is

> Gangrene to the state,
> Earths-curse, hels-blisse, soules-soile, & Angels hate,
> Smoothed Damnation, smothered infamie,
> Horror to Age, and youths calamity…
> It's you damn'd prostitutes that soyle this land,
> With all pollutions, haling downe the hand
> Of vengeance and subuersion on the State,
> Making her flowrie borders desolate.
> It's you that ruine ancient families,
> Occasion bloodshed, pillage, periuries.
> Its you that make the wicked prodigall,
> Strips him of fortune, heritance, and all,
> Its you that makes new Troy with factions bleede,
> As much or more then euer old Troy did.
> Its you (sin-branded wantons) brings decay,
> To publique states. (Brathwaite, 1887, pp.150–1)

## THOMAS DEKKER'S TEARS OVER LONDON

A final interesting observer of the manners and morals of Shakespeare's England is the London-born dramatist and pamphleteer Thomas Dekker (c. 1570–c. 1632). Famous as a playwright, Dekker is also the finest reporter of London life at the beginning of the 17th century. His pamphlets are the most vivid first-hand accounts written before Defoe, and they demonstrate a remarkable knowledge of the city in which Dekker's own existence was balanced between popular success and financial ruin. A reader of Dekker will be reminded of Chaucer and Dickens almost as often as of Greene and Nashe, and this is a tribute to his selective art which brings together urban realism, macabre imagination, ironic humour and moral indignation.

The journalist and the poet appear, in varying proportions, almost everywhere in Dekker's prose. He is the great chronicler of the London plagues in a series of pamphlets beginning with *The Wonderful Year* (1603), in which reports of the grimmest horror are interspersed with passages of the purest fantasy and descriptive beauty. Another series deals with the English underground of vagabonds, thieves and professional cheaters, the first pamphlets being *Newes from Hell* (1606) and *The Seven Deadly Sinnes of London* (1606), later followed by *The Bellman of London* (1608), *Lanthorne and Candlelight* (1608), and *The Gulls Hornebooke* (1609).

In *Lanthorne and Candlelight*, Dekker devotes 24 chapters to 'abuses and villainies' as they are practised in ordinaries, inns, marketplaces, and prisons. Dekker's report on these social cankers contains an interesting chapter entitled 'The Infection Of the Suburbes'. In this section, a visitor from hell makes a tour of the country and winds up in London and its suburbs, where he is delighted to find that prostitution and promiscuity are rampant. Syphilis is described by Dekker as a scourge rivalling the plague, a 'devouring monster' that destroys whole cities by ruining the health of its inhabitants. In spite of this threat to the public, however, the disease is 'laughed at' by the citizens, just as its agents of infection are condoned by the authorities.

Once more alehouses are described as disseminating centres of venereal infection, for Dekker's infernal visitor observes that in the suburbs there are 'More Ale-houses than there are Tauernes in all *Spayne & France*. Are they so dry in the *Suburbs*? Yes, pockily dry' (1884–6, vol.3, p.265). Dekker's eye witness of entertainments in suburban London presents this picture of flourishing and unimpeded prostitution:

> 'What saw he [the *Infernall Promoter*] besides? Hée saw the dores of notorious *Carted Bawdes*, (like Hell-gates) stand night and day wide open, with a paire of Harlots in Taffata gownes (like two painted posts) garnishing out those dores, beeing better to the house then a *Double signe:* when the dore of a poore Artificer (if his child had died but with one Token of death about him) was close ram'd vp and Guarded for feare others should haue beene infected [with the bubonic plague]: Yet the plague that a Whore-house layes vpon a Citty is worse, yet is laughed at: if not laughed at, yet not look'd into, or if look'd into, *Wincked* at.

> The Tradesman hauing his house lockd vp, looseth his customers, is put from worke and vndone: whilst in the meane time the strumpet is set on worke and maintain'd (perhaps) by those that vndoe the other: giue thankes O wide mouth'd Hell! laugh *Lucifer* at this, Dance for ioy all you Diuells.

> *Belzebub* kéepes the Register booke, of al the Bawdes, Panders & Curtizans: & hee knowes, that these Suburb sinners haue no landes to liue vpon but their legges: euery prentice passing by them, can say, *There sits a whore:* Without putting them to their booke they will sweare so much themselues: if so, are not Counstables, Churchwardens, Bayliffes, Beadels & other Officers, Pillars and Pillowes to all the villanies, that are by these committed? Are they not parcell-Bawdes to wink at such damned abuses, considering they haue whippes in their owne handes, and may draw

bloud if they please? Is not the Land-lord of such rentes the Graund-Bawde? & the Dore Kéeping mistresse of such a house of sinne, but his Vnder-Bawd? sithence hee takes twenty pounds rent euery yeare, for a vaulting schoole (which from no Artificer liuing by the hardnesse of the hand could bee worth fiue pound.) And that twenty pound rent, hée knowes must bée prest out of petticoates: his money smells of sin: the very siluer lookes pale, because it was earned by lust.

How happy therefore were Citties if they had no Suburbes, sithence they serue but as caues, where monsters are bred vp to deuowre the Citties themselues?' (pp.265–7)

Dekker's powerful and uncanny metaphor of syphilitic infection and destruction reappears in 1607 in Francis Beaumont's comedy and parody play *The Knight of the Burning Pestle* (Beaumont, 1967), in which syphilis emerges in the mythological shape of a giant monster devouring a number of citizens and storing them in its 'sable cave' (3:359). 'This monster, Barbaroso' (3:319), as the fiend is called, is actually a barber-surgeon in his 'cave', where diseased customers are subjected to a variety of syphilitic cures. Barbaroso is finally conquered by Rafe, the Grocer Errant, who frees a man and a woman and two errant knights from the monster's grip. 'This giant train'd me to his loathsome den', the 1. Knight informs Rafe, 'Under pretence of killing of the itch, And all my body with a powder strew'd, That smarts and stings, and cut away my beard And my curl'd locks…for this my foul disgrace' (3:374–8;382).

On his heels comes the 2. Knight 'whom this foul beast Hath scorch'd and scor'd in this inhuman wise', as the Dwarf of the play tells Rafe (3:389–90). 'I am a knight, Sir Pockhole is my name', the 2. Knight introduces himself,

'And by my birth I am a Londoner, Free by my copy; but my ancestors Were Frenchmen all; and riding hard this way Upon a trotting horse, my bones did ache; And I, faint knight, to ease my weary limbs, Light at this cave, when straight this furious fiend, With sharpest instrument of purest steel, Did cut the gristle of my nose away, And in the place this velvet plaster stands.' (3:393–402)

The third figure to be released from the monster's 'dreadful cave' (3:361) is a Man imprisoned 'in a tub that's heated smoking hot' (3:418). 'I am an errant knight that followed arms With spear and shield', he begins his story,

'and in my tender years I stricken was with Cupid's fiery shaft And fell in love with this my lady dear And stole her from her friends in Turnbull Street And bore her up and down from town to town, Where we did eat and drink and music hear, Till at the length, at this unhappy town We did arrive, and coming to this cave, This beast us caught and put us in a tub, Where we this two months sweat, and should have done Another month if you had not reliev'd us.' (3:434–45)

'This bread and water hath our diet been', the Woman amplifies, 'Together with a rib cut from a neck Of burned mutton. Hard hath been our fare. Release us from this ugly giant's snare' (3:446–9).

## DEKKER'S CALL FOR A REGULATION AND LICENSING OF VICE

'Cities soonest destroy themselues', ruminated Dekker in *The Dead Tearme* (1606), with reference to the 'sins' of adultery, fornication, and whoredom (Dekker, 1884–6, vol.4, p.53). 'Vices in a common-wealth are as diseases in a body', he warned his countrymen,

> 'if quickly they be not cured, they suddenly kill. They are Weedes in the fayrest Garden, if eare they take roote, you pull them not vp, they spoyle the wholesome Hearbes and Flowers, and turne the Ground into a Wildernesse. There is no destruction so fearefull to a Citty, as that destruction which a Citty brings vpon it selfe: and neuer is it more néere a fall, then when it maketh much of those sins, which like Snakes lie in the bosome of it, and sucke out the bloud.' (p.53)

Monstrous and poisonous imagery of syphilitic infection reappears in Dekker's final description of prostitution in his propaganda pamphlet, where the indignant author condemns the trading in human flesh, at the same time as he points out the devastating effects on public health of general promiscuity.

'The setting vp of a whore-house, is now as common as the setting vp of a Trade', he fumed in *The Dead Tearme*,

> 'yea, and it goes vnder that name. A stocke of two beds and foure wenches is able to put a Lady *Pandaresse* into present practise, and to bring them into reasonable doings. In these shoppes (of the world, the flesh, and the deuill) soules are set to sale, and bodies sent to shipwracke: men and women as familiarly goe into a chamber to damne one another on a Featherbedde, as into a Tauerne to bée merrie with wine. But for al this it goes vnder the name of *The sweet sin*, and of all, they are counted *Wenches of the old Religion*, and for all their dancings in Tauernes, ryots in Suppers, and ruffling in Taffities, yet A cloyster of such *Nunnes* standes like a *Spittle*, for euery house in it is more infectious then that which hath a *Redde Crosse* ouer the dore.[*]

> Such as *Smithfield* is to horses, such is a *House of these Sisters* to women: It is as fatal to them, It is as infamous. The Bawds, *Pettie* Bawds, and *Panders* are the Horse-coursers that bring Iades into the market: wher they swear they are frée from diseases, when they haue more hanging on their bones then are in a French Army…Since therfore so dangerous a Serpent shootes hisranckling stinges into both our bosomes, let vs [London and Westminster] not (as desperate of our owne estates) open our breasts to receiue them, and so be guilty to our own destruction, but rather prouide us of Armor to resist the malice of her poyson.' (Dekker, 1884–6, vol.4, pp.58–9)

The last paragraph of this passage makes it clear that Dekker is concerned about the serpent of syphilitic infection and its detrimental effects on the social and political structure of the country. In his campaign against whoredom and promiscuity, Dekker in an interesting way lines up with Nashe in his demand for a regulation of prostitution. Apparently his attitude is influenced by his observation of cheap prostitutes in the streets and his realization of the concomitant spread of venereal diseases on a grand scale. 'As Buls and Beares are for small pieces of Siluer to be bayted, so are these', he writes of the prostitutes of London.

> 'As at common *Outropes*, when housholds-stuffe is to bée sold, they cry *Who giues more*. So stand these vppon their thresholdes, not crying *Who giues more*, (only) but *Who giues any thing*. But that it stands not with the Maiesty of our state, nor with the Lawes of our *Religion*, It were as good, nay better, to giue fréedom and liberties to

---

[*] This was the sign of a plague-ridden house. All the doors and windows were kept closed, and a watchman stood by to ensure the strict confinement of the inhabitants. Elizabeth I ordered a gallows to be erected at Windsor for the execution of any person who concealed a case of plague (Forbes, 1971, p.123).

the setting vp of a common *Stewes*, as heretofore on the *Banck*…it hath béene vsed.'
(pp.55–6)

## HENRY II'S REGULATION OF THE STEWS OF SOUTHWARK IN 1161

Thomas Dekker at this point breaks off his sermon to indulge in a nostalgic
flashback to a time when regulation of prostitution was a way of containing the
spreading of veneareal disease. 'In those dayes Orders were established to keepe this
Sin within certaine boundes', he asserts, 'but now it breakes beyond all limits' (p.56).
In a two-column list, Dekker then proceeds to summarize a number of regulatory
measures introduced in 1161 by an act of Parliament in order to control prostitution
and its medical consequences.

*Thomas Dekker's Case for and against Prostitution Summarized in Two Columns:*

'It was then enacted by a parliament [in 1161]…that the *Bordello* or common *Stewes*
on the *Bancke-side*, should obserue these constitutions:

| | |
|---|---|
| *First*, no *Stew-holder*, or his wife was to compell any single Woman to stay with them against her will, but to giue her leaue to come and go at her pleasure. | Orders for the Stewes. |
| *Secondly* that no *Stew-holder* should kéepe any Woman to board, but shée to boord abroad, or where shée lysted. | Our suburb Bawdes keep Ordinaries for all commers. |
| *Thirdly*, to take for a *Courtezans*\* Chamber not aboue 14. pence by the wéeke. | \*The price of sin is raysed, & so are the rents. |
| *Fourthly*, not to kéepe open doores\* vpon Holy-dayes. | \**Noctes atque dies non.* [Days and nights not (closed)]. |
| *Fiftly*, not to kéepe any single woman in his house on the Holy-dayes, but the *Bailiffe* to sée them voyded out of the Lordship. | Officers now haue siluer eies and cannot see. |
| *Sixtly*, that no single woman should be detayned in any such house against her wil, hauing an intent to forsake that course of life. | Few Turnecoates in houses of this Religion. |
| *Seauenthly*, that no *Stewholder* was to giue entertainment to any Woman of any order in Religion, or to any man's wife. | As well Puritane as Protestant are welcome. |
| *Eyghtly*, that no Courtezan was to receiue hire of any man to lye with him, but she was to lye all night with him till the next morning. | Now they work like Bakers night and day. |
| *Ninthly*, that no man was to be drawne by violence, or be inticed by any impudent and whorish allurements into any Stew-house. | Now they vse plaine dealing. |

*Tenthly,* that euery *Brothely* or *Stew-house* was to bée searched wéekely by Constables and other Officers.

They are searched daily.

*Lastly,* that no Stew-holder should lodge in hys house any Woman that had the dangerous infirmity of burning, &c.

*Iamque vrit flamma medullus.* [Now the flame burns with a full blaze].

These (amongst others) with penalties and punishments vppon the breach of any one of them, were the ordinances of these times, but nowe (thankes to the negligence of this age) though sharper Lawes doe threaten to strike this sinne, yet they do but threaten, for they seldom strike, or if they strike, it is with the backe of the sworde of Iustice.' (pp.57–8)

## GONORRHEA IN MEDIEVAL ENGLAND

Dekker's source for knowledge of the parliamentary act of 1161 is John Stow's *A Survey of London* which had just been published (in 1598 and 1603) and which Dekker quotes fairly closely (Stow, 1908, vol.2, pp.54–5). John Stow in turn builds on a document from the reign of Henry II (1154–89) called 'Ordinaunces Touching the Gouerment of the Stewholders in Southwarke under the Direction of the Bishop of Winchester' (1161). The original document, which was presumably in Latin, has long been lost, but the later version of it contains 32 Latin rubrics and 52 paragraphs in English. For the first time in Europe, licensed brothels were here established under royal sanction with a prelate to manage them. In this way a steady revenue was guaranteed to both Church and State while venereal disease was brought under loose or tentative control.

The moral qualms about such an arrangement were not too severe among the clergy because of the ambivalent attitude of the Church towards prostitution. While fornication was condemned – especially among the clergy – no penalties were laid down for prostitutes in the Apostolical Canons since they were understood to fulfil a social function. As Thomas Aquinas (1227–74), the *Doctor angelicus* of the Medieval Church, wrote one hundred years later: 'Prostitution in the towns is like the cesspool in the palace: take away the cesspool and the palace will become an unclean and evil-smelling place' (Henriques, 1963, p.45).

The parliamentary act of 1161 forbade brothel-keepers to retain 'women with the hidden disease' (*mulieres habentes nephandam infirmitatem*) and stated 'that noo stueholder kepe noo woman withynne his hows that hath any sikenes of brennynge but that she be putte oute uppon the peyne of makyng a fyne unto the Lord of xxs [20 shillings]' (Burford, 1976, p.49). The 'sickness of burning' or 'dangerous infirmity of burning' alluded to in later variants of the Ordinance is most probably a reference to gonorrhea. The fiery metaphor would be an apt expression of the inflammation of the urethra in gonorrhea which causes severe pain on urinating – sometimes with blood in the urine – and a general feeling of malaise with headaches and a high temperature. 'Chaudepisse' was the name given by the French to the disease, a term which was taken over by the middle and upper classes in England, while the lower classes called it the 'brenning' or the 'burning'.

A later reference to gonorrhea in medieval sources is found in the writings of Richard II's (*regnebat* 1377–99) physician, John Arderne (*floruit* 1379), who believed that relief of the urethral burning would cure the disease, and accordingly invented a lead lotion to be injected up the urethra by syringe (Beckett, 1718, p.844). Another manuscript written about the year 1390 has a prescription for 'Brenning of the Pyntyl [penis], yat men clepe ye Apegalle' (p.845). A gall was a running sore, and 'ape' a diminutive of 'apron', a popular euphemism for the part the apron covered – hence the expressions, 'to lead apes in hell' for sexual seduction and 'tied to apron strings', for being dependent on sexual favours.

A mid-15th-century compendium of remedies for various ailments termed *Liber de diversis medicinis* prescribes the following 'For þe chawdpys: Take an vnce of benedicta [an electuary] & halfe an vnce of þe jewse of rose & menge to-gedir & vse þam thryse or iiij sythes in þe weke & ilk [each] a tym bot a sponefull at anes [once]' (Ogden, 1938, p.45).

'Clap' replaced 'chaudepisse' late in the 16th century, and the earliest written use of the term is in the second edition of *The Mirror for Magistrates* (1574), in which a moralizing poem reads:

> We nothing feare, the hurte of falling downe:
> Or litle rome, in lady Fortunes lap,
> We giue no hede, before we get the clap:
> And then to late, we wishe we had bene wise:
> When from the fall, we would and cannot rise.
>
> (Campbell, 1938–46, vol.2, p.118)

Although gonorrhea was familiar in England by the 15th century, syphilis seems to have arrived as a sudden shock in the 1490s. A reflection on the event is seen in a later copy of Henry II's regulation of the stews of Southwark, preserved in the Harleian MSS (Harley MS 1877). As metioned above, the original document of the parliamentary act of 1161 has long been lost, but three copies of it in English are known. That known as MS e Mus. 229 in the Bodleian Library at Oxford is the oldest and most complete, dating back to about 1463. (It is reproduced in full in Burford, 1976, pp.44–50.) The other two copies are the Harley MS 1877, dated about 1580, and the Harley MS 293, dated shortly after 1600. In the two later manuscripts, the preambles differ, and in one case the Latin rubrics are omitted. In other details, however, the later manuscripts closely follow the older text.

The Harley MS 1877 alone mentions a number of additions and amendments to the medieval regulations. The only major amendment concerns the 'perilous disease of the brennynge' mentioned in the 32nd paragraph of the original and likely to be a reference to gonorrhea. Sometime during the four centuries from 1161 to 1580 (the most probable time being about 1500) the penalty for keeping an infected woman had been increased from the original 20 shillings to the staggering sum of 100 shillings (Burford, 1976, p.50). This adjustment points to the presence of the syphilitic epidemic and to the desperation of the prophylactic measures taken by the authorities, which in 1506 went so far as to order the closing of the stews in Southwark. Another interesting feature is the fact that the 'dangerous infirmity of burning' mentioned by the Harleian manuscript would now seem to have been applied also to *syphilis*. As we shall demonstrate in a later chapter, 'burning' soon became a slang expression for syphilitic infection, at the same time as a strange development of medical history turned syphilis and gonorrhea into different manifestations of the same venereal disease (see pp.256–8).

## CONCLUSION

We have quoted various literary sources bearing on prostitution and the spread of syphilis in Elizabethan and Jacobean England. The picture rendered by Greene, Whetstone, Nashe, Rowlands and Dekker is that of a sprawling metropolis in which the authorities were struggling with a many-headed monster made up of prostitution, alcoholism and venereal disease and maintained by powerful economic interests, general promiscuity and public apathy. The present study has asked whether this picture is a correct one and whether it is possible to trust these pamphleteers as sources of social and medical information.

The above authors are, of course, primary sources in the sense that they were all contemporary with the events they attempted to describe and had, thereby, an intimate knowledge of life both in the English capital and in its rural surroundings. The problem is that their pamphlets represent a mixture of fact and fiction and that a satirical and moralistic, even Puritanical, attitude saturates many of them. The scholar is thus forced to allow for the satirist's exaggeration and the moralist's prejudice, just as he has to take into account the fictional element in what purports to be a journalistic report of stark reality.

These questions must be considered, then, in the light of what other writers and sources, whom we generally take to be more objective, have to say about prostitution and the spread of syphilis in Elizabethan and Jacobean England. In the following section, we shall also see how these sources compare with William Clowes's sinister picture of a contemporary scene governed by unimpeded prostitution, widespread promiscuity, rampant syphilis, and public indifference.

# 6

# PROSTITUTION IN ENGLAND

A Swiss physician, Thomas Platter, visiting London in 1599, made the following observations in his diary on life in the English capital:

> 'Since the city is very large, open, and populous, watch is kept every night in all the streets, so that misdemeanour shall be punished. Good order is also kept in the city in the matter of prostitution, for which special commissions are set up, and when they meet with a case, they punish the man with imprisonment and fine. The woman is taken to Bridewell, the King's palace, situated near the river, where the executioner scourges her naked before the populace. And although close watch is kept on them, great swarms of these women haunt the town in taverns and playhouses.' (Platter, 1937, pp.174–5)

Platter's picture of a capital attempting to curb prostitution but overwhelmed by the magnitude of the job may serve to modify Nashe's controversial description of the metropolitan suburbs as little better than 'licensed stewes' operating with the connivance of the magistrates. While this was doubtless an exaggeration, Rowlands came probably closer to the truth when asserting that 'the cause why so innumerable harlots and Curtizans abide about London' was not so much the absence of good laws but rather 'that good lawes are not looked vnto'. Rowlands's observation prompts speculation that the allegedly phenomenal increase in prostitution was not only a product of metropolitan expansion and the ceaseless drift of rootless migrants to London, but was also a product of the failure of Tudor and Stuart policy and administration to enforce the penal code against prostitutes, bawds, and other offenders.

## PROSTITUTION IN LONDON

The unequal struggle with the monster of prostitution may be illustrated by an enquiry organized by the Lord Mayor of London in 1633, which shows that prostitution had by then spread to all districts of the metropolis. The Lord Mayor instructed his Aldermen and their deputies in the City's 26 Wards to imprison all prostitutes arrested in taverns and alehouses and also to bring to punishment all occupiers and keepers of such houses. They were further ordered to exercise control that the bath establishments in different parts of the town were not visited by prostitutes, and see to it that the baths specially reserved for women were not frequented by young men or people of ill-fame. Owners of the above establishments who disobeyed these orders were liable to a £20 fine (Stow, 1633, pp.673–7).

A final interesting paragraph reveals one of the ways in which fresh supplies were procured for the insatiable flesh market of London. 'Ye shall also enquire', the Lord Mayor advised his Aldermen,

'if there bee dwelling within your Ward any Woman-broker, such as resort unto mens houses, demanding of their Maid-servants if they doe like of their services: if not, then they will tell them they will help them to a better service, and so allure them to come from their Masters to their houses, where they abide as Boorders untill they bee provided for. In which time it falleth out, that by lewd young men that resort to those houses, they be oftentimes made Harlots to their utter undoing, and the great hurt of the Common-wealth: wherefore if any such be, you shall present them, that order may be taken for reformation.' (p.681)

## AREAS OF PROSTITUTION IN STUART LONDON

While the most notorious of suburban red-light districts was the Bankside in Southwark, south of the Thames, others were found in the northern suburbs of London. In a speech to the House of Commons on July 9, 1625, the godly Devonshire MP Ignatius Jourdain informed an unsurprised house 'that divers places, viz. Clerkenwell, Pickehatch, Turnmill St., Golden Lane, Duke Humfrey's at Black-friars, are places of open bawdry' (*Commons Journals*, vol.1, p.807).[*]

Certain areas of London were notorious for prostitution in the age of James I. One of these was Saffron Hill, especially Charterhouse Lane, where a Quarter Sessional record of 1623 stated that

'notorious and common whores…are entertained into divers houses for base and filthy lucre sake akreweing to the private benefett of the Landlords and Tenauntes of such houses by the meanes of such women, Who doe usually sitt at the doores of the said houses, And by their wanton and impudent behaviour doe allure and shamefully call in unto them such as passe by that way, to the great corruption of youth.' (Jeaffreson, 1886–8, vol.2, p.171)

According to another Quarter Sessional record of 1627, the suburban areas of

'Cowcrosse…Tur[n]milstreete, Charterhouselaine, Saffronhill, Bloomesbury, Petty-coatelane, Wapping and Ratcliffe and divers other places within this county are pestered with many immodest, lascivious and shamelesse weomen generally reputed for notorious common and professed whoares, whoe are intertayned into victualing or other houses suspected for bawdry houses and other base tenement for base and filthy lucre and gaine to the landlords and tenauntes, whoe usually both in the day and night tyme sitt at the doores of such houses, exposing and offering themselves to passengers.' (vol.3, p.13)

The end of the ordinance issued through the Middlesex Court on the King's behalf requested all suspected bawds and harbourers to be presented before the court and proceeded against, and persistent offenders' places to be closed down. The ordinance also called on all the inhabitants of the above areas to

*    Quoted by K. Thomas in Pennington and Thomas, 1978, p.274.

'be overseers of all the said officers for the tyme being, and not only incite and stirr them up to be vigillant and careful in the due execucion and performance of this service, but alsoe from tyme to tyme as occasion shall serve bee ayding, assisting, counselling and directing to the said officers in the same to informe this Court or some of his Majesties Justices of peace of this county, of all or any disorder, abuse, neglecte, connivence or corrupcion, committed or suffered by the said officers or any others from tyme to tyme, as they tender his Majesties service, the good government of this country, and their owne good, tranquillity and peace.' (p.14)

These observations were an indication that the local arm of the law – 'the constables and headboroughs and other officers' mentioned by the document (p.13) – could be negligent, lenient or directly bribed, and that the citizens could help them to carry out their duties in a way that would ensure their 'own good, tranquility and peace'.

Further testimonies of prostitution are found in the Middlesex Quarter Sessional records between 1613 and 1616 which reveal that at least 11 brothels in Clerkenwell fell foul of the law during that period. In the nearby areas of Cow Hill and Saffron Hill the number of detected brothels is not so easily ascertainable, but may have been even greater. In Wapping, east of the Tower, a Thamesside district known for its numerous sailors and shipyard workers, at least three of the five brothels mentioned in the Quarter Sessional records of the period 1613–1616 were operated by sailors' wives during their husbands' absence at sea (Ashton, 1983, p.14).

Charterhouse Lane and Saffron Hill were not specifically mentioned by Ignatius Jourdain, but Turnmill Street emphatically was. Here was the most notorious street for brothels north of the Thames, a place whose inhabitants were characterized in the preamble to a royal order of 1623 as

'the many lewd and loose percons dwelling neere unto the skirts of the city of London within the County of Middl.[lesex] in Turnemill Street and other places, who keepe common and notorious brothell houses and harboure and entertaine divers impudent and infamous queanes &c.' (Jeaffreson, 1886–8, vol.2, p.177)

'When this Streete was builded', wrote Donald Lupton in 1632,

'surely *Mars* and *Venus* were in a Coniunction. Here are very few men, but they are well arm'd: Nay the Woemen haue receiued presse-money, & haue performed the Seruice: woemen though the colder vessels by Nature, yet these are the hotter by Art.' (Lupton, 1632, p.53)

The end of the order of 1623, issued through the Middlesex Court on the King's behalf, tightened up the bail requirement for persons accused of bawdry and whoredom to ensure that the sureties were substantial persons, 'two sufficient householders, whereof one of them be a subsidie man' (Jeaffreson, 1886–8, vol.2, p.177). Before that year there are many records of the Courts issuing writs against dozens of sureties to appear because the accused had skipped bail – and so had the sureties.

According to the poet Henry Vaughan (1622–95), the Strand and Fleet Street were also areas of flourishing prostitution in London. In a poem written in 1646 entitled *A Rhapsodie*, Vaughan gave a description of the moonlit and alluring capital along the banks of the Thames, visited by him and his friend in a state of alcoholic elation. 'Should we go now a wandring', he addressed his friends,

> we should meet
> With Catchpoles, whores, & Carts in ev'ry street:
> Now when each narrow lane, each nooke & Cave,
> Signe-posts, & shop-doors, pimp for ev'ry knave,
> When riotous sinfull plush, and tell-tale spurs
> Walk Fleet street, & the Strand, when the soft stirs
> Of bawdy, ruffled Silks, turne night to day;
> And the lowd whip, and Coach scolds all the way;
> When lust of all sorts, and each itchie bloud
> From the Tower-wharfe to Cymbelyne, and Lud,
> Hunts for a Mate, and the tyr'd footman reeles
> 'Twixt chaire-men, torches, & the hackny wheels:
> Come...Drink deep; this Cup be pregnant; & the wine,
> Spirit of wit...make us all divine. (Vaughan, 1957, p.11)

## LONDON'S LANDLORDS INVESTING IN PROSTITUTION

In 1587 a troubled citizen of London observed that its streets

> 'swarme with beggers, that no man can stande or staie in any churche or streate, but
> presently tenne or twelve beggers comme breathing in his face, many of them having
> theire plague sores and other contageous disseases running on them, wandring from
> man to man to seke relefe, which is very daungerous to all hir maiesties good subiects,
> and the very highe waie to infecte the whole kingdomme.' (Tawney and Power,
> 1924, vol.3, p.241)

The writer of these lines was a social critic named John Howes, who in a treatise entitled *A Famyliar And Frendly Discourse Dialogue Wyse Setting Foorthe a Number of Abuses Comytted in the Governemente of the Poore within This Cittie* (1587) attempted to analyze the causes of poverty and begging in the sprawling metropolis. One of the causes of such social evils, Howes pointed out, was 'the myserable covetousnes of the Landlords of Alleyes in London, whoe ar not only carelesse in receaving of Tenaunts into theire fylthie houses, but allso gredely exacting and raysing of greate rents vpon the poore, with other harde condicions, which ar not tollerable in a Christian common wealth' (p.427). The author instanced the slum lords' traffic of telling their tenants that 'You must fetche your bread, beeare, butter and cheese, wood and coale of vs' (p.427). By these means, the tenants were gradually turned into debtors and finally evicted after they had pawned their last clothes to pay the rents and bills. 'Bakers, Bruers, victuallers or allie maisters', Howes indignantly pointed out, 'ar the very Catter-pillers and supporters of all these myscheifes' (p.428).

Five years later another citizen of London launched a fierce attack on the landlords of his time and demonstrated that prostitution also formed part of their unscrupulous exploitation of their fellow-men. 'By their auarice Religion is slandered', the printer and playwright Henry Chettle (c. 1560–1607) wrote in his *Kind-Harts Dreame Conteigning Five Apparations with Their Invectives against Abuses Raigning* (1592),

> 'lewdnes is bolstered, the suburbs of the Citie are in many places no other but darke
> dennes for adulterers, theeues, murderers, and euery mischiefe worker: daily expe-
> rience before the Magistrates confirmes this for truth.' (Chettle, 1923, p.46)

'There is great abuse', Chettle went on,

> 'for in euery house where the venerian virgins are resident, hospitalitie is quite exiled, such fines, such taxes, such tribute, such customs, as (poore soules) after seuen yeares service in that vnhallowed order, they are faine to leaue their sutes for offerings to the olde Lenos [bawds] that are shrine-keepers, and themselues (when they begin to break) are faine to seeke harbour in an Hospitall: which chaunceth not (as sometime is thought) to one amongst twentie, but hardly one amongst a hundred haue better ending.' (pp.40–1)

In *Newes from Hell* (1606), Thomas Dekker observed that 'all the Scriueners ith' towne' were busy 'with drawing close conueyances betweene *Landlords* and Bawdes, that now sit no longer vpon the skirtes of the Cittie, but…giue more rent for a house, then the proudest *London* occupier of them all' (Dekker, 1884–6, vol.2, p.93). According to Robert Crowley, leasemongering, which piled rent upon rent on each piece of property, was particularly prevalent in London, where nine-tenths of all houses were sub-let down a chain of tenants, so that rents rose sky-high (Hurstfield, 1979, pp.32–3).

## LONDON'S MERCHANTS INVESTING IN PROSTITUTION

The great property development on the Bankside started in about 1570 and got into stride at the turn of the century, after which it turned into a gold rush between 1600 and 1660, when nearly every garden was overbuilt with rows of jerry-built tenements. Alehouses or brothels – usually both – proved the most profitable objects of investment, and also the London merchants were quick to recognize the golden opportunities offered by this area of consumption and entertainment. In Dekker's play *If This Be Not A Good Play* (1612), a London merchant named Barterville is reviewing his investments and earnings with a number of his servants when suddenly his clerk Bravo enters the office with a bag of money, and is asked by the first servant:

1. SER.   What payment's this?

BRAVO   The pension of the stews, you need not untie it, I brought it but now from the sealer's office: there's not a piece there, but has a hole in't, because men may know where t'was had, and where it will be taken again; bless your worship? Stew-money sir, stew-prune cash, sir.

BART.   They are sure, though not the soundest paymasters. Read what's the sum.

1. SER.   But bare two hundred crowns.

BRAVO   They are bare crowns indeed sir, and they came from animals and vermin that are more bare: we that are clerks of these flesh-markets have a great deal of rotten mutton lying upon our hands, and find this to be a sore payment.

BART.   Well, well, the world will mend.

BRAVO   So our surgeons tell 'em every day; but the pox of mendment I see.

BART.   Do not your gallants come off roundly then?

BRAVO   Yes sir, their hair comes off fast enough, we turn away crack'd French crowns every day. (2,2:54–71)

The ravages of syphilis are aptly described by Bravo's lines, in which the clerk's punning on the French coin and the bald patch caused by syphilis (alopecia) is accompanied by a slang reference to 'rotten mutton', or syphilitic whores. ('Stale mutten' is another expression used in *The Roaring Girl*,3,2:169–70, just as similar phrases are found in *If This Be Not A Good Play*,4,2:86; *1 The Honest Whore*,2,1:107; and *2 The Honest Whore*,2,1:255–6.)

### ENTERTAINMENT MOGULS INVESTING IN PROSTITUTION

In addition to the landlords and the merchants of London, there are indications that the entertainment moguls of the Bankside also invested in prostitution, realizing that brothel-owning was as profitable as the theatre. Philip Henslowe (d. 1616), the best-known impresario of the Elizabethan theatre, and his son-in-law Edward Alleyn (1566–1626), the most celebrated actor of the day, owned a number of brothels along the Bankside. So, too, did Francis Langley (1548–1602), the owner of the Swan Theatre.

Those brothels run by Alleyn appear to have been of a particularly superior type, as evidenced by the many pictures and other *objets d'art* which were catalogued before they were sent to embellish the manor Alleyn had bought in West Dulwich, Surrey in 1603.* Glorious as the end of Alleyn's career may seem, the beginning of it was marked by the dangers inherent in the prostitution trade. In 1593, Henslow's stepdaughter, Joan Woodward, received a letter from her newly-wed husband, Edward Alleyn, who on May 2, 1593, wrote to 'E. Alline on the Bankside': 'Mouse, I littell thought to hear that which I now hear by you, for it is well knowne they say that you wear, by my lorde maior's officer, mad[e] to rid[e] in a cart, you and all your felowes' (Rendle, 1877, p.ix). At the time of writing, whipping, carting and the cucking-stool were the punishment for women who engaged in prostitution.

When Alleyn's wife died in 1623, her property went into the marriage settlement of his second wife, the young Constance Donne, daughter of John Donne, the Dean of St. Pauls's. In Alleyn's will of 1625, he left his second wife The Unicorn Inn in Southwark and The Barge, The Bell, and The Cocke on the Bankside, all well-known brothels of the time (see, p.61) (Bald, 1970, pp.485–6). When Constance died, the revenues from The Bell, The Barge, and The Cocke went to charities according to her will (Rendle, 1877, p.xii; see also Hosking, 1952, pp.227 and 236).

Francis Langley, perhaps the most unscrupulous entrepreneur of the time, moved in on the Bankside, in 1589, when he bought the old manor of Paris Garden. According to Donald Lupton, this area 'may better bee tearmed a foule Denne than a Fayre Garden. Its pittie so good a piece of grounde is not better imploited...Money which was got basely (is here) spent lewdly. The swaggering Roarer, the cunning Cheater, the rotten Bawd, the swearing Drunkard, and the bloudy Butcher haue their Rendeuouz here' (Lupton, 1632, p.67). In 1594, Langley borrowed £1,650 on the security of his various properties to build tenements for rent and the Swan playhouse on his new estate. Langley's activities on the Bankside may safely be

---

*     See George Warner: *Catalogue of MSS & Muniments at Dulwich College*, 1891. See further Burford, 1973, pp.185–6; Burford, 1973, pp.41, 55 and 100; Burford, 1976, p.154.

assumed to have covered both entertainment and prostitution, for throughout his career he was involved in a number of very shady deals, and contemporary sources show him constantly at odds with authority (Ingram, 1978, *passim*).

By 1630 we have evidence that the manor of Paris Garden was functioning as a brothel (see below), but by that time Langley had long ago been forced to sell his estate. The Paris Manor passed out of Langley's hands in 1601 and did not regain prominence until 1632 when the manor house was probably the site of the brothel called 'Hollands' Leaguer'.

## 'HOLLAND'S LEAGUER': A HIGH-CLASS BROTHEL OF STUART LONDON

Thomas Dekker's indignant queston, 'Is not the landlord of such rents the ground-bawd?' is a gibe at the merchants of prostitution, who had representatives even at Court and in the Church. In 1161, when Henry II promulgated his 'Ordinance touching upon the government of the stews in Southwark', a large part of the suburb had been under the control of the Bishop of Winchester for over half a century, and the house rents from the brothels in that area formed a valuable part of episcopal income.

The Reformation party viewed these 'stews' as yet another abomination of popery, and to inflict a severe blow upon the clergy Henry VIII confiscated the property of the Church, which made an end of its profits from prostitution and brothels (1536). However, the many rich and powerful landlords and property speculators who bought the confiscated Church lands continued the old business of prostitution under the guise of 'private enterprise'. In 1578 Elizabeth I, at the request of Henry Carey, the first Lord Hunsdon, granted the lordship and manor of London's Paris Gardens to Robert Newdigate and Arthur Fountaigne, who in turn demised the manor house to Lord Hunsdon. Between 1580 and 1601, the legal maneuverings between Lord Hunsdon, Newdigate, Fountaigne, and Francis Langley are confusing, but apparently they were worthwile, for at one time £6000 was paid for the lease (Barnard Jr., 1970, p.41).

Incidentally, the old manor house of Paris Gardens is the only brothel of the period for which posterity has been provided with a historical record. The brothel in question was a high-class establishment founded at the beginning of the 17th century and later remembered under the posthumous title of 'Hollands Leaguer' (Figure 26). The primary sources from which we know of its history are Laurence Price's ballad *Newes from Hollands Leager* (1632), Shackerley Marmion's play *Hollands Leaguer* (1632), and Nicholas Goodman's pamphlet *Hollands Leaguer: or, An Historical Discourse of the Life and Actions of Dona Britanica the Arch-Mistris of the wicked women of Eutopia. Wherein is detected the notorious Sinne of Panderism, and the Execrable Life of the luxurious Impudent* (1632).[*] All of the works appeared in the year 1632, and they describe a siege undertaken by London officers of the law against a certain Elizabeth Holland and her bordello in a fortified mansion on the Bankside.

Goodman's story of 'Dona Britanica' is in part a parable of the history of the English Church during the first years of the reign of Charles I (*regnebat* 1625–49),

---

[*] All three sources are printed in *Hollands Leaguer by Nicholas Goodman*, a critical edition by Dean Stanton Barnard Jr. The Hague-Paris, 1970.

in which it is described as being first seduced by Catholicism and then sullied by Puritanism. Goodman's theological allegory, however, is also a transparent tale of 'the luxurious Impudent' and of 'the Arch-Mistris' of prostitution, Dona Britanica, or Elizabeth Holland. According to the story told by Goodman's pamphlet, the woman's first attempt in the trade had been in '*an old ruined Castell newly repaired*' (Barnard Jr., 1970, p.67) and situated in the City. 'Of this house by contract, she got possession', Goodman goes on,

> 'and her purse being well filled, and wide open, emptied itselfe to giue it adornment, there wanted nothing for *State*, nothing for *Magnificence*, nothing for *Delight*, nothing for *Beauty*, nothing for *Necessity*, howsoeuer the bones that lodg'd in it were rotten and vnwholesome, yet the *Monument* itselfe was wondrous *Gaudie*, and hansome; there was nothing now for her to search for, but *liuing furniture*.' (pp.67–8)

This Dona Britanica successfully 'brought vp by whole sale from the Countrey' (p.68), and soon her high-class brothel became a flourishing business: 'Her visitants came flocking so fast for entertainment, that her *Kitchin* was like *Aetna*, euer flaming…and her *inward* and priuate *Lodgings*, like *Hell* itselfe, where wicked creatures lay bathing themselues in *Lust*' (p.68).

Goodman further records that Dona Britanica's enterprise came to a sudden end because of the indignation of the City's puritanical fathers. 'And now the noyse of these offences haue awakened Authority and that ioyning with piety, both send forth their Ministers to apprehend her', the pamphlet relates, while her imprisonment is described as being in 'A place like Bridewell' or 'A place like New-gate' (p.69).[*]

Her imprisonment, however, proved a short interlude in Britanica's spectacular career, for by virtue of her wealth and powerful connections she managed to bribe her way to escape and soon set up business in a more grand and sanitary manner than before. 'Out of the *Citie*, only divided by a delicate *Riuer*', Goodman continues his tale, 'there was many handsome buildings, and many hearty neighbours…Like the Banck-side' (Barnard Jr., 1970, p.75). In this area, Dona Britanica finally found 'a *Fort, Citadell*, or *Mansion House*' environed with '*Bulwarkes, Riuers, Ditches, Trenches*, and *Outworkes*, which hem'd in the *Orchard, Gardens, Base-courts*, and *Inferiour Offices*' (pp.75–6) (Figure 26).

Dona Britanica had learned from experience 'That to sinne wisely, was to sinne safely' (p.61), and therefore her new high-class brothel saw a number of innovations. In Shackerley Marmion's play, the Bawd of 'Hollands Leaguer' says that 'I have So much ado to keep my family sound, You would wonder at it' (p.105). In Goodman's

---

[*]    This is one of a number of contemporary suggestions that the traders in the flesh, no longer content to operate in the suburbs, had become emboldened to establish themselves in the City itself. In *Newes from Hell* (1606), Dekker mentions the 'Bawdes, that now sit no longer vpon the skirtes of the Cittie, but iett vp and downe, euen in the cloake of the Cittie, and giue more rent for a house, then the proudest *London* occupier of them all' (Dekker, 1884–6, vol.2, p.93). In *Lanthorne and Candlelight* (1608), Dekker points out that the suburban prostitute who takes to operating in the City has radically to alter her habits. 'If before she ruffled in silkes', he asserts, 'now is she more ciuilly attird then a Mid-wife. If before she swaggred in Tauernes, now with the Snaile she stirreth not out of dores. And where must her lodging be taken vp, but in the house of some cittizen…As for example *she* wil lie in some *Scriueners house*, & so vnder the collour of comming to haue a *Bond* made, she herselfe may write *Nouerint uniuersi*' (Dekker, 1884–6, vol.3, p.268. *Cf. Westward Hoe*, 5, 4: 251–66).

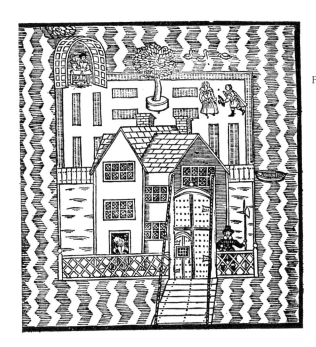

*Sleeping in my orchard, A serpent stung me* (*Ham.* 1,5:35–6).

Figure 26. The woodcut from Nicholas Goodman's pamphlet *Hollands Leaguer* 1632 (Barnard Jr., 1970, p.52) shows the moat of the stately house and the guard at the drawbridge with the peephole where customers could be scrutinized before admittance. Amorous dalliance is taking place in the shady arbour at the back of the garden, while a gentleman greets his chosen girl in the garden and another customer with beplumed hat fondles one of the women in the front room.

pamphlet a passage alludes to the same endeavour by the bawd of the same house: 'As shee hath plenty of meanes, so she will have plenty of attendants, and hereupon presently shee contracts and hyres sundry retayners; as first, a *Surgeon* that tooke care of her *Spittle*, then a *Tyre-woman* of Phantasticall Ornaments, a *Sempster* for Ruffes, Cuffes, Smocks, and wastcoates, and a *Taylor* for cloathes, of all shapes, and all fashions…She had [also] three household Officers, a *Cooke*-wench, a *Laundry-lasse*, and a Girle Scullian' (pp.77–9).

The high-class brothel run by Dona Britanica functioned until 1631–2 when the rising tide of Puritanism made the authorities clamp down on the establishment in a raid which was fiercely resisted by the owner and her inhabitants. The beleaguering of the stately brothel-fortress gave it immortality as 'Hollands Leaguer', and, as we have seen, the event was commemorated in a ballad, a pamphlet, and a play.

## THE 'DRABS' VENOM-KISS', 'THE STRUMPET'S PLAGUE' (OTHELLO 4,1:96)

By the time Clowes wrote his treatise on *morbus gallicus* and Nashe, Rowlands and Dekker published their plays, poems, and pamphlets, even the most uninformed of Englishmen were aware of prostitution as the source of the spread of syphilis among the population. 'Whores and whoremongers [are] trading for the Pox', Rowlands stated in *The Night Raven* (1629) (Rowlands, 1880, vol.2, p.3), while Dekker in *1 The Honest Whore* presented 'The lecher's French disease' side by side with 'the harlot's poison' (3,2:41–2). 'A pox poison em!' curses Sir Bounteous Progress in

Middleton's *A Mad World, My Masters* (1605–6) (2,7:129), while Nathan Richards in his epigraph to the same author's play *Women Beware Women* (1657) speaks of the 'drabs'...venom-kiss' (Middleton, 1885–6, vol.6, p.235).

Writing in a similar vein, John Earle in his *Microcosmographie* (1633) says of libertines and lascivious persons that 'They are men not easily reformed', adding that 'The pox onely converts them, and that onely when it kills them' (Earle, 1633, '37.A Lascivious Man').

The poison metaphors quoted above reveal the fear surrounding syphilis and the general awareness of its dangers to health. 'Eschew vile *Venus* toyes', *The Mirror for Magistrates* warned in 1574, 'she cuttes of[f] age, And learne this lesson of (and teach) thy frende: By pocks, death sodaine, begging, harlots ende' (Campbell, 1938–46, vol.2, p.128). A similar warning, with a typical misogynist twist, was given by the poet John Lane (*floruit* 1620) in his lamentation *Tom-Tel-Troths Message, and His Pens Complaint*, which was published in 1600. Attempting a description of the allegorical figure of 'lewde Lecherie', he stated that

> Her loue is lust, her lust is sugred sower,
> Her paine is long, her pleasure but a flower...
> Thousands of whores maintained by their wooers,
> Entice by land, as Syrens doe by Seas,
> Which, being like pathwaies or open doores,
> Infect mens bodies with the French disease:
> Thus women, woe of men, though wooed by men,
> Still adde new matter to my plaintife pen.
>
> (Lane, 1876, lines 644, 647–8, 655–60)

The most 'plaintive pen' of the period undoubtedly belongs to Thomas Dekker, who never wearies of denouncing promiscuity and exposing prostitution as one of the major social evils of his time. In *1 The Honest Whore*, Dekker's Count Hippolito delivers a long diatribe on the prostitute which has the effect of converting Bellafront from her wicked trade – the conversion of a whore being an Elizabethan common-place in drama and in prose pamphlets.[*]

In the course of his tirade, Hippolito presents his own (and Dekker's) hatred for the whore:

---

[*] In his *A Disputation between a Hee Connycatcher and a Shee Conny-catcher* (1592), Robert Greene devotes the final section to 'The Conversion of an English Courtezan'. This is a first-person narrative about a girl turned wanton because, as in the morality plays, her parents 'spared the rod and spoilt the child'. The chapter describes the girl's whorish affairs and her final conversion at the hands of an honest clothier who reminds her that God is forever watching this world and that whores are eternally damned. She is affected by his talk, gives up whoredom, marries the clothier, and lives happily ever after (Greene, 1881–6, vol.10, pp.256–76). The classic tear-jerker is Thomas Cranley's (*floruit* 1635) *Amanda, or the Reformed Whore* (1635), in which a gentleman in the Fleet Prison spots a woman below whom he recognizes as a prostitute. He sends her a letter to which she replies, and afterwards she gets another letter that finally converts her. One of the gentleman's most forceful arguments to dissuade the woman from her wicked trade is the high risk she runs of contracting syphilis: 'There's a disease that is the plague of whores, Which rooteth in the marrow and the bones; Within thee and without thee full of sores; That, that I say will take thee all at once, And make thee to reduplicate thy grones: That Morbus Gallicus will fill thy veines, And gnaw into thy bowels and thy reines' (Cranley, 1635, p.66).

> You have no soul, that makes you weigh so light;
> Heaven's treasure bought it:
> And half-a-crown hath sold it; for your body
> Is like the common shore, that still receives
> All the town's filth. The sin of many men
> Is within you; and thus much I suppose,
> That if all your committers stood in rank,
> They'd make a lane in which your shame might dwell
> And with their spaces reach from hence to hell. (I,2,1:324–30)

For Dekker, the question which Robert Greene's thief and whore discuss with almost amiable irony is dark and depressing and can admit of only one answer: the whore is a much greater danger to the commonwealth than the thief, for

> there has been known
> As many by one harlot maimed and dismembered
> As would ha' stuffed an hospital...
> A harlot is like Dunkirk, true to none,
> Swallows both English, Spanish, fulsome Dutch,
> Black-beard Italian, last of all the French,
> And he sticks to you, faith, gives you your diet,
> Brings you acquainted, first with Monsieur Doctor
> And then you know what follows.

BELLAFRONT     Misery.
                 Rank, stinking, and most loathsome misery.

HIPPOLITO     Methinks a toad is happier than a whore;
                 That with one poison swells, with thousands more
                 The other stocks her veins: harlot? fie, fie! (I,2,1:331–3;354–62)

'Her veynes', echoes Francis Lenton in his description of 'A Prostitute or Common Whore', 'are fill'd with seuerall sorts of poysons, which swell till they burst out into some loathsome excrement; and then, all that know her, hate her; and all that lusted after her, now loath her' (Lenton, 1631, '24. A Prostitute or Common Whore').

An abundance of contemporary primary sources leaves no doubt that it was the 'poison' of syphilitic infection that induced both medical and lay writers to take the glamour out of prostitution and wenching. The superstructure of theology was never wanting in these efforts directed at behavioural change, but the medical aspect of the moralist's numerous warnings was never missing. This may be demonstrated with particular clarity in Barnabe Rich's denunciation of harlots and whoremongers in *My Ladies Looking-Glasse* from 1616, in which he asserted that

> 'As the *harlot* destroieth his soule that doth frequent her, so she is a plague to the flesh, more infectious to the body then the common pestilence, and carries more diseases about her, then is in an *hospitall*. And as the knowne *whoremonger*, is but of a rotten reputation, so he is most commonly as full of loathsome diseases; or let it be that *God* sometimes doth suffer *whoremongers* to liue, till they may stroke there gray and hoarie haires, yet they neuer escape the filthy diseases of botches, byles, aches, inflammation, & of that loathed disease of the french poxe, a little gilded ouer by the name of the gowt, or sometimes of the sciatica: & besides a corporall stroke

of *heauens* hand in this life, the *whoremonger* shal feele the fearefull addition of an eternal woe in the *fire* of *hell.*' (Rich, 1616, p.36)

Even in John Taylor's humorous poem *A Whore* from 1630, the author's listing of the various slang expressions for a prostitute contains a concluding couplet in which the jester-poet turns moralist by pointing out the dismal end of the syphilized strumpet. 'As *Whores* are of a seuerall cut', he informs the reader,

> So fitting Titles on them still are put:
> For if a Princes loue to her decline,
> For manners sake shee's call'd a *Concubine:*
> If a great Lord, or Knight, affect a *Whore,*
> Shee must be term'd his Honours *Paramore:*
> The rich Gull Gallant call's her *Deere* and *Loue,*
> *Ducke, Lambe, Squall, Sweet-heart, Cony,* and his *Doue.*
> A pretty *wench* she's with the Country-man,
> And a *Kind Sister* with the Puritane,
> She's a Priests *Lemman,* and a Tinkers *Pad,*
> Or *Dell,* or *Doxy* (though the names bee bad)
> And amongst Souldiers, this sweet piece of Vice
> Is counted for a Captaines *Cockatrice.*
> But the mad Rascall, when hee's fiue parts drunke,
> Cals her his *Drab,* his Queane, his *Iill,* or *Punke,*
> And in his fury 'gins to rayle and rore,
> Then with full mouth, he truely call's her *Whore:*
> And so I leaue her, to her hot desires,
> 'Mongst *Pimps,* and *Panders,* and base *Applesquires,*
> To mend or end, when age or Pox will make her
> Detested, and *Whore-masters* all forsake her.
>
> (Taylor, 1636, p.112, 'A Whore')

## The Hot Whore

In his pamphlet *Kind-Harts Dreame* (1592), Henry Chettle expressed an unusual note of compassion for the women who were forced to seek their livelihood by engaging in prostitution. 'Seuen yeares service' was enough to 'break' them, according to Chettle, while Nashe asserted that 'At twenty their liuely colour is lost, theyr faces are sodden & perboyld with French surfets', adding that 'Ere they come to forty, you shall see them worne to the bare bone'. 'The harlot is like a new play, that being thrice presented on the stage, begins to grow staale', Barnabe Rich cynically remarked in *My Ladies Looking-Glasse* (1616), adding that 'the harlot that is once past thirty fiue yeares, is fitter to furnish an Hospitall, then to garnish a bed chamber' (Rich, 1616, p.36).

Venereal diseases and tuberculosis, alcoholism and dissipation were the lot of these women who commanded little mercy or compassion from such writers as Clowes, Nashe, Rowlands and Dekker. Even if they knew of the terrible poverty of the time and also raised their voice against it, they shared the general contempt for the prostitute and her trade, which was condemned on medical, social, moral and religious grounds.

'A Whore is a hie way to the Divell', wrote Sir Thomas Overbury (1581–1613) in his *Characters* (1614). 'The money that she gets is like a Traitors, given only to corrupt her, and what she gets, serves but to pay diseases. Shees ever moor'd in sinne, and ever mending, and after thirtie, shees the Surgions creature' (Overbury, 1936, p.28). 'A very Whore is a woman', he added with a misogynist twist, 'She enquires out all the great meetings, which are medicines for her itching' (p.29).

This was another of the male clichés of the time – the conception of the prostitute as a creature driven by 'unsatiate intemperance' (see p.115) and 'hot desires' (see p.136), ever ready to lure men to lechery and destruction. In his *Newes from Hell* (1606), Dekker says of Hell (London) that 'such daungerous hot shottes are all the women there, that whosoeuer meddles with any of them is sure to be burnt' (Dekker, 1884–6, vol.2, p.98). Similarly, 'a fair hot wench in flame-coloured taffeta' (*1 Henry IV*, 1,2:10) was the kind of woman that was capable of attracting Falstaff, the fat, dissolute knight, whose prostitute girlfriend Doll Tearsheet was so hot that 'she's in hell already and burns poor souls' (*2 Henry IV*, 2,4:335–6). 'Burn' was an Elizabethan metaphor not only for the hotness of sexual passion but also for the infection of syphilis and gonorrhea (see pp.255–68). Typically, these women were seen as responsible for venereal infection and disease, while it did not occur to the Elizabethans that men were equally culpable in this respect.

This is a marked tendency in the early history of syphilis, where much of the moral opprobrium was directed specifically at women and therefore fostered or intensified misogynist attitudes. Von Hutten, for example, sees

> 'this thing [syphilis] as touching women; [it] resteth in their secret places, having in those places litle pretty sores ful of venom, poison being very dangerous, for those [who] unknowingly medle with them. The which sicknese gotten by such infected women, is so much the more vehement & grevous, how they be inwardly poluted & corrupted.' (Hutten, 1533, sig.Avi^v)

Such loaded suggestions are carried a step further by Peter Lowe when concluding that men and children can catch diseases from women who are healthy, but who are menstruating. Distinguishing between syphilitic chancres and those which are not, Lowe says:

> 'There happeneth oftentimes certaine little excressence of flesh like Warts betwixe the gland prepuce, of which there are two sorts. The one proceedeth of the venerian sicknes, the other not: yet neyther of them both for the most part dollorous, but very much troublesome, by reason of the great number of them. The cause of such as are venimous [syphilitic] is the evill indisposition of women accompanied with some infection. Those which are not venimous happen by having to doe with women in the time of their purgations, of which happeneth not only that [the warts], but also many other greevous diseases both to the men, & also the children, which are conceaved at that time, for eyther they become Leapors universally, or some particular part, which we call Elephanciasis.' (Lowe, 1596, sig.B2^r)

Also here a misogynist tone may be perceived in the author's view of women as not only carriers of syphilitic infection but also of a number of crippling and deadly diseases, passed on through their tainted blood. The Bible's idea of original sin as having been introduced by Eve – the first whore – through her fall is probably behind such medical speculations.

Rather surprisingly, the Scottish doctor exonerates the hot whore in the question of syphilitic transmission, because her profession discourages any real 'hotness' of emotion. Citing Fallopius, he claims that 'the cause of thys infection, commeth often of the passion of the minde: for when a woman loueth not that man shee hath to doe with, she heateth not her selfe, but lieth quietly, and so thrusteth not forth the venim, as some whores doe' (sig.B2ᵛ). In contrast to most medical writers who rightly argued that prostitutes were largely responsible for spreading syphilis, Lowe claims that they are less dangerous than other women since 'common women take not so great pleasure, because they [are] accustomed night and day to exercise venerie' (sig.B2ᵛ). Healthy wives or mistresses, on the other hand, who were emotionally involved with their partners would more likely infect them with syphilis because their sensual and passionate thoughts generated excessive body heat, a major cause of the disease according to some physicians (Bentley, 1989, pp.27–31).

## SYPHILIS AND THE PLAGUE

The most extraordinary misconception of syphilitic infection, shared by laymen and physicians alike, was the notion that syphilis rendered an infected person immune from the bubonic plague. The basic medical idea underlying this belief was that two diseased actions could not take place in the same constitution, nor in the same individual at one time. Since diseased actions were incompatible with each other, two fevers, for example, could not together afflict one individual, nor could the pox and the plague be manifest in the same part at once. 'Sergeant Carbuncle, one of the plague's chief officers', observes Lawrence Lucifer in Middleton's *The Blacke Booke* (1604), 'dares not venture within three yards of an harlot, because monsieur Drybone, the Frenchman, is a leiger [resident ambassador] before him' (Middleton, 1885–6, vol.8, p.23).

Needless to say, the fallacy of the mutual antagonism of bubonic plague and syphilis was bound to have disastrous consequences in a century of great epidemics. 'Most unhappily a report got abroad', W.G. Bell records in his history of the Great Plague of 1665, 'that venereal disease gave immunity from Plague…Its results beggared in horror the worst effects of the Plague itself' (Bell, 1924, p.99). The medical falsehood appears to have been widely circulated, and according to J.F.D. Shrewsbury there is no evidence that it was ever denounced by the medical profession. Indeed, there is evidence that some doctors believed it (Shrewsbury, 1970, p.449).

Such natural prophylactics were enthusiastically welcomed by the syphilized members of the London underground who, according to Dekker's *Newes from Gravesend* (1604), were the only ones to regard the renewed outbreak of the bubonic plague in 1603 with equanimity. 'Painted harlots' and 'muffled halfe-fac'de Pandars', Dekker observed in his long poem,

Smile at this plague, and black mischance,
Knowing their deaths come o're from *France:*
Tis not their season now to die,
Two gnawing poisons cannot lie,
In one corrupted flesh together,
Nor can this poison then fly thether:
Theres not a Strompet mongst them all
That liues and rises by the fall,
Dreads this contagion, or her threats,
Being guarded with French Amulets. (Dekker, 1925, pp.99–100)

## CLASS DIVISION OF PROSTITUTES

Evidence of class distinction in the English world of prostitution is found in many sources and follows recognized patterns both ancient and modern. The title-page of Thomas Randolph's *Cornelianum Dolium* (1638) (Figure 27) shows three prostitutes portrayed as belonging to different classes of society. To the left is the street prostitute, in the middle the ordinary prostitute of the brothel, and to the right a high-class prostitute in the dress of a gentlewoman.

In Beaumont and Fletcher's *Loves Cure, or the Martial Maid* (1647), the woman at the bottom of the prostitutes' hierarchy is described as 'A barefoot, lowzie, and diseased whore…shift[ing her] lodgings oftner than a rogue That's whipt from post to post' (4,2; 209). This is the vagrant whore in the countryside and the street-walking prostitute in the towns, a creature of poverty and disease whom Nicholas Breton included in his presentation of 'foure kindes of ugly objects: a scabbie Iade, a mangy dog, a lowsie knave, and a pockie whore' (Breton, 1879, vol.2, p.7).

Higher up the social scale was the urban public whore who operated from an alehouse, tavern or bawdy house, while her counterpart in the countryside emerged as the village whore. At the top of the hierarchy was the high-class prostitute who catered for the bourgeoisie and the upper classes. '*Whoredome* hath many friends in these daies', Barnabe Rich ruminated in 1616, with reference to the courtezans of his time,

> 'a number of fauorites, that giueth her boldnesse whereby shee insinuates herselfe into the world…*Whoredome* scornes to be closed vp in any obscure place, no, shee hath friends to boulster her out, and to support her in the highest and most principall places of the citty. *Harlots* now adaies, do not lurke in by corners as *theeues* are wonted, nor in secret chambers, as *strumpets* haue bin accustomed, nor in close *clossets* as conspiring *Papists*, when they be at their *Masse*; but shee frequents the principall places of the cittie, where shee giues entertainment to those that comes vnto her, that are not of the basest sort, but many times of the best reputed.' (Rich, 1616, p.36)[*]

In *Doctor Merrie-Man* (1609), Samuel Rowlands gives this satirical picture of a high-class prostitute:

---

[*]  cf. also p.383.

I am a profest Courtezan,
That liue by peoples sinne:
With halfe a dozen Puncks I keepe,
I haue great comming in.
Such store of Traders haunt my house,
To finde a lusty Wench,
That twentie Gallants in a weeke,
Doe entertaine the French;
Your Courtier, and your Citizen,
Your very rustique Clowne,
Will spend an Angell on the Poxe,
Euen ready mony downe.
I striue to liue most Lady-like,
And scorne those foolish Queanes,
That doe not rattle in their Silkes
And yet haue able meanes.
I haue my Coach, as if I were
A Countesse, I protest,
I haue my daintie Musicke playes
When I would take my rest. (Rowlands, 1880, vol.2, p.21)

Figure 27. The engraved title-page of Thomas Randolph's Latin play *Cornelianum Dolium* (1638, engraving by W.M.) shows the hero's suffering through a venereal sweating cure ' in a tub that's heated smoking hot' (see p.119). There are only three allusions to 'Cornelius Tub' in English literature, and the origin of the name is obscure. The earliest reference is in Thomas Nashe's novel *The Unfortunate Traveller* (1594), where it says: 'Mother Cornelius tub, why it was like hell, he that came into it neuer came out of it' (Nashe, 1910, vol.2, p.228).

In Middleton's *The Familie of Love* (1608), a physician named Glister jestingly refers to 'one of the hoops of my Cornelius' tub' (3,6:31–2) while witnessing a scuffle between two City lechers. A final reference is found in Cotgrave's *English Treasury of Wit and Language* (1655), where a rather anachronistic epigram tells of Diogenes who 'took his habitation in a tub' and 'took the dyet, sit, and in That very tub sweat for the French disease. And some unlearn'd apothecary since, Mistaking's name, call'd it Cornelius tub' (Brewster, 1958, p.490).

In Randolph's engraving, the syphilitic patient in the tub takes leave of three prostitutes from different social levels while groaning: 'Good by, you Venuses and Cupidos: I am sitting in Venus's bath (solium) – in this tub (dolium) I suffer'. Shakespeare's *Sonnets* ends in the same hot place when the frustrated and 'sick' (153) poet 'hie[s]' (153) himself to Bath to seek 'Against strange maladies a sovereign cure' (153). Describing himself as 'a sad distempered guest' (153), he further presents himself as 'my mistress' thrall' (154) and burnt by 'Cupid' (153) – his hope of a 'healthful remedy for men diseased' (154) proving to be 'a seething bath' (153), or the most common cure of syphilis.

Bath was a famous Elizabethan spa known especially for its treatment of rheumatic and venereal patients. Harrison says of the Cross Bath in the city that 'This bath is much frequented by such as are diseased with leaprie, pockes, scabs and great aches...The common bath...is worthilie called the hot bath, for at the first comming into it, men thinke that it would scald their flesh, and lose it from the bone: but after a season, and that the bodies of the commers thereto be warmed throughlie in the same, it is more tollerable and easie to be borne. Both these baths be in the middle of a little street, and ioine to S. Thomas hospitall' (Harrison, 1586, vol.1, pp.362–3).

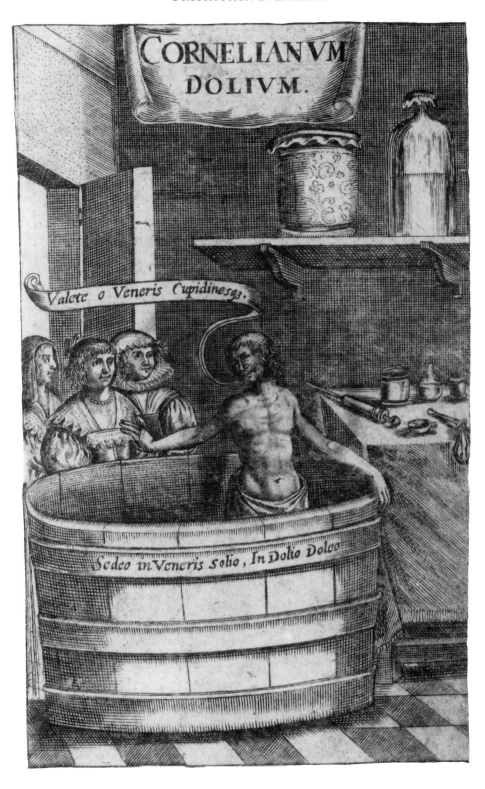

In Ben Jonson's *Bartholomew Fair* (1614), Punk Alice includes Dame Overdo in this sophisticated company and shouts at her:

> 'A mischiefe on you, they are such as you are, that vndoe vs, and take our trade from vs, with your tuft-taffata hanches...The poore common whores can ha' no traffique, for the priuy rich ones; your caps and hoods of veluet, call away our customers, and lick the fat from vs.' (4,5:65–71)

If high-class prostitutes presented a more aesthetic aspect of the flesh trade, their customers were in no position to assume that such women offered any protection against venereal disease. Rowlands's courtezan frankly asserts that twenty gallants are syphilized under her roof and that all social classes are willing to spend 'an angel on the pox' in her arms. In John Ford's *The Fancies Chaste and Noble* (1638), Flavia, in the presence of her second husband, Julio, warns Fabricio, her first husband, that high-class prostitutes present a health risk to be taken seriously. 'You must not loiter lazily', she admonishes him,

> And [lurk] about the town, my friend, in taverns,
> In gaming-houses; nor sneak after dinner
> To public shows, to interludes, in riot,
> To some lewd painted baggage, trick'd-up gaudily
> Like one of us: – O, fie upon 'em, giblets!
> I have been told they ride in coaches, flaunt it
> In braveries so rich that it's scarce possible
> How to distinguish one of these vile naughty packs
> From true and arrant ladies: they'll inveigle
> Your substance and your body, – think on that,
> I say, your body; look to't! (3,2:271–2) (Ford, 1869, vol.2, pp.271–2)

In addition to open prostitution there was its clandestine counterpart in which a woman was kept by one or two men. The dark lady of Shakespeare's *Sonnets* may be placed at this end of the promiscuous hierarchy, for according to the Shakespearean scholar A.L. Rowse she was identical with an Italian beauty by the name of Emilia Bassano who, at the age of 17, was made the mistress of the elderly Henry Carey (c. 1524–96), the first Lord Hunsdon and founder of the Lord Chamberlain's Company, Shakespeare's troupe (see p.182) (Rowse, 1974, pp.99–117). Her appearance in Shakespeare's collection of poems is aptly characterized by E.A.J. Honigmann as that of 'a high-class courtesan' (Honigmann, 1982, p.20).

## Behavioural Change through Fear of Syphilis

The fact that syphilis might be contracted at all social levels of prostitution is demonstrated by Dekker's *The Welsh Ambassador* (1624), in which the victims of venereal infection are depicted as 'a woman...burnt in Smith Field...five carmen burnt in Turnball Street, and four gentlemen in Bloomsbury' (5,3:81–2). Bloomsbury differed from other resorts of the time in being a more fashionable area of prostitution. Thus Dekker in *Penny-Wise, Pound-Foolish* (1631) observes that 'You talke of the poore Cat-a-mountaines in *Turnebull*, who venture vpon the pikes of damnation for single money; and you wonder at the fethered Estridges in *Westminster, Strand, Bloomsbury* etc. how they can liue' (Dekker, 1631, sig.D4^v).

Leantio's meditations in Middleton's *Women Beware Women* (1657) on prostitutes at the higher end of the social scale show that fears of contracting the 'foul disease' had a tempering effect on many a young gallant when feeling the temptations of youth and the flesh:

> When I behold a glorious dangerous strumpet,
> Sparkling in beauty and destruction too,
> Both at a twinkling, I do liken straight
> Her beautified body to a goodly temple
> That's built on vaults where carcasses lie rotting;
> And so, by little and little, I shrink back again,
> And quench desire with a cool meditation. (3,1:95–101)

A still more eloquent expression of a young man's dread of the medical consequences of wenching and whoredom is provided by Richard Brathwaite in one of his poems in *A Strappado for the Divell* (1615). Here the poet contemplates the orgastic delights of 'lust that's cal'd by th' sensuall Epicure, The best of mouing pleasures, and the lure, That for the instance makes our organs rise, Thinking that place wee'r in is Paradice' (Braithwaite, 1887, p.152). Prostitutes as men's means of satisfaction of their sexual desire gives way to the poet's contemplation of the ruinous effects of venereal disease and makes his reason finally triumph over his lust to the point where the very thought of a whore is sufficient to quell all his his body's libidinal stirrings. The prostitute, he asserts,

> Bring forth no fruit at all,
> Saue news from 'th Spittle, or the Hospitall.
> Drie rewmes, catarchs, diseases of despaire,
> Puritane-sniueling, falling of the haire.
> Akes in the ioynts, and ring-worme in the face,
> Cramps in the nerues, fire in the priuy place...
> If best of pleasures haue no other end
> Mong'st earth's delights, then haue we cause t'extend,
> Our pure affections to an higher ayme,
> Then to corrupt the honour of our name.
> For present appetite: I thanke the[e] whoor,
> Thou hast instructted me to haue a power
> Ouer my sence by reason rectified,
> And hast well neere my senses mortefied. (pp.152–3)

CONCLUSION

The pamphleteers' picture of a London scene riddled with widespread prostitution is underscored by the records of a Swiss tourist visiting the city in 1599 and by the legal records of the period, which testify to the presence of numerous urban districts engaged in prostitution. The Lord Mayor's Inquiry of 1633 suggests that the municipal authorities were aware of an escalation in prostitution in the growing city, and that they attempted to get a better grasp on it by inquiries into the actions of

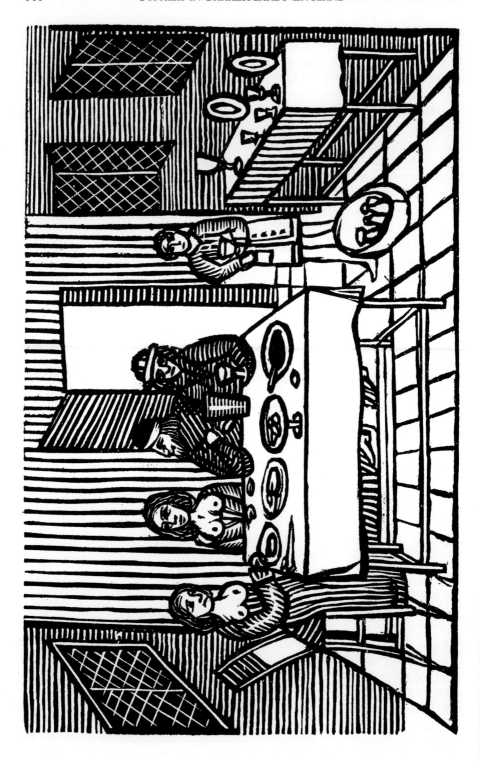

the owners of taverns, alehouses, and bath establishments. Sources also indicate that the authorities could be negligent, lenient or directly bribed, and that Tudor and Stuart policy and administrative practices generally failed to enforce the penal code against prostitutes, bawds, and other offenders.

The pamphleteers' claim that prostitution was maintained by powerful economic interests is confirmed by a number of sources which show that the landlords, merchants and entertainment moguls of the period invested in prostitution, which was commercialized according to the trend of the age. This meant that prostitution was stratified and ranged from high-class brothels to establishments catering to the more common classes of the population. In similar fashion, private enterprise ranged from the high-class courtezan to the street whore, with concomitant variations in price. The average price of a visit to a brothel appears to have been 6 pence – the same price as the costliest theatre ticket.

Sources further show that there was a general awareness of prostitutes as the prime transmitters of syphilis, and that the disease was feared because of its serious threat to life and well-being. Numerous sources show that fear of the 'foul disease'

Figure 28. Woodcut of a brothel, in Viles and Furnivall, 1880, opposite *Contents*, executed from a faded woodcut in *The Roxburghe Ballads* (vol.1, p.346) and illustrating *The Excellent Parable of the Prodigal Child*. Prostitution in London was big business and involved not only its property owners and prosperous merchants but also the nobility and, at least until 1536, the Church. After the development of an entertainment industry in the last quarter of the 16th century, the moguls of the theatre also moved into the flesh trade, seeing it as yet another profitable investment. Thomas Platter, a Swiss physician visiting England in 1599, observed that 'I have never seen more taverns and alehouses in my whole life than in London', adding that 'although close watch is kept on them [the prostitutes], great swarms of these women haunt the town in taverns and play-houses' (Platter, 1937, pp.189, 175). Thomas Nashe's Pierce Penniless tells the Devil that he hopes the whores of London will be speedily carried to hell, 'there to keepe open house for all young Diuels that come, and not let our ayre bee contaminated with theyr six-pennie damnation any longer' (Nashe, 1910, vol.1, p.217).

'I wil give thee sixpence to lye one night with thee', says the soldier Ruf to Meretrix, the prostitute, in Thomas Preston's (1537–98) *Cambises* (1558–70). 'Gogs hart, slave, doost thinke I am a sixpeny iug?', Meretrix retorts, 'No, wis ye, Jack, I looke a little more smug!' At this point another soldier, Snuf, intervenes to treble the price: 'I will give her xviii pence to serve me first' (Manly, 1897, vol.2, pp.171–2). In *Christs Teares* Nashe describes 'sixe-penny whoredome' (Nashe, 1910, vol.2, p.148) as flourishing in the suburbs, though elsewhere in the same passage he asserts that 'Halfe a Crowne [2 sh.6 p.] or little more (or sometimes lesse) is the sette pryce of a strumpets soule' (p.149). This must refer to the price paid for prostitutes at the higher end of the social scale, as indicated also by Thomas Dekker's *2 The Honest Whore* (1630), in which Catharina Bountinall asks Mistress Horseleech, a bawd: 'How many times hast thou given gentlemen a quart of wine in a gallon pot? how many twelve-penny fees, nay two shillings fees, nay, when any Embassadors have been here, how many half crown fees hast thou taken?' (5,2:377–81).

In the field of prostitution the variations in prices paid were probably at least as great as those for the other diversions and entertainments of the bustling metropolis (see Ashton, 1983, pp.3–19). At the end of the reign of James I, however, there are signs that prostitution had become so widespread that it affected the market mechanisms. 'This plenty of Harlots hath done some good in the Common-wealth', Barnabe Rich noted with a sigh of relief in 1617, 'it hath much abated the price of Bawdery; for now a whoremonger may haue his pot of Ale, his pipe of Tobacco, and his pocky whore, and all for his three pence, and that almost in euery by-Lane. A happy thing for poore Knights, that the market is thus beaten downe' (Rich, 1617, p.16).

could be equally as powerful an agent of behavioural change as the religious fear of eternal damnation. There is also an indication that women in general were seen as responsible for venereal infection and disease, and that this belief fostered or intensified misogynist attitudes.

The evidence as a whole seems to confirm William Clowes's depiction of a contemporary scene characterized by unimpeded prostitution, widespread promiscuity, rampant syphilis, and public indifference.

# 7

# HIGH-RISK GROUPS

Next to Antwerp, London was the biggest seaport in Europe and one of its economic centres. Much points to the fact that the English capital was also a centre of syphilitic infection, owing to the vast extent of English trading activities. Sailors and soldiers formed a large part of the influx of foreigners in London, and these sections of European society were the prime transmitters of syphilis after 1492. Sailors and soldiers figured as prominent clients of prostitutes in all European cities and seaports, and the Bankside in London was one such centre of prostitution for single men, who came not only from England but from all over the world. In this way the great European seaport became an important centre for both the reception and transmission of venereal diseases.

In addition to sailors and soldiers, London harboured another population group for whom sex was hard to obtain, with the result that it fuelled the spread of prostitution. This group consisted of young men who came to take up apprenticeships in the various trades, due to the expansion and diversification in metropolitan manufacturing. In contrast to the sexual imbalance in larger towns during the 16th and 17th centuries (see p.99), London was somewhat unusual in that there was a shortage – not a surplus – of women, at least during the first half of the 17th century. According to M.F. and T.H. Hollingsworth, whose results were confirmed recently by R. Finlay, the sex ratio in the city's population was 115 males per 100 females (Holingsworth, 1971, p.134).[*]

This marked surplus of men is explained by the many apprentices working in London. These immigrant youths made up an estimated 15 per cent of the population, and they settled predominantly in the suburbs where prostitution is known to have flourished. The apprentices were forbidden to marry until their terms were completed, which usually meant their late 20s. Brothels and alehouses catered to the sexual needs of this deprived male population, while other commercialized nexuses of social intercourse included taverns, gaming-houses, cockpits, bear gardens, bowling-alleys, barber-shops, and of course theatres. For the females involved in London's equally expanding victualling trade, service sector and domestic industries, the incentives to prostitution were great in a period of declining real wages and contracting opportunities for female labour. A life of prostitution was probably also a way out to women who had fallen on hard times or were unmarried

---

[*]    cf. also Finlay, 1981, pp.19, 139–42.

mothers. As always, prostitution and poverty went hand in hand, as did promiscuity and venereal disease.

While sailors, soldiers, apprentices and vagabonds formed part of a high-risk company, similar high-risk groups with great potential for venereal infection and continued transmission included the student population of the English capital, the members of its royal Court, and, finally, the members of its flourishing literary and dramatic establishment. We shall examine these groups at closer range to see to what extent syphilization might have befallen the social and cultural elite of Tudor and Stuart England. In the following section we shall flash the medical searchlight on some of the greatest luminaries of the Shakespearean age, including the great poet himself.

## THE SYPHILIZATION OF THE GENTRY AND THE ARISTOCRACY

'There's none here but can fight for a whore as well as some Inns-a'-court-man', says Lieutenant Mawworm to Dick Follywit in Middleton's *A Mad World, My Masters* (3,3:147–8) (1605–6). In Samuel Rowlands's *Greenes Ghost Haunting Conicatchers* (1602), the author tells the story of 'A Certaine queane belonging to a close Nunnerie about Clarkenwell [who], lighting in the company of a yong Punie of the Innes of Court, trained him home with her to her hospitall: and there couenanting for so much to giue him his houseroome all night' (Rowlands, 1880, vol.1, p.26). 'To bed they went together like man and wife', he resumes his warning tale, which finishes with the fleecing of the young student by the queane's three accomplices, who leave him in the street as poor as 'an Irish beggar', with only a blanket wrapped around him (pp.25–6).

Figure 29. Detail of view of London, 1616 (Engraving by Claes Janszoon de Visscher (1586–1652), in the British Library). Great material progress was made by the upper classes and the merchants in the Elizabethan Age. The economic development of these sectors of society converged in London, in which the centralization of Court and political life stimulated consumption, while the capital's seaport and the establishment of monopolies drew the merchants to the new economic centre. Organized in companies such as the Merchant Adventurers (1407), the Muscovy Company (1555), the Turkey (later, Levant) Company (1581), the East India Company (1600), and the Virginia Company (1607), the merchants of London established themselves as a powerful and wealthy class, eager to invest their earnings in new enterprises. While the merchants fostered sheep and wool production in the countryside, which led to enclosure and depopulation, they spearheaded London's development into the country's leading manufacturing centre. Expansion and diversification in metropolitan manufacturing helped to expand the suburbs and provided jobs for thousands of immigrants. A large number of these came to take up apprenticeships in the various trades, and they settled predominantly in the burgeoning northern and eastern extra-mural parishes, where the apprenticeship system was laxly enforced (Beier and Finlay, 1986, p.15).

These immigrant youths made up an estimated 15 per cent of the population and they were all single men. As such they formed a high-risk group for the contraction of venereal diseases together with sailors and soldiers. Other high-risk groups consisting of single men included the student population at the Universities and the Inns of Court, the members of the Royal Court, and the leading figures of London's literary and dramatic Bohemia.

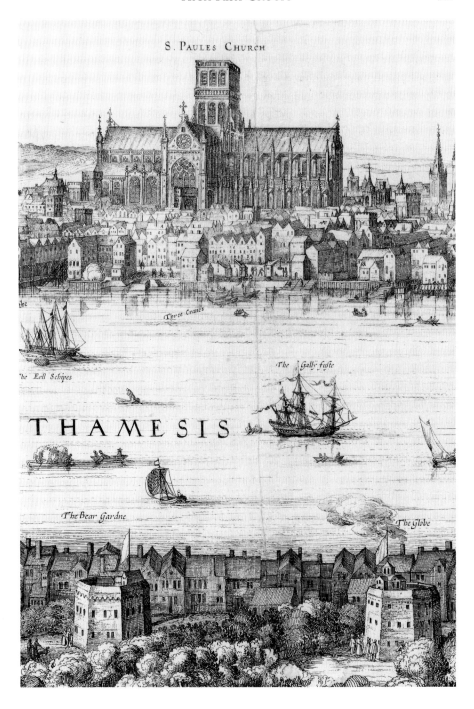

From Shakespeare's plays one could take a third and final example of student life outside the walls of the four great Inns of Court in London. 'You were called "lusty Shallow" then, cousin', the country justice Silence tells his kinsman and colleague, Robert Shallow, who replies:

> 'By the mass, I was called anything; and I would have done anything indeed too, and roundly too. There was I, and little John Doit of Staffordshire, and black George Barnes, and Francis Pickbone, and Will Squele a Cotsole man – you had not four such swinge-bucklers in all the Inns o' Court again. And I may say to you, we knew where the bona-robas were, and had the best of them all at commandment.' (*2 Henry IV*, 3,2:15–23)

As may be gleaned from these examples, the stereotypical Inns of Court student depicted by contemporary dramatists, moralists, poets and satirists, was an idle and fairly dissolute young man, with a marked preference for 'Shakespeare's plaies instead of my Lord Coke' (Lenton, 1631, sig F4ʳ, '29. A Yong Innes a Court Gentleman'). Even if Wilfrid R. Prest, the brilliant historian of *The Inns of Court under Elizabeth I and the Early Stuarts, 1590–1640* (1972), warns us against accepting such a portrait at face value, both because it may be unduly influenced by the escapades of a rakish minority and because it inevitably contains an element of caricature, he also admits that scepticism can be carried too far. There are simply too many examples of the prodigal appetites of the Inns of Court students, particularly their appetites for violence and lechery.

According to Prest, the problems began very early in the history of this learned institution. Between 1480 and 1530, the benchers, the senior members at the Inns, had gained control over the societies, attempting to impose a general discipline on the younger members and to instill respect for their own authority. They punished members for encouraging quarrels between their fellows, for shooting bows and arrows within the house, for letting their shirts hang outside their doublets, and for speaking 'lowde and hyghe at meyle time' (Prest, 1972, p.91). In addition to assaults and brawls, the most common infractions were insolence to the bench and moral misdemeanours. According to Prest, 'The first recorded punishment for sexual misconduct was inflicted in 1478 upon a member who had entertained a woman in his chamber "at the forbidden time"' (p.91). After a rash of similar offences in the late 1480s, the bench decreed that anyone caught fornicating in his room would be fined £5, although the penalty was reduced to £1 if the act was committed in the garden or Chancery Lane.

But from the 1530s on, the gradual expansion of membership and the lack of proctors or tutors made it increasingly difficult for the benchers to continue policing the personal lives of their subordinates. 'Attempts to regulate extramural behaviour ceased altogether during the second half of the sixteenth century', concludes Prest, 'and by the beginning of our period [the 1590s] barristers and students were perfectly free to attend plays or sermons as they chose, to drink in taverns ("the inns-a-court man's entertainment," according to Bishop Earle), and patronise dicing houses or stews at their pleasure' (p.92).

With theatres on both sides of the river, and Alsatia, Ram Alley and the Savoy on their door steps, young gentlemen at the Inns of Court were exposed to the full range of metropolitan temptations and vices. At Oxford and Cambridge the young gallant's

> Tutor was the man that kept him in,
> That he ran not into excess of sinne. (Lenton, 1629, p.3)

But once established in London and its Inns of Court, the student of law had 'crept from the cradle of learning to the court of liberty…from his tutor to the touchstone of his wits…he is his owne man now' (Lenton, 1631, sigF4$^r$, '29. A Yong Innes a Court Gentleman').

According to Prest, the lack of regimen and academical superintendence at the Inns of Court was accompanied by another critical factor which was the tedium of the study of law, that 'most difficult and grave learning, which hath nothing illecbrouse, or delicate to tickle their tender witts', as Sir Thomas Elyot phrased the problem (Elyot, 1880, vol.1, p.136). Many a law student would undoubtedly agree with the gifted and industrious Simonds D'Ewes who at the age of 22 'found still the study of the law so difficult and unpleasant' that he could 'justly account the two years last past among the unhappiest days of my life' (Prest, 1972, pp.141–2).

A classic description of a young student's agony of soul and sexual temptations in his study was provided by the London printer and dramatist John Rastell (c. 1475–1536), who as a young man had attended the Inns of Court in London. In his interlude *The Nature of the Four Elements* (c. 1518), he depicts Humanity pursuing his studies under the supervision of Studious Desire. However, after his first lesson, Humanity is lured away from his cell by Sensual Appetite, who knows a place where a wearied student may regain his spirits. He takes him to a tavern, where the host offers him a variety of services. 'I wolde we had a good stewyd capon', Humanity opens the conversation with an ambiguous twist, to which the Taverner readily replies that 'all capons be gone', but that other fowl may be had, for

|          | I can get you a stewwd hen |
|          | That is redy dyght [prepared]. |
| HUMANITY | Yf she be fat yt wyll do well. |
| TAVERNER | Fat or lene I cannot tell, |
|          | But as for this, I wot well |
|          | She lay at the stewes all nyght. (Rastell, 1979, p.45) |

As it turns out, Humanity has now two tempters on his hand, for Sensual Appetite quickly joins the Taverner's lead by suggesting that

> we wyll have lytell Nell,
> A proper wenche, she daunsith well,
> And Jane with the blacke lace;
> We wyll have bounsynge Besse also,
> And two or thre proper wenchis mo,
> Ryght feyr and smotter [pretty] of face…
> And after that, if ye wyll touche
> A feyre wenche nakyd in a couche
> Of a soft bed of downe,
> For to satisfye your wanton lust,

> I shall apoynt you a trull of trust,
> Not a feyrer in this towne.
> And whan ye have taken your delyte,
> And thus satisfyed the appetyte,
> Of your wyttis fyve,
> Ye may sey than I am a servaunt
> For you so necessary and plesaunt,
> I trowe non suche a lyve. (pp.46, 62)

The triumph of Sensual Appetite over hero and audience is signalled when at this point of the interlude he brings dancers into the hall 'to pipe, to singe, to daunce, to spring, with plesure and delyte...our sprytys to revyve and comfort' (p.63). Luckily for the hero, Nature returns at the end of the interlude to admonish Humanity for his bestial life, and all the plot requires is for Ignorance to be banished and Humanity to repent so that he can be reinstated with his former tutor, Studious Desire.

## WHETSTONE'S WARNING SERMON

Excursions of the kind described by John Rastell, William Shakespeare, Samuel Rowlands and Thomas Middleton reveal that a considerable part of the English intelligentsia may be classed as a risk group in relation to venereal diseases. This was yet another critical aspect of the affluence of Tudor society, in which luxury was spreading with the result that the wealthy men's sons were now attending not only the Universities but also the Inns of Court. These were even more exclusive than the Universities, since they offered no scholarships, and in the early 17th century nine out of ten of the students there came from the aristocracy and the gentry.

The medical and social problems of the promiscuity of this group did not escape the attention of a social critic like George Whetstone. Significantly, he dedicated his *Mirour for Magestrates of Cyties* (1584) not only to the Mayor of London and his Aldermen but also to the Inns of Court in that city. Addressing their permissive behaviour, Whetstone observes that 'It is verie wel knowen, that these famous Houses are the first intertayners of your Lybertie. For (notwithstanding) in your Gouernments, there are many good and peaceable Orders, yet your chiefest Discipline, is by the Purse. Those that are disposed, studdie the Lawes: who so liketh, without checke, maye follow Dalliance' (Whetstone, 1584, Preface, n.p.). Because the law student had ready money and access to the dicing houses and stews, Whetstone saw their license as a threat to English society, particularly to the upper classes and aristocracy.

In his addition to the *Mirour* entitled 'A Touchstone for the Time: exposing the daingerous Mischiefes, that the Dicying Howses...do dayly breede: Within the Bowelles of the famous Citie of London' (title-page), Whetstone warned against the alcoholization, syphilization and social ruining of England's intellectual and social elite. Once again addressing the Inns of Court, Whetstone explained how a young lawyer's riotous living not only wasted his father's money but how it also jeopardized the family heritage and the family line. After a long encomium to the Inns as

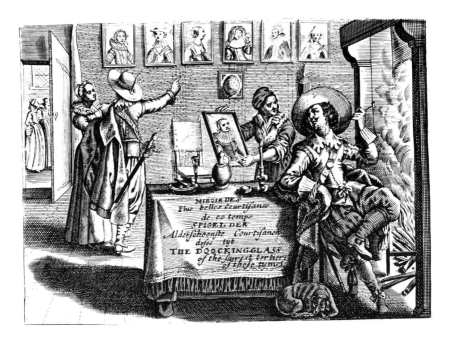

Figure 30. Engraving by Crispijn de Passe II (c. 1597–1670) on the title-page of *Le Miroir des Courtisanes*, Paris, 1630. In addition to *Hollands Leaguer*, another description of one of the luxury brothels of Stuart London survives in *The Times' Whistle* (1614), where the anonymous author denounces the vices of the time and launches a concerted attack on the debauched Court of James I. Referring to the 'bawdes which doe inhabite Troynovant', or London, R.C. (1871, p.86) describes one of the finest and most sophisticated brothels established in the capital by the traders in the flesh. 'If some gallant, whose out side doth holde Great expectation', he begins his report,

> Come to demaund (for soe it often happes)
> To see their choysest beauties, him they bring
> (After request [not] to say any thing)
> Into a privat roome, which round about
> Is hung with pictures; all which goodly rout
> Is fram'de of Venus fashion, femals all...
> That picture which doth best affect the eye
> Of this luxurious gallant, instantly
> Is by some traine brought thether in true shape
> Of lively substance. Then good Bacchus grape
> Flowes in abundance; Ceres must be by,
> For without them ther is noe venerie.
> Provocatives to stir vp appetite
> To brutish lust & sensuall delight,
> Must not be wanting...
> Then after this libidinous collation
> They doe proceed to act their owne damnation.
> Thus is the worthiest citty of our land
> Made a base brothel-house, by a lewde band
> Of shamelesse strumpets...
> Thus City scapes not, nor the Court is free
> From obsceane actes of hatefull luxurie. (pp.87–9)

institutions of learning and honour, Whetstone went on: 'But, by reason of Dicynghouses, and other Alectiues to unthriftinesse, the good Father, which is at charge, to make his Sonne a Lawier, to do his Countrey seruice, throughe the loosnesse of the Sonne (many times) spendeth his money to the vndooyng of his posterytie' (fol.25). According to Whetstone, this financial 'loosnesse' was only the first step along the path to moral and physical corruption, the agents of which were 'Three dangerous gwestes belonging to ordinarie tables: The braue Shifter: the Bawde, and the Broaker' (fol.28ʳ).

'The man that is inticed to be a Dicer', Whetstone concluded his warning sermon to the students of law, 'of his owne accorde wil be a Horemaster...[and then] they go to some blind brothel-house wher (peraduenture) for a Pottle or two of wyne, the imbracement of a paynted Harlot, and the French Pockes for a reckoning, the *Punie* payeth fortie shillings' (fol.26ᵛ).

'Thus, by vnsatiable Ryot, wherof, Dicyng Houses are the fowntaynes', George Whetstone finished his moral tract, 'the welthiest of our yong Gentlemen, are soone learned to synge:

> I wealthie was of late, though naked now you see:
> Three things haue chaunged mine estate. Dice, Wine and Lecherie.'
>
> (fol.27ʳ)

## Syphilis – the 'Court Disease'

A risk group of particular interest to historians and one which appears frequently in the sources is the nobility, particularly its members at Court. The term 'court disease' was coined in Spain, towards the end of the 15th century, as one of the numerous names for the new disease, syphilis. The Valencian physician, Gaspare Torella (1452–1520), doctor at the courts of Pope Alexander VI and Cesare Borgia, noted in 1497 in his book on syphilis that, in southern Spain, the disease was known as 'morbus curialis', because it was always to be found in the vicinity of a court. This connection, enshrined in the name 'Mal de Cour', survived up to the 19th century (Nutton, 1990, pp.18–9).

In John Florio's well-known Italian grammar for Englishmen, *Florios Second Frutes* (1591), the ninth chapter is devoted to a 'pleasantlie discourse of newes, of the court, of courtiers of this day and many other matters of delight' (p.139) – a subject which makes Tiberio remark that 'as soone as they come to the Court, at the first cast, they will spend in lecherie what they had, they will play at dice what they haue, and consume in gluttonie what they may haue'. To which his friend replies: '*Sustine & Abstine*, should be the Courtiers Recipe' (p.147).

Apparently the courtly life of leisure and pleasure was conducive to promiscuity, since 'The childe of Sloath is Lecherie', as Thomas Nashe succinctly observed in *Pierce Penilesse* (1592) (Nashe, 1910, vol.1, p.216). Here he launches an attack on the promiscuity at the court of Elizabeth I while describing lechery, the seventh and last vice corrupting London. 'The Court I dare not touch', he begins, 'but surely there (as in the Heauens) be many falling starres, and but one true *Diana. Consuetudo peccandi tollit sensum peccati.* Custome is a Lawe, and Luste holdes it for a Lawe, to liue without Lawe' (p.216). After describing the promiscuity of such courtly figures as Lais, Cleopatra, and Helen, Nashe concludes his section on lechery by associating these women not only with women of the Court but also with London's prostitutes, relegating the whole sisterhood to hell:

> '*Lais, Cleopatra, Helen*, if your Clyme hath any such, noble Lord warden of the witches and iuglers, I commend them with the rest of our vncleane sisters in *Shorditch*, the *Spittle, Southwarke, Westminster, & Turnbull streete*, to the protection of your Portership: hoping you will speedily carrie them to hell, there to keepe open house for all young Diuels that come, and not let our ayre bee contaminated with theyr six-pennie damnation any longer.' (p.217)

## A SYPHILIZED COURTIER

In similar fashion, the anonymous author (R.C.) of *The Times' Whistle* (1614) launches an attack on the debauched court of James I, which shares with London the sin of 'luxury'. Speaking of prostitution, R.C. observes that neither

> City…nor the Court is free
> From obsceane actes of hatefull luxurie.
> Those men and women that doe make resorte,
> In hope of gaine or honour, to the Court,
> Doe live soe idely, & in such excesse,
> That it must needs produce this wickednesse. (R.C. 1871, p.89)

R.C. illustrates his point by instancing the fate of one courtier named 'Vitellus'. 'He keeps a whore i' th' city', we are informed, for

> Vitellus must have one
> That's a rare piece of the best fashion,
> Although she make these three thinges fare the worse,
> His soule, his body, & his strouting purse.
> His purse, her gay apparel & fine fare
> Have made allready very thin & bare;
> His bodie, her vnwholsome luxurie
> Hath brought to the disease of venery;
> And I much fear this their lewde fashion
> Will bring his soule vnto damnation. (pp.89–90)[*]

While R.C. presents the soul of Vitellus as 'polluted with the rust Of canckered sinne' (R.C., 1871, p.91), his body is obviously diseased by the venereal malady termed 'Gallicus morbus' in an earlier part of the poem (p.80). In this respect, Vitellus joins a number of famous syphilitics of the English court, 'hugely Frenchifide…Yet never crost the seas' (p.80), as the author ambiguously observes. Among the best known examples are Elizabeth I's favourite, the Earl of Essex (1566–1601), and James I's favourite, the Duke of Buckingham (1592–1628).

---

[*]   cf also Rich, 1616, pp.35–6.

## Two Famous Syphilitics: the Earl of Essex and the Duke of Buckingham

Robert Devereux, second Earl of Essex, was one of the political and social stars of the Elizabethan age, famous as a courtier, soldier, and favourite of Queen Elizabeth I. The final years of Essex's life were marked by an obvious, almost physical deterioration of judgement and faculties which culminated in his ill-fated rebellion against the Queen in 1601. His erratic behaviour and irrational outbursts of emotion are explained by Robert Lacey, the Earl's best modern biographer, as due to the effects of late syphilis of the nervous system (Lacey, 1971, pp.201–2).

Contemporary rumours asserted that the Earl of Essex had contracted the pox, and the alleged source of the rumours is significant – Roderigo Lopez, the Queen's chief physician who also ministered to Essex. Lopez's betrayal of his patient's venereal disease aptly explains the extreme vindictiveness with which Essex hounded the prominent Jewish London doctor to death over the alleged conspiracy to poison the Queen (p.201). Another piece of circumstantial evidence is Essex's confession to the clergyman in the Tower before his execution on February 25, 1601: 'I have bestowed my youth in wantonness, lust and uncleanness'.[*] The Scottish physician Peter Lowe probably had good reasons for dedicating his treatise on syphilis to 'The right Honourable Robert Deuorax, Earle of Essex' (Lowe, 1596, title-page).

The syphilis contracted by George Villiers, the Duke of Buckingham, is well-documented and is of literary interest as well because it is an example of the 'revenging copulation' which Shakespeare put to dramatic use in *Othello* and which probably underlies also the 'foul play' destroying the King in *Hamlet*. In 1624 Buckingham, who exercised a virtual dictatorship over English foreign policy from 1618 to 1628, attempted to arrange a marriage between Prince Charles (later Charles I) and the Infanta of Spain. During his negotiations in Madrid, the Duke displayed such wildly promiscuous behaviour that he even courted the beautiful wife of the King's Minister, the Conde de Olivares. The jealous husband and his offended wife conspired with Buckingham's implacable enemy, the Earl of Bristol, England's ambassador to Spain, and together the trio played a nasty trick on the arrogant and lecherous Duke.

According to the anecdote related by Sir Antony Welldon in *The Court and Character of King James* (1650),

> 'Bristoll did not forbeare to put all scorns, affronts, and tricks on him [the Duke], and *Buckingham* lay so open, as gave the other advantage enough by his lascivious carriage, and miscarriage. Amongst all his tricks, he playes one so cuningly; that it cost him al the hair on his head, and put him to the dyet; for it should seem he made court to *Conde Olivores* Lady, a very handsome Lady; But it was so plotted betwixt the Lady, her Husband and Bristoll, that instead of that beauty, he had a notorious Stew sent him, and surely his carriage there was so lascivious, that had ever the Match been really intended for our Prince, yet such a Companion or Guardian, was enough to have made them believe that he had been that way addicted [himself], and so have frustrated the Marriage.' (pp.146–7)

---

[*]  Woods, 1934, pp.106–7. Wechter, 1928, p.720. cf. also Grosart, 1870, vol.4, p.99.

Buckingham's apologists and a number of historians dismiss the anecdote as scandalous gossip, but the facts remain that Buckingham was ill in August 1624 when his wife sent a letter to him in which she replied to a now lost letter from her husband: 'But for one sin you are not so great an offender, only your loving women so well. But I hope God has forgiven you and I am sure you will not commit the like again' (Williamson, 1940, p.136). In the October of 1624, Buckingham was ill of his 'indisposition brought from Spain', and Sir Kenelm Digby, who was in Spain with him, confirms that he 'received some bitter affront in the matter of his mistresses' (p.136). Apparently the warning given to Buckingham by his father-in-law on the eve of the Duke's departure for Spain had been of little avail: 'I know you are in a hot country, therefore take heed of yourself. If you court ladies of honour, you will be in danger of poisoning or killing, and if you desire whores you will be in danger of burning. Therefore, good my lord, take heed' (p.136).

A third medical example from the English court is James I's Lord Chamberlain, William Herbert, third Earl of Pembroke (1580–1630), who was almost certainly a syphilitic as well. This is a point of major interest to students of English literature, because William Herbert is the most probable candidate for the fair youth of Shakespeare's *Sonnets* (1609), which were dedicated by their publisher, Thomas Thorpe, to a certain 'Mr. W. H.'. We shall examine his case more closely later in this study (see pp.179–95).

## The Syphilization of English Students at Home and Abroad

Student life at the universities of Oxford and Cambridge also had its temptations and dangers which contemporary sources did not hesitate to uncover. In *Euphues* (1589), John Lyly, a graduate of Magdalen, Cambridge, charged that there was gaming, drinking, dalliance with women, unseemly attire, wickedness, ill living, and atheism. The common people sent their sons to the university only to 'finde them little better learned, but a great deale worst lyued then when they went, and not onely vnthriftes of their money, but also banckeroutes of good manners' (Lyly, 1902, vol.1, pp.273–6). In *The Repentance of Robert Greene* (1592), the prominent poet and playwright, who was a graduate of Clare Hall, admitted that 'being at the Vniuersitie of Cambridge, I light[ed] amongst wags as lewd as my selfe, with whome I consumed the flower of my youth' (Greene, 1966b, p.19).

Also at Oxford and Cambridge, Studious Desire had to compete with Sensual Appetite, and students who gave in to the latter's temptations and riots ran a fair chance of contracting syphilis – like the fellow of Merton College, Oxford, who in 1511 'was ordered to leave that place because he had the French Pox' (see p.62).

Sources indicate that syphilization was a danger which in particular lay in wait for students going abroad for postgraduate study. 'For as our common courtiers (for the most part) are the best lerned and indued with excellent gifts', William Harrison observed in his *Description of England* (1577–87), 'so are manie of them the worst men when they come abroad, that anie man shall either heare or read of' (Harrison, 1877, p.271). This remark by the learned Elizabethan historian and sociologist highlights a critical aspect of English education abroad. Left on their own, many young noblemen and gentlemen spiced their studies at the various universities of

Europe with visits to brothels and frequentation of prostitutes. The inevitable result was the syphilization of many members of England's social and intellectual elite. Sources on this relationship are scarce, but the few that have survived will be presented in the following.

In Shakespeare's *Hamlet*, Laertes's visit to Paris for purposes of education causes his father Polonius considerable anxiety, for the elder statesman suspects his son of being open to 'such wanton, wild, and usual slips As are companions noted and most known To youth and liberty' (2,1:22–4). As instances he specifies 'drinking, fencing, swearing, quarrelling, drabbing' (2,1: 25–6) – all 'crimes' (2,1:44) to be reported by Reynaldo, who is Polonius's spy on Laertes in the French capital. However, Reynaldo is told to go about his job in a cautious and roundabout manner.

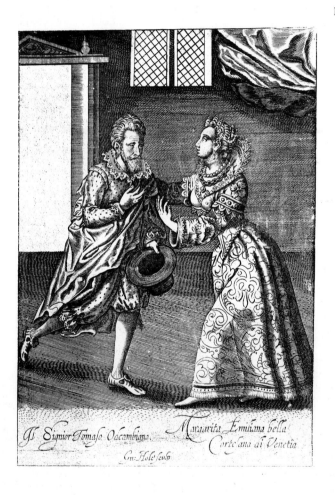

Figure 31. Coryat, 1905, vol.2, p.408, engraving by G.H. The famous Jacobean traveller 'M. Thomas Coryate of Odcombe in Somersetshire' (1577?–1617) pays a visit to a high-class prostitute in Venice, identified by the engraver with a rich courtezan called Margarita Æmiliana, who built a monastery in the city 'to make expiation unto God by this holy deede for the lascivious dalliance of her youth', as Thomas Coryat politely informs the reader (p.388). According to the author's own statement, his Venetian brothel visit to 'one of their noble houses' served partly to 'see the manner of their life, and observe their behaviour', partly to 'convert' a beautiful prostitute 'from a wanton Cortezan to a holy and religious woman' (p.408). Other Englishmen abroad paid similar visits with less pious intentions.

'You must not put another scandal on him, That he is open to incontinency', Polonius instructs his servant. 'That's not my meaning. But breathe his faults so quaintly That they may seem the taints of liberty, The flash and outbreak of a fiery mind, A savageness in unreclaimed blood, Of general assault' (2,1:29–35). Polonius finally tells Reynaldo about the kinds of report he expects from him, such as '"There was a gaming," "there o'ertook in's rouse," "There falling out at tennis," or perchance "I saw him enter such a house of sale" Videlicet a brothel, or so forth' (2,1:58–61).

In voicing these fears, Polonius shared the opinion of many of Shakespeare's contemporaries who mention 'dicing, drinking, and drabbing' as 'the ciuil plagues, that very vnciuily destroy the Sonnes (but not the Sinnes) of the Cittie' (Dekker, 1884–6, vol.2, p.105). And the city of the English capital was not different in that respect from other urban centres in Europe. In 1561, John Bale (1495–1563), the Protestant controversialist, bishop and dramatist, presented an interesting account of the destruction of England's students abroad when succumbing to the motions of 'unreclaimed blood' and the 'slips' of 'youth and liberty'.

Bale's report centres on the student life of a certain Thomas Martin, who is probably identical with a leading English clergyman and a contemporary of Stephen Gardiner, Hugh Weston, and Edmond Bonner. These men came into power during the Marian Restoration of the 1550s, and their support of the old Church forced Bale into exile on the Continent. From here he published his propaganda treatise *A Declaration of Edmonde Bonners Articles* (1561), in which he attacked the Articles just published by the bishop of London, just as he slandered the private lives of 'Gardyner, Bonner, whyte Weston, Feckenham and Wymbestay, most filthy lecherous locustes…whose abhominable lyues we partely knowe by theyr Bastardes of both kindes, and partelye by their botches & breche burninges' (Bale, 1561, fol.58^(r–v)).

This is one of several syphilitic innuendoes in Bale's controversial pamphlet, whose libellous reports should be treated with a certain caution. However, other sources testify to the moral looseness of the leading figures of the Marian Restoration (see p.78), and so Bale's testimony is not to be dismissed as a source entirely without historical or medical interest. It is in the beginning of his pamphlet that Bale quotes a report from France which concerns the undergraduate life of Thomas Martin and several other English students at the University of Bourges.

'[Here is] A testimony geuen forth by Fraunces Baldwin Attrebatius, a Doctor of the ciuil law, and publike reader at *Bituris* [Bourges], a vniuersity in Fraunce, concerning the baudy behauiour, and lecherous life of the foresayd Doctor Martin, such time as studied in the same vniuersity.

Doctour Martyne, being an Englishman, did soiourne or dwel in the vniuersitye of Bourges in the house of one called Boi' [Boium], being a most filthy priest, blynde of one eye, and all his bodye full of lothesome leprosye, and stynkinge frenche poxe…the moste vyle whoremonger, that was in al the whole towne. For, he kepte at home at his house and that openly a most abhominable harlote. Yea, hys house, was nothinge elles but a common stewe, and a schoole of all kynde of impudencye and fylthye vnclenlynesse. There did the sayde Martyne lyue swetely and pleasauntely, eatynge and drynkinge euerye daye, at one borde with the same harlot. And (which is more shameful) he kept in that broderell howse or stewe, certain yonge Englyshe gentilmen, committed to his charge, whom how myserably, this bawde, and rather a marrer or destroyer of children, then an instructour, dyd by suche example and company corrupte those yonge gentylmen, let his chiefe disciple and scholare, the nephew of sir Thomas More beare wytnesse, who folowing the example of his hoste, and of his scholemaster dyd walow himselfe in all kynde of fylthye abhomination, hauntinge all the harlots howses that were in the city of Bourges and abidinge continuallye in such scholes of vnclenlynesse: Although many honest men, and doctours of that vniuersitye, did take greuouslye this abhominable filthinesse, and did therefore blame the same Martine very sore.' (fol.42ᵛ-43ʳ⁻ᵛ)

Later in his pamphlet, Bale alludes to the syphilitic infection contracted by Thomas Martin when referring to the clergyman as 'the popes generall surgeon for Winchestre gese bytinges in his cleargie' (fol.51ʳ) – 'Winchester goose' being a popular slang expression for a syphilitic prostitute from Southwark or for a person infected with the pox (see pp.214–9).

## SYPHILIS AMONG THE MEMBERS OF LITERARY AND DRAMATIC BOHEMIA

The last high-risk group to be considered in this chapter is that which was formed by the members of London's literary and dramatic Bohemia. At a time when syphilis was spreading rapidly in the Elizabethan capital, the number of cases probably increasing geometrically, a leading figure from the artistic community stepped forward to disclose the dissolute lives of himself and his cohorts – 'that vncleane generation of vipers', as he called them (Greene, 1966a, p.36) – and the fearful consequences of 'lust and lecherie' (Greene, 1966b, p.7).

His name was Robert Greene (1560?–92), and like Shakespeare, his contemporary, he was one of the most famous playwrights and poets of his time. Greene's dreadful warning was entered in the Stationers' Register on September 20, 1592, three weeks after his death on September 3 at the age of 32. Shortly afterwards his pamphlet was published by one of his literary executors, Henry Chettle, under the title *Greenes Groatsworth of Witte, Bought with a Million of Repentance* (1592). The subtitle explained the purpose of the pamphlet as that of 'Describing the follie of youth, the falshood of make-shifte flatterers, the miserie of the negligent, and mischiefes of deceiuing Courtezans. Written before his death and published at his dyeing request' (Greene, 1966a, title-page, p.3).

'Blacke is the remembrance of my blacke workes, blacker than night, blacker than death, blacker than hell' (p.41), Greene opened his confession, adding that his countrymen ought to 'Learne wit by my repentance (Gentlemen) and let these few rules following be regarded in your liues' (p.41). The author then proceeded to admonish the reader to make it his first rule to fear God, and next to obey the following precepts:

'2 Beware of looking backe, for God will not bee mocked; and of him that hath receiued much, much shal be demaunded.

3 If thou be single, and canst abstain, turne thy eies from vanitie; for there is a kinde of women bearing the faces of Angels, but the hearts of Deuils, able to intrap the elect if it were possible.

4 If thou bee married, forsake not the wife of thy youth to follow straunge flesh; for whoremongers and adulterers the Lord will iudge. The doore of a harlot leadeth downe to death, and in her lips there dwels destruction; her face is decked with

odors, but she bringeth a man to a morsell of bread and nakednes: of which my selfe am instance.' (p.41)

*Greenes Groatsworth of Witte* was followed in the same year by another pamphlet which carried the title *The Repentance of Robert Greene Maister of Artes* (1592). The subtitle explained the pamphlet as a confession 'Wherein by himselfe is laid open his loose life, with the manner of his death' (Greene, 1966b, title-page, p.3). This time Greene addressed himself 'To all the wanton youths of England', whom he earnestly entreated to make a 'reformation of [their] wilfulnes' (p.5) and 'pride':

> 'Companion to this vice [pride], is lust and lecherie, which is the viper, whose venome is incurable, and the onely sinne that in this life leadeth vnto shame, and after death vnto hell fire: for he that giueth himselfe ouer to harlots, selleth his soule to destruction, and maketh his bodie subiect to all incurable diseases.' (p.7)

After this cautionary preface, Robert Greene went on to give a detailed account of his own life after proceeding BA at Cambridge 1578–9. It appears that he then left England for postgraduate study in Italy and Spain, where he reports seeing and practising 'such villainie as is abhominable to declare' (p.20). Back in England, Greene informs the reader that 'being new come from Italy, (where I learned all the villanies vnder heauens) I was drownd in pride, whoredome was my daily exercise, and gluttony with drunkennes was my onely delight' (p.23). He confesses that 'I were sundry times afflicted with many foule and greeuous diseases, and thereby scourged with the rod of Gods wrath', but his repentance was short-lived, and, in his own phrase, he 'went again with the Sow to wallow in the mire' (p.10).

## GREENE'S DREADFUL END

In *The Repentance of Robert Greene*, the author also provides the reader with informa-tion of a more personal character, telling the story of how 'I married a Gentlemans daughter of good account, with whom I liued for a while: but forasmuch as she would perswade me from my wilfull wickednes, after I had a child by her, I cast her off, hauing spent vp the marriage money which I obtained by her' (Greene, 1966b, p.24). This happened in about 1586 after Greene had taken his MA in 1583 from Clare Hall, Cambridge. Settled in London where he worked as a poet and play-wright, Greene took for his mistress 'a sorry ragged queane' (Harvey, 1884–5, vol.1, p.169) who was the sister of Cutting Ball, a thief who ended his days at Tyburn. The woman bore Greene a son, ironically named Fortunatus, who would die young and only by a miracle could have escaped being born a congenital syphilitic.

Soon his father was himself to realize 'that vices haue ill endes as well as sweete beginnings' (Greene, 1966b, p.5). Rumours in London had it that Greene's death on September 3, 1592, was brought on by a surfeit of pickled herrings and Rhenish wine, enjoyed in the company of Thomas Nashe and other of Greene's cronies (Harvey, 1884–5, vol.1, p.162, 170). However, according to the poet's own account of his last days, his death would rather seem to have been an effect of tertiary syphilis with gummae. While Greene lay dying – 'deeplyer serched with sicknes than euer heretofore', 'sicknesse, riot, Incontinence hau[ing] at once shown their extremitie', according to his own report (Greene, 1966a, p.6) – he wrote a letter to his deserted wife and begged her forgiveness. Since a venereally infected husband would pass on the disease to his spouse and probably also to his child, Greene's final supplications to his wife may be viewed against a background of more than ordinary marital offence:

> 'That I haue offended thee highly I knowe, that thou canst forget my iniuries I hardly beleeue: yet perswade I my selfe, if thou saw my wretched estate, thou couldst not but lament it: nay certainly I know thou wouldst. All my wrongs muster themselues before mee, euery euill at once plagues mee. For my contempt of God, I am contemned of men: for my swearing and forswearing, no man will beleeue me: for my gluttony, I suffer hunger: for my drunkennes, thirst: for my adultery, vlcerous sores. Thus God hath cast me downe, that I might be humbled: and punished me for example of other sinners: and although he strangely suffers me in this world to perish without succor, yet trust I in the world to come to find mercie, by the merites of my Sauiour to whom I commend thee, and commit my soule.

Thy repentant husband for his disloyaltie, Robert Greene.' (p.51)

A medical report of Greene's last illness was also provided by Cuthbert Burby, the publisher of one of Greene's posthumous pamphlets, from whom we learn that Greene 'said that al his paine was in his belly', and that 'his belly sweld, and neuer left swelling vpward, vntill it sweld him at the hart and in his face' (Greene, 1881–6, vol.12, p.184). This might indicate that yet another cause of Greene's death could have been dropsy due to a cirrhosis of the liver, the final result of chronic alcoholism.

During the last month of his life, Greene was lodging with his mistress and their bastard son in the house of a shoemaker of Dowgate, one Isam, and his wife. From Mrs. Isam, the scholar Gabriel Harvey (1545?–1630) succeeded in obtaining a report of the poet's last days, 'for she loued him derely [and] told me of his lamentable begging of a penny pott of Malmesy: and, sir reuerence how lowsy he, and the mother of Infortunatus were (I would her Surgeon found her no worse, then lowsy)' (Harvey, 1884–5, vol.1, p.171). Harvey further learned from Mrs. Isam that on the poet's death she had crowned him with a garland of bays, in accordance with his last wish (p.172).

Harvey finishes his research of Robert Greene's career and works with a commemoration remarkable for its harshness and hostility. 'Who in London hath not heard of his dissolute, and licentious liuing', Harvey sums up the Bohemian's life, 'his fonde disguisinge of a Master of Arte with ruffianly haire, vnseemely apparell, and more vnseemelye Company…his riotous and outragious surfeitinge; his continuall shifting of lodginges: his plausible musteringe, and banquettinge of roysterly acquaintaunce at his first comminge; his beggarly departing in euery hostisses debt; [and] his infamous resorting to the Banckside, Shorditch, Southwarke, and other filthy hauntes' (pp.168–9).

## Two More Syphilitics of Greene's Entourage

Gabriel Harvey provided posterity with yet another portrait of a contemporary Bohemian, whom he viewed in a still more hostile light than Greene. This was the poet and pamphleteer Thomas Nashe, who had attacked Harvey's family and now tasted a savage counterattack in the latter's *Four Letters* (1592). Here Nashe was described with Greene as 'either meere Paper-bugs and inckehorne-pads: or a great deale worse...as the Ring-leaders of leaud Licentiousnes' (Harvey, 1884–5, vol.1, p.223).

In an ensuing polemical pamphlet entitled *Pierces Supererogation* (1593), Harvey listed Nashe among 'the slaues of that dominiering eloquence, that knoweth no Art but the cutting Arte; nor acknowledgeth any schoole, but the Curtisan schoole' (vol.2, p.52). 'Would it were not an infectious bane, or an incroching pocke' (p.52), Harvey added with a malicious innuendo at what he later termed Nashe's 'brothell Muse' and 'bawdye, and filthy Rymes, in the nastiest kind' (p.91).

Four years later Nashe was in for yet another attack on his aggressive journalism and dissolute living, this time by the barber-surgeon Richard Lichfield at Trinity College, Cambridge, where Nashe had studied as a young man. In a pamphlet entitled *Have with You to Saffron-Walden* (1596), Nashe had written about 'olde Dicke of Lichfield' that the barber-surgeon for all his 'dexteritie' had received no 'requitall' except for 'some few *french crownes*, pild Friers crownes, drye shauen' (Nashe, 1910, vol.3, p.6). Richard Lichfield retorted by disclosing that Nashe had lost his facial hair through syphilis – 'by chacing after whores, his beard away hath chast' (Harvey, 1884–5, vol.3, p.36; see also pp.38–9).

In his *Groatsworth of Witte* (1592), the dying Greene had addressed his 'olde consorts, which haue liued as loosely as my selfe' (Greene, 1966a, p.43), a statement which is commonly taken to refer to the poets Christopher Marlowe, Thomas Nashe, and George Peele. Christopher Marlowe (1564–93) was the greatest talent before Shakespeare and a known homosexual who proclaimed that 'all they that love not tobacco & Boyes are fooles' (Campbell and Quinn, 1966, p.500). Like the other members of literary and dramatic Bohemia, he lived a short and dangerous life: in 1593 he was stabbed to death in a tavern brawl at the age of 29. George Peele (1556–96) was another promising playwright whose life was cut short at the age of 30 by dissipation and disease. According to the literary historian Francis Meres (1565–1647), the cause of Peele's death was syphilis. 'As Anacreon died by the pot', he wrote in *Palladis Tamia* (1598), 'so George Peele by the pox' (Meres, 1938, fol.286$^v$).[*]

The greatest luminary of the Elizabethan and Jacobean stage was of course William Shakespeare, who must be viewed as a leading member of literary and dramatic Bohemia during the years he lived in the capital. This particular way of living was not only a consequence of his profession and of his separation from his family, but also one that suited certain features of his own personality. The chief evidence of Shakespeare's Bohemian tendencies is *Willobie His Avisa, Shakespeare's Sonnets*, John Manningham's contemporary talk of a more ephemeral intrigue, and the gossip in Oxford about Mistress Davenant. We shall examine this evidence in the chapters on Shakespeare (see pp.175–254).

CONCLUSION

High-risk groups for the contraction of syphilis were those composed of single young men, and, especially, of those who were sailors or soldiers or vagabonds.

---

[*]   See also Prouty, 1952–70, vol.1, pp.108, 113, 127.

Evidence shows that these groups were instrumental in the spread of syphilis during the period. Another high-risk group emerges with the numerous apprentices in London – also single young men – who were concentrated in the suburban districts where prostitution is known to have flourished. A third high-risk group surfaces with the student population at the Universities and the Inns of Court in London. Evidence is produced to show that syphilization occurred in these circles, both at home and abroad.

The members of the Royal Court were yet another high-risk group, and evidence shows that even high-ranking members of the nobility such as the Earl of Essex and the Duke of Buckingham were probably syphilitics.

The final high-risk group examined in this chapter is that which was formed by the leading members of London's literary and dramatic Bohemia, and available evidence indicates that Robert Greene, Thomas Nashe, and George Peele were also syphilitics.

# 8

# THE PROMISCUOUS CITY AND ITS STAGE REPRESENTATION

A German traveller visiting England around 1602 quoted a saying that 'England is a paradise for women, a prison for servants, and a hell or purgatory for horses', adding by way of explanation that 'the females have great liberty and are almost like masters, whilst the poor horses are worked very hard' (Harrison, 1908, p.1xx).

In 1599, another visitor from the Continent, the Swiss physician Thomas Platter, presented a similar impression of English women, and in particular those of London. 'There are a great many inns, taverns, and beergardens scattered about the city', he wrote in his diary,

> 'where much amusement may be had with eating, drinking, fiddling and the rest, as for instance in our hostelry, which was visited by players almost daily. And what is particularly curious is that the women as well as the men, in fact more often than they, will frequent the taverns or alehouses for enjoyment. They count it a great honour to be taken there and given wine with sugar to drink; and if one woman is invited, then she will bring three or four other women along and they gaily toast each other; the husband afterwards thanks him who has given his wife such pleasure, for they deem it a real kindness.' (Platter, 1937, p.170)

## THE COURTSHIP OF THE SEXES IN LONDON

Such *joie de vivre* and such liberal customs explain the worried letter which a gentleman sent a female member of his family in 1603 on the occasion of her movement to the capital. 'Your Sex (Cousin) is of it selfe prone and propense vnto pleasure', he told her, 'and *London* is a place fuller of prouocatiues to Sinne: your Beauty shall there hourely meete with forcible temptations, though haply in the harmlesse country the fortresse of your chastity found no assaylants' (Breton, 1879, vol.2, p.7). Life in the City obviously presented a more dangerous environment to a young woman than life in the countryside, not only because of the capital's many entertainments but also because of its greater opportunities for sexual encounters.

The courtship of the sexes in the bustling metropolis found its most colourful expression in fashion, which made the tailors of London the busiest of craftsmen. In his *Itinerary* (1617), Fynes Moryson says of his countrymen that 'they haue in this one age worne out all the fashions of *France* and all the nations of *Europe*...If I should begin to set downe the variety of fashions and forraign stuffes brought into

*England* in these times, I might seeme to number the starres of Heauen and sands of the Sea' (Harrison, 1908, pp.278, 280). Moryson especially noticed a fashion among his female countrymen which considerably enhanced their sexual attraction. 'Gentlewomen virgins weare gownes close to the body, and aprons of fine linnen', he observed, 'and often ruffes, both starched, and chaines of pearle about the necke, with their brests naked…the young married Gentlewomen no lesse then the Virgins, shew their breasts naked' (pp.281–2).

Figure 32. The woodcut shows the bubonic plague as depicted on the title-page of Thomas Dekker's pamphlet *A Rod for Runawayes* (1625). The most deadly medical scourge in England during the 16th and 17th centuries, the plague regularly decimated the population and struck the country with particular virulence in the years 1504–5, 1514–5, 1526, 1530–2, 1536–8, 1542–3, 1548, 1551, 1558, 1563, 1593, 1597, 1603, 1608–10, 1625, 1636, and 1665 (Shrewsbury, 1970, pp.157–538). It is a testimony to the contagiousness and spread of syphilis during the same period that the disease was frequently compared to the plague and endowed with such epithets as the 'French pestilence' or the 'Naples pestilence' (Marston, 1966, pp.31, 72). In Middleton's *The Phoenix* (1603–4), the Jewish Wife is presented as 'one of those For whose close lusts the plague ne' er leaves the city. Thou worse than common! private, subtle harlot!' (5,1:227–9). 'If she enter here, the house will be infected', Bellamont asserts of a promiscuous woman in Webster's and Dekker's *Northward Hoe* (1607), 'the plague is not half so dangerous as a Shee-hornet' (5,1:367–8). Dekker's plays and pamphlets teem with references to syphilis, which in *Westward Hoe* (1605) is described as a disease that is 'as catching as the plague, though not all so general' (4,1:83–4).

In *The Seven Deadly Sinnes of London* (1606), written only three years after the catastrophe of 1603, Dekker admonishes his native city: 'Sicknes was sent to breathe her vnholsome ayres into thy nosthrils, so that thou, that wert before the only Gallant and Minion of the world, hadst in a short time more diseases (then a common Harlot hath) hanging vpon thee; thou suddenly becamst the by-talke of neighbors, the scorne and contempt of Nations' (Dekker, 1884–6, vol.2, pp.10–1). The reason: 'O London, thou art great in glory, and enuied for thy greatnes: thy Towers, thy Temples, and thy Pinnacles stand vpon thy head like borders of fine gold, thy waters like frindges of siluer hang at the hemmes of thy garments. Thou art the goodliest of thy neighbors, but the prowdest; the welthiest, but the most wanton. Thou hast all things in thee to make thee fairest, and all things in thee to make thee foulest: for thou art attir'de like a Bride, drawing all that looke vpon thee to be in loue with thee, but there is much harlot in thine eyes. Thou sitst in thy Gates heated with Wines, and in thy Chambers with lust' (Ibid., pp.10–1. Cf. also Thomas Lodge and Robert Greene: *A Looking Glasse for London and England* (1598) (5,5:2265–72). (Greene, 1905, vol.1, p.214).

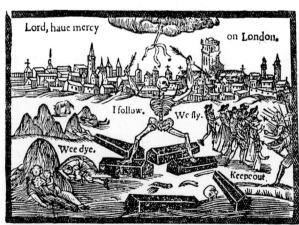

Printed at London for *Iohn Trundle*, and are to be sold at his Shop in Smithfield. 1625.

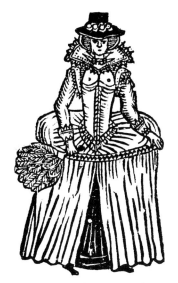

Figure 33. The woodcut adorns a ballad entitled *The Cruel Shrow* and shows a gentlewoman dressed in the fashion of the time, with broad-brimmed felt hat, ruff, corset and farthingale (vertugale) (*Roxburghe Ballads*, vol.3, p.175). The woman's heavy armour of wired clothes is subtly broken by 'those milk paps That through the window-bars bore at all men's eyes', as the protagonist of Shakespeare's *Timon of Athens* observes (4,3:117–8). The tempting aspect of the décolletée fashions of Elizabethan and Jacobean England was emphasized by Lewis Wager's interlude *The Life and Repentaunce of Marie Magdalene* (1566), in which Pride, Cupidity and Carnal Concupiscence tell the wanton girl of the New Testament:

> Your garments must be so worne alway
> That your white pappes may be seene, if you may.
> If young gentlemen may see your white skin,
> It will allure them to loue, and soone bryng hem in.
> Both damsels and wiues vse many such feates.
> I know them that will lay out their faire teates,
> Purposely men to allure vnto their loue. (Wager, 1904, pp.28–9, lines 588–94)

It was the lot of one of the Puritans of the time, Stephen Gosson (1554–1624), to point out a dangerous aspect of too sexy fashions and too much freewheeling in an urbanized society:

> These naked paps, the deuils ginnes,
> to worke vaine gazers painfull thrall...
> These Holland smockes, so white as snowe
> and gorgets braue, with drawn work wrought:
> A tempting ware they are you know,
> wherewith (as nets) vaine youth are caught.
> But manie times they rue the match
> When poxe & pyles by whores they catch!
> (Gosson, 1595, sig.A4ʳ. See also Camden, 1975, p.224)

The fashion was an old one, for as early as 1565 the poet and surgeon John Hall (1529?–66) observed in his *Court of Vertue:*

> When I was a boy, I nowe well remember,
> (Though I at that tyme of age were but tender)
> That women theyr breastes dyd shew & lay out.
> And wel was that mayd whose dugs then were stoute.
> Which vsance at fyrst came vp in the stues,
> Which mens wyues and daughters after dyd vse. (Hall, 1961, p.351)

The seductive intent of the new fashion was also surmised by Nashe who, in *Christs Teares over Jerusalem* (1593), complained that 'Theyr breasts they embuske vp on hie, and theyr round Roseate buds immodestly lay foorth, to shew at theyr handes there is fruite to be hoped' (Nashe, 1910, vol.2, p.137). 'What shold we thynk of the women that in London we se?', another shrewd observer of the fair sex, Robert Crowley, wondered around the middle of the 16th century:

> For more wanton lokes,
> I dare boldely saye,
> Were neuer in Iewyshe whores,
> then in London wyues thys daye.
> And if gate and garmentes
> do shewe any thynge,
> Our wiues do passe their whoris
> in whorelyke deckynge...
> Hyr face faire paynted,
> to make it shyne bryght,
> And hyr bosome all bare,
> and most whorelyke dight. (Figure 33)

'I haue tolde them but trueth', the Puritan Crowley concludes his epigram with a flourish, 'let them saye what they wyll; I haue sayde they be whorelike, and so I saye styll' (Crowley, 1872, pp.44–5). The 'whorelike' impression conveyed by London's women was noted by other observers, although the behaviour of the men does not appear to have differed in any conspicuous way from that of women.

This appears with particular clarity in a new theatrical craze in London's flourishing world of entertainment known as Jacobean City Comedy. The new genre provides an interesting look at the promiscuous habits of the citizens of the English capital, just as it conveys information about the medical consequences of such habits. In one of these city comedies, a country wench's father speaks of London as 'This man devouring city...where I spent My unshapen youth, to be my age's curse' (*Michaelmas Term*,2,2:20–2).

## JACOBEAN CITY COMEDY: MONEY AND SEX MAKE THE WORLD GO AROUND

Around the turn of the century, the gory tragedies, patriotic chronicle-plays and romantic comedies of the Elizabethan stage gave way to a new genre known as Jacobean City Comedy. This genre offered a true to life presentation of London society and brought with it a new immediacy and freshness, providing the audience with theatrical versions of themselves, and furnishing an outlet for satiric descriptions of contemporary events. The lasting success of citizen comedies was due in part to the fact that Londoners could find in these plays a mirror of society with its fads and fashions, errors and follies, vices and ambitions, lust and greed.

Jacobean City Comedy presents a society devoted to trade, profit, promiscuity and unprincipled competition, the latter including the game between the sexes. The stage of the citizen comedies is one of warehouses and whorehouses, vaults and granaries, docks and banks, inns and prisons and – now and then – a church. The stock characters are those of whores and rogues, ambitious merchants and grasping usurers, reckless prodigals and swaggering gallants, flirtatious women and pleasure-hating puritans. In addition to their financial intrigues and legal tricks, the majority of the comedies are concerned with promiscuity in a variety of forms, ranging from lechery and whoredom to fornication, adultery and cuckoldry. The plots never weary of describing seducers' attacks on women's chastity and wives' cuckolding of their husbands.

If money makes the world go round, sex is the pleasure of its whirligig. In the mercantile society described in Jacobean City Comedy, money and sex are often merged, as in Jonson's *The Devil Is an Ass* (1616), where Meercraft asserts that

> money's a whore, a bawd, a drudge;
> Fit to run out on errands: let her go.
> *Via, pecunia!* (2,1:38)

Not surprisingly, Jonson also states in his *Staple of News* (1626) that 'Pecunia' is 'The talk o' the time! the adventure of the age…The Venus of the time and state' (1,2:183–4;2,1:210).

By about 1605, City Comedy becomes established with such plays as Jonson's *Volpone*, Marston's *The Dutch Courtesan*, Middleton's *Michaelmas Term*, and Dekker's and Webster's *Westward Hoe* and *Northward Hoe*. (The two last plays proved such a success that they inspired the parody *Eastward Hoe* (1605) by Chapman, Jonson and Marston, who cashed in on the farcical river journey taken by London character types as described by Dekker and Webster). *Westward Hoe* (1604) and *Northward Hoe* (1605) and Middleton's *The Familie of Love* (1608) represent the flower of Jacobean City Comedy and are highly representative of the new genre. An examination of the plots of the three comedies will serve to acquaint the reader with the ingredients of the new theatrical craze.

The mainplot and subplot of *Westward Hoe* are linked by the Italian merchant Justiniano, who, furious at his wife's supposed infidelity, determines to unmask the immorality of all city wives. Disguised as a writing-master, Justiniano provides the wives of three London merchants with gallants and arranges secret meetings for them. The wives at first respond with an eagerness that confirms the merchant's low estimation of their morals, and the tone of these early scenes is one of joking acceptance of immorality.

The women agree to go to 'Brainford' (the modern Brentford) with their gallants and spend the night there, but they prove to be willing only to flirt with the men. Their sense of mischief which led them to Brainford also leads them to lock the doors when the three gallants finally arrive:

> 'They shall know that citizens' wives have wit enough to outstrip twenty such gulls; though we are merry, let's not be mad; be as wanton as new married wives, as fantastic and light-headed to the eye, as feather-makers, but as pure about the heart, as if we dwelt amongst 'em in Blackfriars.' (5,1:159–63)

Meanwhile, their husbands are on their way to Brainford, hot with indignation and led by Justiniano. However, when they get there, the tables are turned on them as they were on the gallants. Not only are their suspicions proved groundless, but their own clandestine visits to the brothel of the bawd Birdlime are revealed. 'Have we smelt you out, foxes?', their wives laugh with glee, 'Do you come after us with hue and cry when you are the thieves yourselves?' (5,4:236–8).

The subplot of the comedy has an added twist in the attempt of a lecherous old Earl to seduce Mistress Justiniano, who has been abandoned by her husband and is afraid that she may be forced to accept the Earl's proposition in order to survive. Like so many of her female contemporaries, Mistress Justiniano's attitude to vice is merely a reluctant acceptance of it as better than starvation (1,1:203–5). But when she sees the Earl, she is revolted by the picture of aged lechery he presents – 'I wonder lust can hang at such white hairs' (2,2:83) – and with indignation she rejects him. During their second meeting, the profligate Earl is shamefully outwitted by Justiniano, disguised as a woman and masked, and the comedy ends on a note of repentance and reconciliation between the marital partners.

In *Northward Hoe* (1605), Dekker and Webster once more picture the freewheeling life of London's fun-loving citizens, sugared over with the final triumph of virtue over vice. Once more they present a comedy of attempted cuckoldry and adulterous intrigue and its cast is the familiar parade: citizens, gallants, wives, and a whore and her entourage. The sex-formula is the same as that of its predecessor – 'all is but a merriment, all but a May game' (*Westward Hoe*, 5,4:278) – and once again moral pronouncements and trickery are blended and sex seen as a game with predictable rules: 'March then, this curse is on all lechers thrown, They give horns and at last, horns are their own' (4,1:281–2).

The lecher in this play is the gallant Greenshield who has been paying court to Mistress Mayberry, a citizen's wife. Typically, Greenshield's primary motive is not love for the woman but a desire to translate into action his cynical belief that all city wives are lecherous. When she refuses him, Greenshield takes a mean sort of revenge by pretending to Mayberry that he has actually lain with his wife. As proof he produces Mistress Mayberry's ring which he has obtained by force after his vain attempt to seduce her. This drives citizen Mayberry to a frenzy of jealousy, but Mayberry is finally convinced by his wife's denial of the charge, and the rest of the action is taken up with his comic revenge on Greenshield. This unpleasant lecher is proved a cuckold himself by his wife Kate, who takes up an affair with Featherstone, Greenshield's companion. Kate's adultery is presented as a laughing matter and as a means of defeating her husband in the game of sex. The play gives the amusing presentation of adultery as a good joke against a bad husband, along with a straightforward dramatization of a chaste wife.

In Middleton's comedy *The Familie of Love* (1608), adultery runs riot. Practically the only characters who do not attempt or commit it are the lovers Gerardine and Maria who are not married and so have to make do with fornication. Bedding other people's wives is a game that everyone tries to play, and the only standards that have any meaning are those of success or failure in the game.

In Jacobean City Comedy, lecherous gallants who attempt seduction generally come off badly. This is seen in particular in the play's two representatives of the type, Lipsalve and Gudgeon. Initially, the two gallants confidently express the conviction of other promiscuous men in the city that sex may be had everywhere and with females of all ages:

> Since every place now yields a wench;
> If one will not, another will:
> And, if what I have heard be true,
> Then young and old and all will do. (1,2:48–51)

However, when their eyes fall on the beautiful and flirtatious Mistress Purge, a citizen's wife, they find that the game is more difficult to play that they imagine. Outwitted by rival and more successful lechers, their deepest humiliation comes at the hand of Glister, a barber-surgeon whom they consult for advice on how to win Mistress Purge. He tricks them into performing an elaborate conjuring ritual during which they whip each other soundly, but Glister's motives are not those of moral correction; he resents the gallants' designs on Mistress Purge because he is sleeping with her himself.

Adultery, fornication, and whoredom are such common features of Citizen Comedy that prostitutes sometimes figure as protagonists in the plays. In Dekker's *The Honest Whore*, the prostitute Bellafront is the heroine of the play, and in Marston's *The Dutch Courtesan* (1605), the prostitute Franceschina functions as the centre of dramatic action. The discussions about prostitution in the opening scenes of the latter play present the institution as inseparable from city life and indicate commercial exploitation itself as having two sides: that of venereal disease, hypocrisy, degradation and crime on the one hand, and amusement, easy profits, and physical gratification on the other. There is insistence in these discussions regarding prostitution that business is business, that life in London is hard, and that a puritanical obsession with sexual vice only helps obscure the equally harsh facts of other kinds of business and trade.

Cocledemoy, a knavish and witty citizen in *The Dutch Courtesan*, aptly observes that

> 'no trade or vocation profiteth but by the loss and displeasure of another – as the merchant thrives not but by the licentiousness of giddy and unsettled youth, the laywer but by the vexation of his client, the physician but by the maladies of his patient – only my smooth-gumm'd bawd lives by others' pleasure, and only grows rich by others' rising. O merciful gain! O righteous income!' (1,2:42–8)[*]

Another of the figures in the play, young Freevill, points out that survival must come first in the struggle for life in the urban jungle, and frankly presents an ironic view of prostitution as a model for all forms of city enterprise:

> 'Every man must follow his trade, and every woman her occupation. A poor, decayed mechanical man's wife, her husband is laid up; may not she lawfully be laid down when her husband's only rising is by his wife's falling? A captain's wife wants means, her commander lies in open field abroad; may not she lie in civil arms at home? A waiting gentlewoman, that had wont to take say to her lady, miscarries or so; the court misfortune throws her down; may not the city courtesy take her up? Do you know no alderman would pity such a woman's case?' (1,1:94–103)

---

[*] Quoted after John Marston: *The Dutch Courtesan*, edited by M.L. Wine. Regents Renaissance Drama Series. London, 1965.

For all his praise of bawds and whoredom, the promiscuous Freevill cannot help concluding his observations on prostitution by underscoring the inherently danger-ous nature of women who 'sell the pleasure of a wanton bed' (1,1:122):

> 'They will give *quid* for *quo*: do ye protest, they'll swear; do you rise, they'll fall; do you fall, they'll rise; do you give them the French crown, they'll give you the French – *O justus justa justum!'* (1,1:115–8)

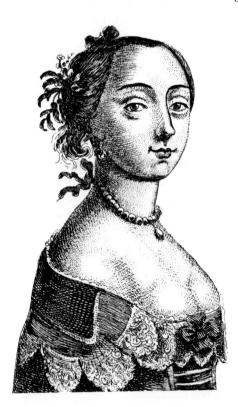

Figure 34. Seventeenth century engraving in the Mansell Collection (reproduced in Burford, 1973, p.48). Middleton's poem *Microcynicon* (1599) anticipates the preoccupation of Ja-cobean City Comedy with appearance and reality, hypocrisy and vice, glamour and dis-ease, outward show and inner rottenness. In the poem, Middleton launches a fierce attack on the call girls of his time, beautiful and charming like the above picture of one of them ('Sophia Broom, 5 guineas per night'). 'List, ye profane, fair-painted images', he apostro-phizes them with scorn,

Ill-favour'd idols, pride anatomy,
Foul-colour'd puppets...
Where sin, the mistress of disgrace,
Hath residence and her abiding place;
And sin, though it be foul, yet fair in this,
In being painted with a show of bliss;
For what more happy creature to the eye
Than is Superbia in her bravery?
Yet who more foul, disrobèd of attire?
Pearl'd with the botch, as children burnt
                with fire;
That for their outward cloak upon the skin,
Worser enormities abound within.
      (Middleton, 1885–6, vol.8, pp.123–4)

A stronger version of the same theme is found in Cyril Tourneur's *The Revenger's Tragedy* (1608), where the dramatic climax is the scene of revelation in which Vendici makes an arrangement to revenge himself on the old, licentious Duke. Vendici's betrothed had some years earlier committed suicide rather than submit to the Duke, and when the Duke commissions Vendici, now disguised as Piato, to find a young girl for him, Vendici fetches the skull of Gloriana, his dead beloved. He dresses it in rich, hanging silks, veils it and smears its lips with poison. Revenge is accomplished by leading the Duke to this 'bony lady' (Tourneur, 1878, vol.2, p.86) and encouraging the old lecher to kiss her after convincing him that she is beautiful. The stark symbolism of the kiss and the skull is meant to render the true image of lust: beauty is no more than a skull dressed in gorgeous coverings, the illicit embrace is not life clasping life but death touching death, and the lecherous kiss is the seal on the death warrant.

An example of such justice is Malheureux, Freevill's friend, who is brought to final despair through his relations with Franceschina, the prostitute heroine of the play. 'That I, a man of sense', he complains, 'should conceive endless pleasure in a body whose soul I know to be so hideously black!' (3,1:235–6). To which Freevill makes the appropriate reply: 'That a man at twenty-three should cry, "O sweet pleasure!" and at forty-three should sigh, "O sharp pox!"' (3,1:237–8).

Syphilis as the agent of divine justice also surfaces in Jacobean City Comedy, in which urban promiscuity and gaiety are often followed by the retributive trio of 'pox…barber surgeons and…diet-drink' (*The Dutch Courtesan*, 1,2:22–4). A similar connection between dissipation and medical chastisement is expressed in Rowlands's parody of the genre in *Diogines Lanthorne* (1607), in which the old philosopher in his tub one day spots a number of these stock characters in the crowded streets of the city:

> 'Oh tis *Prodigallitie* and his whore, a Gentleman and a Gentlewoman, they are walking towards the suburbs of a Bawdiehouse for their recreation: younder rides the Bawde in her Coach before, and they two come leysurely (with the pox) behinde, but will all meete together anone to make worke for the Chirurgion, who will answer their loose bodyes with the squirt.' (Rowlands, 1880, vol.1, p.6)

The medical consequences of whoredom and promiscuity are also strongly on the mind of the prodigal hero of Middleton's *A Trick to Catch the Old One* (1608), in which Witgood at the end of the play renounces the follies and vices of his youth. Having got his girl and recovered his social respectability, the redeemed prodigal assumes a kneeling position as the curtain falls to make this confession on behalf of himself and all promiscuous inhabitants of the Jacobean capital:

> And here for ever I disclaim
> The cause of youth's undoing, game…
> Soul-wasting surfeits, sinful riots,
> Queans' evils, doctors' diets,
> 'Pothecaries' drugs, surgeons' glisters;
> Stabbing of arms for a common mistress;
> Riband favours, ribald speeches;
> Dear perfum'd jackets, pennyless breeches;
> Dutch flapdragons, healths in urine;
> Drabs that keep a man too sure in:
> I do defy you all.
> Lend me each honest hand, for here I rise
> A reclaim'd man, loathing the general vice. (5,2:191–205)

'Pox was the reality which undermined many of the pretensions of urban life and symbolized its vice and falsity', Margaret Pelling observes in a central paragraph of her study of the barber-surgeons of London – an observation which may also be applied to many of the medical and moral lessons taught by the authors of Jacobean City Comedy.

'It lay in wait as the common punishment of peers who wasted their substance, foolish gentlefolk who left the country for the city, and city tradespeople with social aspirations. Felons and beggars were branded by the iron, or had their ears lopped; the physical effects of the pox served in like manner to punish other kinds of social transgression. When it emerged from its hiding places in the body, pox often betrayed the difference between appearance and reality, between bravado and pretended distinction and the common rottenness inside.' (Pelling, 1986, pp.104, 99)

## CONCLUSION

Contemporary sources indicate that women in England, and in particular in London, had considerable freedom and that liberal mores prevailed in the sprawling metropolis. Jacobean City Comedy also reflects this liberal attitude in that it depicts the freewheeling life of a bourgeois society enjoying a growing economic prosperity while regarding sex as yet another area of consumption and unprincipled competition.

Promiscuity and prostitution were salient features of the new theatrical craze, which to a certain extent reflected the conditions of society in general. Promiscuity was furthered by economic prosperity, social inequality, increasing consumption, and the rise of an entertainment industry which also commercialized prostitution.

A factor contributing to the loosening of morals was the social disintegration rampant in the expanding cities – above all London – where overcrowding, unemployment, poverty and crime furthered prostitution and its concomitant spread of venereal diseases. Jacobean City Comedy also depicts this situation with its numerous references to brothels, pox, barber-surgeons, and medical treatments for venereal disease.

# 9

# SHAKESPEARE AND HIS CIRCLE

One is tempted to include *Willobie His Avisa* (1594) in the genre of Jacobean City Comedy although the collection of poems is neither a Jacobean product, nor located in the city, nor written as a comedy. However, *Avisa* anticipates the new literary trend by its cast of lechers placed in a bourgeois and mercantile setting, and by its love games and adulterous intrigues, which serve the author as a vehicle for satiric vision and moral comment.

## WILLOBIE HIS AVISA

The book was entered in the Stationers' Register on September 3, 1594, under the title *Willobie His Avisa. Or the True Picture of a Modest Maid, and of a Chast and Constant Wife.*[*] The publication was so popular that it went into six editions in forty years, but the success of *Avisa* does not appear to have been appreciated by the authorities. They disliked the book so strongly that it was included in the category of books to be burned in June 1599, in the 'bishops' bonfire' of Archbishop Whitgift. The books burned on that occasion were such works as *Pygmalion, The Scourge of Villainy*, Davies's *Epigrammes* and *The Fifteen Joys of Marriage*. These works were primarily pornographic or contained personal satire of an offensive nature, and *Avisa* was apparently classed in the second category. *Willobie His Avisa* (1594) is a third-rate moral poem of love's labours lost and is composed under the immediate influence of Shakespeare's narrative poems *Venus and Adonis* (1593) and *The Rape of Lucrece* (1594). *Willobie His Avisa* adopts the well-known rhyme scheme of *Venus and Adonis*, but secures a faster movement by cutting the five-foot meter to four feet and by throwing the narrative more conspicuously into dialogue. Organized in short 'cantos', the poem introduces a more essential novelty by replacing mythological voluptuousness with the love adventures of a real woman, Avisa, 'vertues birde' (Willoby, 1966, p.21). With its flat and boyishly immature verse, *Avisa* emerges as a typical undergraduate production – also apparent in the poem's strange blend of high morals and lewd adventures.

The authorship of *Willobie His Avisa* seems purposely wrapped in a mantle of mystification and self-contradiction. The work is introduced by a student of Oxford,

---

[*] Willobie His Avisa (1594) is quoted after the reprint in Elizabethan and Jacobean Quartos, no.9, edited by G.B. Harrison. Edinburgh, 1966.

Hadrian Dorrell, in an Epistle Dedicatory 'To all the constant Ladies & Gentle-women of England that feare God'. This is followed by an 'Epistle to the gentle & courteous Reader' in which Hadrian Dorrell relates how not long since

> 'my very good frend and chamber fellow M. Henry Willobie, a yong man, and a scholler of very good hope, being desirous to see the fashions of other countries for a time, departed voluntarily to her Maiesties seruice. Who at his departure, chose me amongst the rest of his frendes, vnto whome he reposed so much trust, that he deliuered me the key of his study, and the vse of all his bookes till his returne. Amongest which (perusing them at leysure,) I found many prety & witty conceites, as I suppose of his owne dooing. One among the rest I fancied so much, that I haue ventered so farre vpon his frendship, as to publish it without his consent.' (p.5)

In addition to Henry Willobie and Hadrian Dorrell, two more Oxford students seem to have been attached to the riddling production. Dorrell's two epistles are followed by two commendatory poems, the first one signed 'Abell Emet', 'in commendation of Willobies Auisa', the second one signed 'Contraria Contrarijs: Vigilantius: Dormitanus', 'in praise of Willobie his Auisa, Hexameton to the Author' (pp.18–9). It is in the latter poem that we find the earliest direct mention of a work by Shakespeare in English literature:

> Yet *Tarquyne* pluckt his glistering grape.
> And *Shake-speare*, paints poore *Lucrece* rape. (p.19)

While everything points to the fact that *Avisa* seems to have originated in Oxford student circles, it is obvious that it was published with the aim of satirizing and scandalizing certain persons of great importance, so great, in fact, that the scandals about them were still commercially worth retailing forty years later.

     A good deal of heated controversy went on over the intention of the book, and in the 'Apologie' of the second edition of *Avisa* it appears that Hadrian Dorrell finally stuck out his neck to 'show the true meaning of *Willobie His Avisa'*, or the real intention of those behind the book:

> 'This plaine Morall deuice was plotted only for the repression and opening of *Vice*, and to the exaltation and triumph of *Vertue*...For it seemeth rather to me that the Author intending some rare exploit, endeuoured to describe the doubtful combat, that is daily fought betweene Vice and Vertue, two princes of great power. And to that end he chose out two of the most approued Captaines of both the Campes to trie the quarrell. Out of the one hee tooke *Luxuriam*, Lecherie, which as we see, swayeth the minds of the greatest men, and commandeth largely. Out of the other, he opposeth *Castitatem*, Chastitie, a souldier rarely seene (in these dayes) to resist the enemies Push.' (p.239)

After this edifying sermon, Hadrian Dorrell-Henry Willobie sets out to relate the story of an inkeeper's beautiful and charming wife, who is beleaguered by a number of 'lawlesse suters' (p.244) 'in pursuit of their fancied fooleries' (p.244) – a set of 'lust-led youth' (p.21) seeking only the satisfaction of their 'fleshly concupiscence' and 'wicked pleasures' (pp.243–4).

A STORY OF 'LUST-LED YOUTH, OF WICKED LOVE'[*]

Among the many suitors in the spicy poem is a certain amorous young man called 'H.W.' who 'more furiously inuaedeth his loue, & more pathetically indureth then all the rest' (p.8). His ardent suit is encouraged by his 'familiar frend' (p.116), a certain 'W.S.', who is more closely described in a prose passage placed under Canto XLIII. Here the two libertines are presented in metaphorical terms relating to medicine and to venereal diseases and their treatment:

> 'H.W. being sodenly infected with the contagion of a fantasticall fit, at the first sight of A [visa] pyneth a while in secret griefe, at length not able any longer to indure the burning heate of so feruent a humour, be wrayeth the secresy of his disease vnto his familiar frend W. S. who not long before had tryed the curtesy of the like passion, and was now newly recouered of the like infection; yet finding his frend let bloud in the same vaine, he took pleasure for a tyme to see him bleed & in steed of stopping the issue, he inlargeth the wound, with the sharpe rasor of a willing conceit, perswading him that he thought it a matter very easy to be compassed, & no doubt with payne, diligence & some cost in time to be obtayned. Thus this miserable comforter comforting his frend with an impossibilitie, eyther for that he now would secretly laugh at his frends folly, that had giuen occasion not long before vnto others to laugh at his owne, or because he would see whether an other could play his part better then himselfe, & in vewing a far off the course of this louing Comedy, he determined to see whether it would sort to a happier end for this new actor, then it did for the old player. But at length this Comedy was like to haue growen to a Tragedy, by the weake & feeble estate that H.W. was brought vnto, by a desperate vewe of an impossibility of obtaining his purpose, til Time & Necessity, being his best Phisitions brought him a plaster, if not to heale, yet in part to ease his maladye. In all which discourse is liuely represented the vnrewly rage of vnbrydeled fancy, hauing the raines to roue at liberty, with the dyuers & sundry changes of affections & temptations, which Will, set loose from Reason, can deuise. &c.' (pp.115-7)

In the course of their friendly conversation, H.W. pours out his amorous troubles to W.S., whom he calls 'my faythfull frend, That like assaultes hath often tryde' (p.119). The elder and more experienced friend then proceeds to give him good advice as to how Avisa may be brought down. 'She is no Saynt, She is no Nonne, I thinke in tyme she may be wonne' (p.121), the 'old player' consoles his friend, recommending persistence, gifts, and flattery – 'wicked wiles to deceaue witles women' (p.122), as amplified by the marginal note. After his words of consolation, W.S. disappears from the scene, and his worldly-wise advice, whether offered ironically or not, is naturally of no avail to H.W. in his fruitless pursuit of Avisa, the paragon of wives.

The odd conjunction of the initials 'W.S.' and the references to 'Comedy', 'Tragedy', 'Will' (the poet's pet name in the *Sonnets*), a 'new actor' and an 'old player' is to many scholars irrefutable evidence of Shakespeare's identity. This is further strengthened by the allusion to *The Rape of Lucrece* by 'Vigilantius Dormitanus' in the commendatory verse and by the words in which W.S. attempts to console H.W.: 'She is no Saynt, She is no Nonne, I thinke in tyme she may be wonne'. This is certainly a parody of well-known lines from *1 Henry VI* (5,3:78–9), *Richard III*

---

[*]  Willoby, 1966, p.21

(1,2:232–3), and *Titus Andronicus* (2,1:82–3) – all plays which first appeared on the London stage in the period 1590–94.

The identification of H.W. has not presented scholars with insurmountable difficulties either, for Shakespeare's poems *Venus and Adonis* and *The Rape of Lucrece*, whose rhyme scheme *Avisa* imitates, were both dedicated to Henry Wriothesley, third Earl of Southampton (1573–1624) and William Shakespeare's youthful patron – only twenty years old at the time of the registration of *Avisa*. (According to the poem, H.W. is a 'headlong youth' (p.129) who says of himself that 'If yeares I want, why I will stay' (p.138). 'The love I dedicate to your Lordship is without end', the poet exuberantly proclaims in the *Lucrece* dedication from 1594 – the year of the publication of Avisa: 'What I have done is yours, what I have to do is yours, being part in all I have devoted yours'.*

The Oxford students' picture of William Shakespeare is clearly that of a Bohemian and libertine who is the ringleader of an aristocratic jetset specializing in the courtship of beautiful ladies. This picture is underscored by the fact that Shakespeare's poems and plays from this period reveal him as an expert on the subject of romantic love – with *Venus and Adonis* (1593), *The Rape of Lucrece* (1594), *Love's Labour's Lost* (1594–5), and *Romeo and Juliet* (1594–5) as classic expressions of romantic love and unbridled passions.

### Shakespeare's Sonnets: 'Love Is My Sin' (142)

*Shakespeare's Sonnets* (1609) shows him in the same light as *Avisa*, only the poet is here accompanied by another young aristocrat with the initials 'W. H.'. There is general agreement that this figure is identical with the fair youth of the *Sonnets* and that Shakespeare's poems describe the youth to be a boyish aristocrat to whom his admirer feels socially inferior (36).

Shakespeare's sonnets are passionate, directed to specific persons and seemingly autobiographical. They indicate that their author had deep-seated emotional attachments to a 'dark lady' and to a 'beauteous and lovely youth' (54) whom he praises in words that seem to raise friendship to a level more Greek than English.

The heterosexual love story of the *Sonnets* is told by the sequence of poems 127–152, and the story they tell is about the poet's 'Poor soul, the centre of my sinful earth' (146). The poet's mistress in the *Sonnets* is an unknown gentlewoman playing the virginals (128) and appearing as a dark beauty (132) with 'raven black' (127) 'mourning eyes' (132). Known in literature as the 'dark lady', she also emerges as a married woman, a wife who 'In act [her] bed-vow broke' (152), as did the poet himself, to engage in an illicit sexual affair. They are both presented as adulterous

---

\*    Willoby, 1966, pp.216–7. The smoke screen produced by *Avisa* to hide the identity of 'H.W.' even includes the poem's spurious author, called Henry Willobego at the head of Canto XLIV (ibid., p.115). Yet Hadrian Dorrell professes his own uncertainty about the identification of 'H.W.' with the author of the poem (ibid., p.8), just as 'H.W.' is once more wrapped in a mantle of mystification at the end of the episode (ibid., p.170). Donald W. Foster, who has written on the initials 'W.S.' in literature printed during the years 1570–1630, identifies *Avisa's* 'W.S.' with William Shakespeare, but thinks that the poem's 'H.W.' is identical with a real Henry Willoughby who studied at Oxford 1591–94 (Foster, 1989, pp.187–91). G.B. Harrison identifies 'H.W.' with Henry Wriothesley, Earl of Southampton, and 'W.S.' with William Shakespeare (Willoby, 1966, pp.213–20).

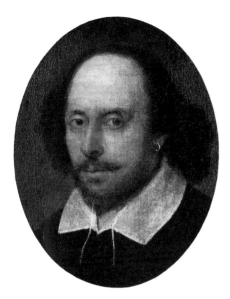

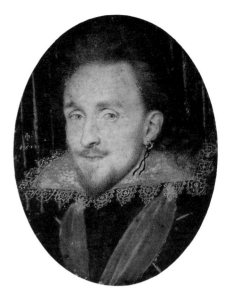

Figure 35. John Taylor (c. 1608): William Shakespeare. Chandos portrait. National Portrait Gallery, London.

Figure 36. Isaac Oliver: William Herbert, 3rd Earl of Pembroke. The Folger Library.

*Shakespeare's Sonnets* was published in 1609 by Thomas Thorpe, who furnished them with a dedication 'To the onlie begetter of these insuing sonnets Mr. W. H.', whom Chambers identifies with William Herbert, third Earl of Pembroke (1580–1630). Significantly, Heminges and Condell dedicated the First Folio (1623) to Herbert and his brother Philip, Earl of Montgomery, because, as they explain in the dedication, both men 'haue beene pleas'd to thinke these trifles something, heeretofore; and haue prosequuted both them, and their Authour liuing, with so much fauour' (Chambers, 1930, vol.2, p.228).* The dedication of the Folio to William Herbert instead of Henry Wriothesley, Earl of Southampton and Shakespeare's patron, who was still alive, is the major point in the argument identifying Pembroke as Mr. W. H. The other argument is age. Southampton (1573–1624) was too old to be called a 'boy' (108,126) by the middle of the 1590s, and so William Herbert, born in 1580, is the best candidate for the fair youth of the *Sonnets*, who would be 14–15 when they began c. 1594–5 and who would grow into sexual maturity in the following 'Three winters…[and] three summers' (104) described by the *Sonnets*. Iconographical evidence also points strongly toward William Herbert as the 'lovely boy' (126) of the *Sonnets*. John Taylor's portrait of the middle-aged William Shakespeare and Isaac Oliver's miniature of the young William Herbert bear out the close physical similarity between the two men, an important point because the fair youth emerges as a strong self-projection in the *Sonnets*: ''Tis thee, myself, that for myself I praise, Painting my age with beauty of thy days' (62).

In addition to the physical resemblance between the loving poet and his adored youth, the poet's self-projection appears to have been further supported by the fact that the two men also shared their first name. This is another important point because the punnings on the name Will in Sonnets 135 and 136 are pointless unless the fair youth's name was, like the poet's, Will. As far as one may infer from the portraits, William Shakespeare and William Herbert were even of the same psychological type – that of introverted intuition.

---

* Objections that Thomas Thorpe would dare address William Herbert as 'Master' are countered by Martin Seymour-Smith in his introduction to *Shakespeare's Sonnets* (1963, pp.18–19).

and promiscuous lovers, the woman's lips having 'sealed false bonds of love as oft as mine, Robbed others' beds' revenues of their rents' (142). The background of 'sinful loving' (142) of this liaison colours the partners' protestations of 'love' (138,152), 'truth' (138,152) and 'constancy' (152), which have to be built on a secret pattern of mutual deception and falsehood: 'When my love swears that she is made of truth, I do believe her though I know she lies…Therefore I lie with her, and she with me, And in our faults by lies we flattered be' (138).

The adulterous and promiscuous setting is treated as a matter of fact here as elsewhere (141,152), just as the sense of 'sin' expressed by Sonnets 141 and 142 is neither that entertained by a guilty husband nor a contrite Puritan, but that admitted by a leading member of literary and dramatic Bohemia, frankly confessing that 'Love is my sin' (142). The lady's moral qualms and 'Hate of my sin, grounded on sinful loving' (142) are therefore to be dismissed as hypocritical since his adulteries are at least matched by hers. In short, the violent fluctuations of mood and the 'despair' (144) characterizing the relationship are not to be explained by any pangs of moral conscience. They are due to the spell that the dark lady casts on him and to the sufferings of his 'foolish heart' (141) when betrayed by her looseness, deceits and 'cruel' (131, 133, 140, 149) actions.

One of these acts of deceit is the seduction of the poet's adored young friend after having made his acquaintance. 'Beshrew that heart that makes my heart to groan For that deep wound it gives my friend and me', the poet addresses the dark lady in an outburst of despair, 'Is't not enough to torture me alone, But slave to slavery my sweet'st friend must be?' (133).

The promiscuity of the dark lady and her affair with the fair youth bring the poet to a state of despair. 'Tell me thou lov'st elsewhere', he implores her in Sonnet 139, 'but in my sight, Dear heart, forbear to glance thine eye aside' (139). In Sonnet 137 he presents her as a 'bay where all men ride' (137) and as 'the wide world's common place' (137). In Sonnet 135 she is made to appear as a woman 'whose will [libido] is large and spacious' (135), just as she is associated with 'things of great receipt' (136) and presented as a capacious female absorbing a throng of lovers, in which the poet is but an insignificant number:

> Among a number one is reckoned none.
> Then in the number let me pass untold,
> Though in thy store's account I one must be;
> For nothing hold me, so it please thee hold
> That nothing me, a something sweet to thee. (136)

Having experienced both the 'heaven' and the 'hell' of sexual passion (129), the poet of Sonnet 144 realizes that he and the fair youth are truly playing with fire in descending into the 'hell' (129,144) of their common love object:

> Two loves I have, of comfort and despair,
> Which like two spirits do suggest me still;
> The better angel is a man right fair,
> The worser spirit a woman coloured ill.
> To win me soon to hell, my female evil
> Tempteth my better angel from my side,

> And would corrupt my saint to be a devil,
> Wooing his purity with her foul pride.
> And, whether that my angel be turned fiend,
> Suspect I may, yet not directly tell;
> But being both from me, both to each friend,
> I guess one angel in another's hell.
> Yet this shall I ne'er know, but live in doubt,
> Till my bad angel fire my good one out. (144)

The concluding couplet, perceived as ambiguous by modern readers, was not difficult to decipher for an Elizabethan. In the slang of the time, 'hell' meant vagina, and 'fire out' was to infect with syphilis or gonorrhea (the two venereal diseases having been regarded as one in Shakespeare's time, see pp.255–8).

Epigram 15 in Samuel Rowlands's *The Letting of Humours Blood* (1600) was evidently written in imitation of this sonnet and shows that Rowlands was acquainted with Shakespeare's 'sugred Sonnets among his priuate friends', as Francis Meres informs us in *Palladis Tamia* (1598) (Chambers, 1930, vol.2, p.194). Rowlands's version of Sonnet 144 brings out the original's venereal implications:

> Amorous *Austin* spendes much Balleting,
> In rimeing Letters, and loue Sonnetting.
> She that loues him, his Ynckehorne shall be paint her,
> And with all *Venus* tytles hee'le acquaint her:
> Vowing she is a perfect Angell right,
> When she by waight is many graines too light:
> Nay all that do but touch her with the stone,
> Will be depos'd that Angell she is none.
> How can he proue her for an Angell then?
> That proues her selfe a Diuell, tempting men,
> And draweth many to the fierie pit,
> Where they are burned for their en'tring it.
> I know no cause wherefore he tearmes her so,
> Vnlesse he meanes shee's one of them below,
> Where *Lucifer*, chiefe Prince doth domineere:
> If she be such, then good my hartes stand cleere,
> Come not within the compasse of her flight,
> For such as do, are haunted with a spright.
> This Angell is not noted by her winges,
> But by her tayle, all full of prickes and stinges.
> And know this lustblind Louer's vaine is led,
> To prayse his Diuell, in an Angels sted. (Rowlands, 1880, vol.1, p.21)

Perhaps the two concluding Sonnets 153–54 of the entire collection refer to the dark lady, since they follow immediately upon the group of poems addressed to her. In that case it appears that also the poet himself might have been 'fired out' by the promiscuous love object of the amorous triangle. In Sonnets 153–54, the 'sad distempered' poet, who has been burnt by 'Cupid' (153) and his 'mistress' (153), goes to Bath to seek a 'cure' (153) which strongly suggests syphilis (see p.140).

Figure 37. *Parthenia or the Maydenhead of the First Musicke That Ever Was Printed for the Virginalls* (London, 1613, title-page). Who was the mysterious dark lady of Shakespeare's *Sonnets*? Scholars have put forward a number of suggestions ranging from Queen Elizabeth to a negro prostitute in London known as Lucy Negro, Abbess de Clerkenwell. Less fanciful suggestions are two ladies of Elizabeth's court, Elizabeth Vernon, whom the Earl of Southampton married in 1598, and Mary Fitton, whom William Herbert refused to marry in 1601. But both are dismissed by E.K. Chambers for a very simple reason: 'Neither of these can, of course, be the Dark Lady, a married woman, who broke her bed-vow (152) to take first Shakespeare and then his friend' (Chambers, 1930, vol.1, p.565). If one is to find the dark lady, one must search for a woman who fulfils these requirements: (1) she must be a married woman; (2) she must be promiscuous; (3) she must be an 'Italian' type of woman; (4) she must be musical and able to play the virginals – 'those dancing chips O'er whom thy fingers walk with gentle gait' (128); and (5) she must belong to Shakespeare's social circle.

In 1974 the Shakespearean scholar A.L. Rowse came up with the best suggestion so far: Emilia Lanier. He found her in the diaries of Simon Forman, a popular physician and astrologer in Shakespeare's London with many clients from all classes of Elizabethan society. Shakespeare's landlady around 1600, Mrs. Mary Mountjoy, consulted Forman in 1597, and Emilia Lanier visited him several times in the same year. She wanted to know if her husband, who had gone with Essex and Southampton on an expedition to the Azores, would be knighted on his return or not, and thus if 'she should be a lady or no' (Rowse, 1974, p.100). Forman was taken with the charming lady, and his diary strongly suggests that he had entered into a sexual relationship with her. He records that 'she hath had hard fortune in her youth. Her father died when she was young; the wealth of her father failed before he died, and he began to be miserable in his estate' (p.99). Emilia's father was a royal musician of Italian origin, Baptista Bassano, whose family had come to England from Venice in the reign of Henry VIII. Baptista Bassano married an English woman by the name of Margaret Johnson, and Emilia Bassano was born of their union about 1569–70. When her mother died in 1587, she was left at seventeen to take the chances of life, endowed with nothing but her Italian looks and, no doubt, her skill on the virginals. Not long after, the elderly Henry Carey (c. 1524–96), the first Lord Hunsdon and founder of the Lord Chamberlain's Company, Shakespeare's troupe, took Emilia Bassano as his mistress. On May 17, 1597, Forman records that 'she was paramour to my old Lord Hunsdon that was Lord Chamberlain and was maintained in great pride; [but] being with child she was for colour married to a minstrel' (p.99). This happened in 1593 when Emilia and her son Henry – evidently named after his father – were taken over by a French musician named Alfonso Lanier. When Emilia Lanier consulted Forman in 1597, she had been married four years, and the old Lord Chamberlain had kept her long. 'She was maintained in great pomp', Forman entrusts his diary, adding that 'she is high-minded' and that 'she hath many false conceptions' (p.99).

Forman's entry on September 2, 1597, provides a fuller character-sketch of her and shows her considerable sexual attraction, her strong social aspirations, and her strained relations with her husband. 'She hath been favoured much of her Majesty and of many noblemen, hath had great gifts and been much made of – a nobleman that is dead hath loved her well and kept her. But her husband hath dealt hardly with her, hath spent and consumed her goods. She is now very needy, in debt and it seems for lucre's sake will be a good fellow, for necessity doth compel. She hath a wart or mole in the pit of the throat or near it' (p.100). The last we hear of Emilia Lanier in Forman's diary is on January 7, 1600, when the physician-astrologer wants 'to know why Mrs Lanier sent for me; what will follow, and whether she intendeth any more villainy' (p.102).

This woman could easily be the temperamental, capricious and promiscuous dark lady of Shakespeare's *Sonnets*, who seduced the young and inexperienced nobleman William Herbert, 'Wooing his purity with her foul pride' (144). Shakespeare's acquaintance with Emilia Lanier fits well with the date of composition of *Love's Labour's Lost* (1594–5) in which the play's greatest sonneteer, Berowne, falls desperately in love with Rosaline, described by the King as 'black as ebony' (4,3:243). The event also fits well with the founding of the Lord Chamberlain's Company in 1594 under the patronage of Lord Hunsdon, a company of which Shakespeare was a leading member. On this occasion the poet could have met the nobleman's former mistress and fallen in love with her. At that time Emilia Lanier had just been married off to Alfonso Lanier, a match which Shakespeare may refer to in Sonnet 150 where he states that his love for her had originated in pity: 'If thy unworthiness raised love in me, More worthy I to be beloved of thee'.

Two years after the publication of Shakespeare's *Sonnets* in 1609, Emilia Lanier issued a volume of verse, *Salve Deus Rex Judaeorum*, from which we learn of her religious conversion. Only the love of Christ, not of men, is able to save human beings. 'Sweetness that makes our flesh a burden to us, Knowing it serves but to undo us' (p.115), must be replaced by the love of Christ: 'What pride hath lost, humility repairs… lodge him in the closet of your heart Whose worth is more than can be showed by art' (pp.115, 111). Her poems teem with echoes of Shakespeare's plays, and of particular interest is an

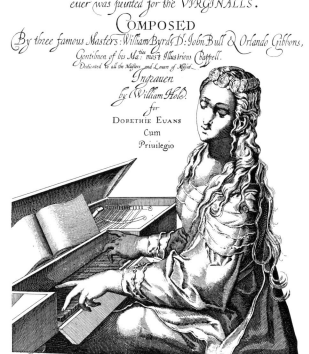

PARTHENIA

or

THE MAYDENHEAD

of the first musicke that *euer was printed for the VIRGINALLS.*

COMPOSED

*By three famous Masters: William Byrd, D: John Bull & Orlando Gibbons, Gentilmen of his Ma:ties most Illustrious Chappell. Dedicated to all the Maisters and Lovers of Musick*

Ingrauen by William Hole. for DORETHIE EVANS Cum Priuilegio

Printed at LONDON by G: Lowe and are to be soulde at his howle in Loathberry.

address in prose in which she passionately defends women against men's defamation of them, referring in this connection to 'evil-disposed men' who 'like vipers, deface the wombs wherein they were bred' (p.112). Emilia Lanier appears to have reached old age and to have died as a 'pensioner' in London at the end of the Civil War (p.117).

## TWO LIBERTINES: W.H. AND W.S.

In Sonnet 104 Shakespeare looks back on his friendship with the fair youth and states that he had made his acquaintance some three years earlier: 'Three April perfumes in three hot Junes burned, Since first I saw you fresh, which yet are green' (104). If the three years' period the sonnet encompasses starts with the late autumn of 1595 (see p.189), it runs through the winters of 1595–6, 1596–7, 1597–8, and the springs and Junes of 1596, 1597, and 1598, to the autumn of 1598 (Chambers, 1944, p.129).

The love sonnets to the dark lady would belong to the immediately preceding period of 1594–5, her seduction of the fair youth taking place in 1596 or 1597, after the poet had begun his friendship with the young aristocrat. The same crucial period surfaces in Rowland Whyte's letter of April 3, 1597 to Sir Robert Sidney, William Herbert's uncle, in which the youth appears to have spent his time in London during 1596 and the first quarter of 1597 (Gebauer, 1987, p.27). This is also the time when Shakespeare's star was at its zenith in London as a playwright and when the figures of Falstaff and his young friend, Prince Hal, were born out of a sense of gaity, fulfilment and *joie de vivre* which was probably the poet's own.

In his poems to the dark lady, Shakespeare reveals a sexual relationship which is presented as illicit and adulterous and as part of a promiscuous pattern of behaviour shared by the poet and his mistress alike (141,142). The poet's relations to his 'bad angel' (144) and 'female evil' (144) open the door to a background hinted at in the Sonnets addressed to the fair youth (18–126).

Here the poet appears to suffer ill-fame, admitting to 'vulgar scandal stamped upon my brow' (112) and referring to 'my bewailèd guilt' (36). Similar suggestions of some well-known 'shame' (36, 72, 112, 129), 'stain' (109), or 'abuse' (121) occur elsewhere in the sonnets, just as the poet acknowledges 'my sportive blood' (121) and 'my deeds' (121) – a word which seems throughout the Sonnets to denote some sort of sexual vice (34,61, 69,94,131,150). (Eric Partridge in Shakespeare's Bawdy (1968) informs us that 'do it, do the deed, do the deed of darkness, do the deed of kind' was an Elizabethan euphemism for having sexual intercourse (p.95)). 'In my nature reign All frailties that besiege all kinds of blood' (109), he sums up his case, appearing to waiver between humility (88, 111) and the self-assertion of '*No, I am that I am*' (121) in spite of public condemnation of his behaviour.

In the *Sonnets*, Shakespeare's 'frailties' clearly emerge as those belonging to his 'sportive blood' (121) and the sensual sphere. 'Love is my sin', he confesses in Sonnet 142, 'my sin, grounded on sinful loving' (142). Like Antony who succumbed to the charms of his dark Egyptian, Shakespeare's weakness appears as 'love of love and her soft hours' (*A&C*,1,1:44). The freewheeling and promiscuous nature of this kind of love is evidenced by the use of such words as 'sport' and 'deeds' for it in the *Sonnets*. 'Sport' in the sense of amorous or 'filthy sport' (*Avisa*,1594, p.102) is found in many places in Shakespeare, not only in the plays (*Titus*,2,3:75–9;5,96; *Measure*,3,2:120–1; *Othello*,2,1:228–9;3:17–8) but also in *Venus and Adonis* (1.105–6).

In the *Sonnets*, likewise, 'sport' has a clear sexual meaning throughout the cycle. 'Some say thy fault is youth, some *wantonness*, Some say thy grace is youth and gentle *sport*' (96), the poet confides to the fair youth in Sonnet 96, adding that there are also people who are not so kind, 'Making *lascivious* comments on thy *sport*' (95). Apparently, the youth is not unacquainted with the coursing of '*sportive* blood' (121), and there are strong indications in the *Sonnets* that in this respect he is following in the footsteps of his friend and tutor.

The youth is described as having been at first chaste, 'contracted' only to his 'own bright eyes' (1), feeding his 'light's flame with self-substantial fuel' (1). We are told that he has presented 'a pure unstainèd prime' (70), passing untainted the temptations of youth. He has been a person 'unmovèd, cold and to temptation slow'

(94). However, the youth's chaste reserve has obviously been broken by the poet's mistress, who, 'Wooing his purity with her foul pride' (144), manages to seduce him into a sexual relationship. The poet shows pain, both at the youth's association with the dark lady (133,134,144) and at his mixing in a false society (67).

Soon we observe the youth's involvement in a hinterland of 'shame' (34,95) and 'ill report' (95) which has the same air of surrounding scandal as the society in which his poet friend moves. The author of the *Sonnets* cannot but voice his fears that his idealized youth may become contaminated by the gay society to which he himself belongs. The poet complains that the young man is ruining his good name by a 'sport' (95,96) which is not only 'sensual' (35), but which is described twice as 'lascivious' (40,95) and as 'sin' (35,95), 'soil' (69), 'riot' (41), and 'liberty' [licentiousness] (41).

The word 'deed' figures prominently in this context. In Sonnet 34 the '*ill deeds*' (34) of the fair youth appear in a context of sexual 'offence' (34), which is attended by the youth's 'shame', 'sorrow', and 'repent[ance]' (34) at his 'sensual fault' (35). 'They [that] look into the beauty of thy mind', the poet goes on to tell the youth in Sonnet 69, 'they measure [it] by thy *deeds;* Then, churls, their thoughts, although their eyes were kind, to thy fair flower add the *rank* smell of *weeds;* But why thy odor matcheth not thy show, The *soil* is this, that thou dost *common* grow' (69). In Sonnet 94 the poet continues the same metaphor, observing that 'the summer's flow'r is to the summer sweet, Though to itself it only live and die' (94). 'But if that flow'r with *base infection* meet', he warns the youth, 'The *basest weed* outbraves his dignity: For sweetest things turn sourest by their *deeds*; Lilies that *fester* smell far worse than *weeds*' (94).

In the sonnets addressed to the dark lady, the word 'deed' is brought within the same libidinal sphere of meaning. 'In nothing art thou black save in thy *deeds*' (131), the jealous and frustrated poet tells his promiscuous love object in Sonnet 131, 'and thence this *slander*, as I think, proceeds' (131). 'Who taught thee how to make me *love* thee more, The more I hear and see just cause of *hate?*' (150), he finally asks her. 'Whence hast thou this becoming of things *ill*, That in the very *refuse* of thy *deeds* There is such strength and warrantise of skill That, in my mind, thy *worst* all best exceeds?' (150).

As in the case with the dark lady, it is the fair youth's '*deeds*' that lead the poet to doubt 'the beauty of thy mind' (69), contrasting his 'fair flower' (69) with 'the *rank smell of weeds*' (69) and '*canker vice*' (70). 'For *canker vice* the sweetest buds doth love' (70), the poet goes on to explain, 'And *loathsome canker* lives in sweetest bud' (35). In *Venus and Adonis* the love goddess mentions 'This *canker* that eats up love's tender spring' (1.655), while Luciana in *The Comedy of Errors* asks her sister's adulterous husband: 'Shall, Antipholus, Even in the spring of love, thy love-springs *rot?*' (3,2:2–3). In *Romeo and Juliet* Friar Lawrence explains that where 'rude will', or fleshly desire, 'is predominant Full soon the *canker death* eats up that plant' (2,3;24–6). And in Sonnet 99 an overweening rose related to the fair youth is punished with 'A *vengeful canker eat[ing] him up to death*' (99).

*Hamlet* brings conclusive evidence that by his canker metaphor Shakespeare means venereal disease. Just before his departure for Paris, Laertes, in a Robert Greene-like sermon, warns his sister Ophelia against any kind of promiscuous behaviour. 'The *canker* galls the infants of the spring Too oft before their buttons be disclos'd', he points out to her, 'And in the morn and liquid dew of youth *Contagious blastments* are most imminent. Be wary then: best safety lies in fear. Youth to itself rebels, though none else near' (1,3:39–44). The gist of Laertes's advice is that youth is particularly susceptible to diseases and thus its own worst enemy when listening to the message of the blood. For this reason, young girls cannot be too careful and ought to keep themselves 'Out of the shot and danger of desire' (1,3:35).

Shakespeare's collocation in 'canker vice' of a floral word of corruption ('canker') and a sexual word of dissolution ('vice') may therefore be taken to carry a syphilitic innuendo. Because of their common derivation, similar spelling and sound, as well as overlapping meaning, canker may be used to imply chancre. Cotgrave explains *Chancre* as 'A Canker' and under the entry *Chancreux* writes: 'Cankarie, cankared; full of cankers. *Bosse chancreuse*. A cankered byle; pockie sore, Winchester goose', i.e., a syphilitic chancre.

In *The Evolution of the Term Chancre and Its Relation to the History of Syphilis* (1949), Harry Keil traces the origin of the word chancre to *cancer*, which in the 17th century was used by various medical authors to describe venereal lesions on the secret parts. In particular French writers, employing Latin as the medium of scientific communication, often described the primary venereal lesions as 'cancerous', whereas the translations into the vulgar French tongue recorded these alterations as 'chancrous'. Keil finds the earliest use of the term chancre in the English medical language in Harris's translation of de Blegny's book on the Venereal Disease (1676), in which the word appears as a translation of the Latin original's *cancer* for the primal syphilitic lesions. De Blegny's *ulcera et cancri luis* is thus rendered by Harris as 'venereal ulcers and chancres' (Keil, 1949, p.413).

However, even before that time the term had arrived on the wings of racy and bawdy literature written in the first part of the 17th century. Thus, in the poem called *The Flyting*, penned by a Scotsman, Alexander Montgomerie (1605), reference is made to the chancre, and evidently the term has the broad connotation of a venereal ulcer. Somewhere between 1640 and 1680, Samuel Colville wrote a poem entitled *The Whig's Supplication*, in which he exclaims: 'The French...They first brought shankers o'er the Alps'. Within this period, also, John Wilmot Rochester (1647–80) refers to the shanker (Keil, 1949, p.412).

A medical ambiguity in Shakespeare's use of the term 'canker vice' is therefore a strong probability and is supported by the sinister undercurrent of the cautionary sonnets addressed to the fair youth. While Sonnet 40 calls him 'Lascivious grace, in whom all ill well shows' (40), Sonnet 95 sums up the 'sins' (95) of the 'straying youth' (41) in this way:

> How sweet and lovely dost thou make the shame
> Which, like a canker in the fragrant rose,
> Doth spot the beauty of thy budding name!
> O, in what sweets dost thou thy sins enclose!
> That tongue that tells the story of thy days,
> Making lascivious comments on thy sport,
> Cannot dispraise, but in a kind of praise;

> Naming thy name blesses an ill report.
> O, what mansion have those vices got
> Which for their habitation chose out thee,
> Where beauty's veil doth cover every blot,
> And all things turns to fair that eyes can see
> Take heed, dear heart, of this large privilege;
> The hardest knife ill-used doth lose his edge. (95)

Given the widespread occurrence of syphilis among Elizabethans, this passage in all likelihood alludes to the dangers of syphilitic infection incurred by promiscuous living in London and frequentation of its brothels. A similar sinister allusion appears in John Davies of Hereford's sombre punning on similar imagery in his 96th Epigram *Upon English Proverbes*:

> 'Phryne makes much but of her painted sheath:'
> And yet tis but the very gate of Death:
> For all those blades that therein cleanly go,
> Are soild, and spoild, the sheath is painted so.
> (Davies, 1878, vol.2, p.43. 'Upon English Proverbes,' Epigram 96)

Another reference to knives that may be spoilt be being ill-used is found in Beaumont and Fletcher's *The Coxcomb* (1608–9). Here a lewd tinker, when robbing a female victim, is tempted to make her his whore: 'A pretty young round wench, well bloudded, I am for her, Theeves'. But he is promptly tempered by his trull Dorothy, who warns him: 'Coole your Codpiece, Rogue, or I'll clap a spell upon't, shall take your edge off with a very vengeance' (2,1:330).

For all the humour and irony of Shakespeare's warning to his young friend, the concluding couplet of Sonnet 95 carries the same message as Robert Greene's advice to 'all the wanton youths of England' in *The Repentance of Robert Greene*. Another sign of warning imagery appeared many years later in Shakespeare's *Timon of Athens* (1607–8), where the protagonist, during his embittered talk with Apemantus, mentions the possibility that, under certain circumstances, 'thou wouldst have plunged thyself In general riot, melted down thy youth In different beds of lust, and never learned the icy precepts of respect, but followed The sugared game before thee' (4,3:257–61). A similar ring may be perceived in Sonnet 67, where the poet, despairing of the youth's behaviour, muses:

> Ah, wherefore with infection should he live,
> And with his presence grace impiety,
> That sin by him advantage should achieve
> And lace itself with his society? (67)

### THE HERBERT-FITTON SCANDAL OF 1601

The promiscuous behaviour of the fair youth of the *Sonnets* is yet another feature pointing to William Herbert, who was not above the sort of behaviour that Shakespeare attributes to the friend. The young earl's sexual debut with the dark lady of the *Sonnets* opened a career famous for its promiscuity and dissolution. In *The History of the Rebellion and Civil Wars in England*, Edward Hyde, the Earl of Clarendon, wrote that William Herbert 'indulged to himself the pleasures of all kinds, almost in all excesses. Whether out of his natural constitution, or for want of his domestic discontent and delight, (in which he was most unhappy, for he paid much too dear for his wife's fortune by taking her person into the bargain,) he was immoderately given up to women.' (Gebauer, 1987, p.161)

A similar picture is presented by the clergyman T.C. who, in his sermon at the burial of Pembroke in 1630, told the audience:

'I am loth to giue him [Pembroke] more, then hee would haue giuen himself; though I call him iust, yet I dare not say he was perfect; though righteous, yet not without sinne: I should lie, and I say not, *non est humilitas*, but *non est veritas*, there were no truth in me; he knew that the way to heauen by innocency was long sithence blocked vp, and therefore he tooke another course, and our hope is, he is arriu'd there by the way of penitencie; hee that was so often, so daily, so duely, every morning and

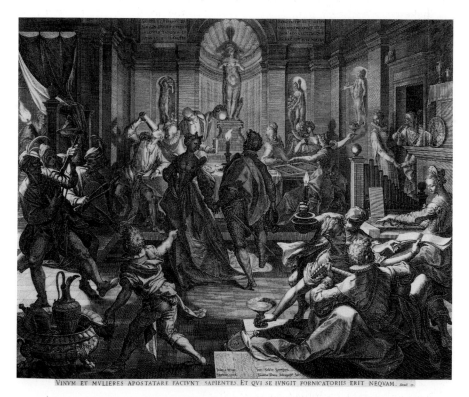

Vinvm et mvlieres apostatare facivnt sapientes. Et qvi se ivngit fornicatoriis erit neqvam.

Figure 38. The promiscuous behaviour of the aristocratic youth of the *Sonnets* would be liable to have taken place in establishments of a higher order. A centre of the sex trade, London offered a number of brothels for the upper classes of society, much like the one shown in the engraving entitled *Carnival* by Johan Sadeler (1588) (Den kongelige Kobberstiksamling, Copenhagen). Venus presides over the pleasure palace (background), while members of the aristocracy engage in love-making, game-playing, drinking, dancing and listening to music. At the entrance, right, a high-class prostitute gives her purse to an elderly bawd, behind whom is seen a waiting visitor. To the left a pair of jesters are about to join the party. 'Vinum et mulieres apostatare faciunt sapientes, et qvi se jungit fornicatoriis erit neqvam', reads the Latin caption, quoting Sirach 19:2. ('Wine and women make men of understanding to fall away, and he that cleaveth to harlots will be beneath contempt.')

euening vpon his knees to God, for the pardon of the sinnes of his youth, I doubt
not, and for preuenting the sinnes of his age, did acknowledge he was a grieuous
sinner.' (pp.162–3)

One of the greatest 'sins of his youth' sparked a national sex scandal in 1601, the
circumstances of which we shall examine more closely in this section. The fact is
that the young William Herbert was one of the most eligible bachelors in the
aristocratic circles of the 1590s. In 1595, when William Herbert was only fifteen,
sources show that his father, the second Earl of Pembroke, attempted to negotiate
the marriage of his son to Sir George Carey's daughter, Elizabeth Carey. This was
a match intended to bring together two of the greatest aristocratic families in
Elizabethan England, for George Carey's father was Henry Carey, first Lord
Hunsdon and the Queen's Lord Chamberlain and first cousin. In addition, Pembroke
was ailing and wanted the future of his earldom and estates decided.

Shakespeare's first 17 sonnets are an appeal to the 'lovely boy' (126) to marry
and beget children, an 'embassage' many critics believe to have been inspired by
the noble youth's parents. Shakespeare's commission by the cultivated Pembroke
household to make William Herbert 'affect' the partner selected for him is a strong
probability, and perhaps the Pembrokes were joined in their efforts by the Careys.
Shakespeare was well known to both families, since George Carey was the son of
Lord Hunsdon, in whose company Shakespeare was then a leading member; at the
same time he was familiar with the Earl of Pembroke, to whose company he had
probably belonged at an earlier date. 'If they wanted a plausible man to stimulate
the imagination of young Herbert', E.K. Chambers observes, 'they could hardly
have made a better choice' (Chambers, 1944, p.127).

A FREEWHEELING BACHELOR

However, the efforts of the commissioned poet to join the fair youth in the bonds
of matrimony failed for, on November 22, 1595, Rowland Whyte, a correspondent
to Sir Robert Sidney, William Herbert's uncle, disclosed the catastrophic news that
'The Speach of Marriage between 900 [W.H.] and qq [Elizabeth Carey] is quite
broke of, by his not liking' (Gebauer, 1987, p.23).

Gebauer thinks it likely that, after the abortive marriage negotiations in November–December 1595, the young man returned to the capital after his first visit there
in the late autumn of 1595, spending the following year and the first quarter of
1597 there. He had probably got a taste for the bustling life of the metropolis, and
Rowland Whyte's letter of April 3, 1597 shows him to be in contact with the Earl
of Essex and, hence, with the Court circle (p.27).

Here a number of further attempts were made at the end of the 1590s to join
him in the bands of matrimony. In 1597 a match was suggested with Bridget Vere,
daughter of Edward, Earl of Oxford, and granddaughter of Lord Burghley. But, like
the first attempt in 1595, this scheme also broke down, financial discrepancies being
once more given as the reason for the abortive negotiations. On October 22, 1597,
Rowland Whyte wrote to Sir Robert Sidney:

'For the matter of 9000 [William Herbert] it is upon a sudden quite dashed, and in the opinion of the wise by great fault in 2000 [Pembroke], who makes the occasion of the breach to be a refusal of the portion offered by 900 [Burghley]. 2000 [Pembroke] will have 3000 £ in money and 500 £ a year in possession, else will he not bargain. 13 [unidentified] grieves at it, for he foresees the harm will ensue.' (HMC, Isle, vol.2, p.297; Gebauer, 1987, p.29)

In the autumn of 1598 there was further talk of a marriage with the 20-year-old Elizabeth, daughter of Sir Thomas Cecil, and grand-daughter of Lord Burghley – and the wealthy widow of Sir William Hatton who had died the year before (1597). Apparently the failure of this scheme was due to no fault of William Herbert's, for before the year was over the much-coveted widow had married the 47-year-old Sir Edward Coke, the Queen's attorney. According to a sworn statement by one Mary Berham on April 30, 1599, ten weeks after the marriage, at the beginning of Lent 1599, Lady Hatton gave birth to a son who had been begotten by one of her servants (CSP, Dom. 1598–1601, p.189; Gebauer, 1987, p.32).

In 1599 Rowland Whyte attempted to bring Herbert to the altar with a niece of Charles Howard, Earl of Nottingham, mainly because Nottingham, as Lord Admiral, could advance Sir Robert Sidney's affairs. But on August 16, 1600, he had to admit that he did not 'find any Disposicion at all in this gallant young Lord to marry' (Gebauer, 1987, p.41). William Herbert was much too fond of the freewheeling life he lived in London, and in the period 1599–1600 he entered into an intimate relationship with a young woman at Court by the name of Mary Fitton (c. 1578–1647). She was one of the great beauties of her day, and at the age of 17 she had been sent to the Court by her father, Sir Edward Fitton. An undated source probably originating in 1602 reports 'that Mistress fytton was in great favour and one of her majesties maids of honor' (p.43). However, it was this very position that proved the undoing of Mary Fitton and William Herbert who, in 1601, were involved in the greatest sex scandal in the reign of Elizabeth I. The disgraceful episode prompted the furious Queen to imprison William Herbert, who had just become third Earl of Pembroke, and afterwards to banish him from Court for the rest of her life.

### WILLIAM HERBERT'S ILLNESSES 1598–1600

Very few sources on the life of William Herbert survive from this period, but one of them tells of an illness contracted in June 1598 when William's father writes to Sir Robert Cecil: 'If my son had not been distempered in his body he should have come up to do my duty and his own to her Majesty. But as it is I must for some few days stay [by] him till he perfectly recover' (HMC, Salisbury, vol.8, p.219; Gebauer, 1987, p.32). More than a year later, when William Herbert had gone up to Court, Rowland Whyte on September 12, 1599, informs Robert Sidney that 'Lord Herbert is blamed for his weak pursuing of her Majesty's favour. Want of spirit is laid to his charge, and that he is a melancholy young man' (HMC, Isle, vol.2, p.390).

More than three months later, on December 22, 1599, Rowland Whyte writes to Sir Robert Sidney that 'My Lord Harbert is not come vp [to London] according to his Apointment, and writes vnto me, that he is sicke of an Ague' (Collins, vol.2, p.152). On January 5, 1600, Whyte informs his master that 'My Lord Harbert is [still] sicke of his Tertian Ague at Ramesbury.' (p.156). The following dates in Rowland Whyte's extant correspondence to Sir Robert Sidney are interesting from a medical point of view:

'January 12, 1600. From Ramesbury something wilbe said. My Lord Harbert is recovered, and purposes to be here vpon Tuesday next; my Lord Southhampton, my Lord Effingham, and Sir Charles Danvers, are at Ramesbury [visiting him]...Mrs. [Mistress] Fitton is sicke, and gon from Court to her Fathers.' (p.158)

'January 19, 1600. My Lord Harbert coming vp towards the Court, fell very sicke at Newsberry, and was forced to goe backe again to Ramisbury...My Lady Pembroke desires you to send her speedely ouer some of your excellent Tobacco.' (pp.161–2)

'January 24, 1600. My Lord Harbert...is fallen to haue to haue his Ague again, and no Hope of his being here, before Easter, which I am sorry for.' (p.164)

'January 26, 1600. Even now I open a Lettre from my Lord Harbert to me, who saies, that he hath a continuall Paine in his Head, and finds no Manner of Ease, but by taking of Tobacco. He wills me to comend hym to you, and to signifie, that you cannot send hym a more pleasing Gifte then excellent Tobacco. The like Request I made from my Lady Pembroke.' (p.165)

'February 2, 1600. The Lord Harburt is very ill at Ramesbury.' (HMC, Isle, vol.2, p.435)

'February 9, 1600. The tobacco for Lady Pembroke is delivered. Lord Herbert is well amended.' (p.437)

'February 21, 1600. My Lady [Robert Sidney's wife, Barbara] goes often to my Lady Lester, my Lady Essex, and my Lady Buckhurst, where she is exceeding welcom; she visited Mrs. Fitton, that hath long bene here sick in London, and lately she was with Sir Walter Rawley, and his Lady, who indeed did most kindly vse her.' (Collins, vol.2, p.168)

According to the sources quoted above, William Herbert could have had an unidentified disease in June 1598 and contracted syphilis at the end of 1599, or he could have been syphilitically infected in June 1598 and suffered a relapse of his condition in 1599–1600. For various reasons the latter alternative seems the stronger probability because Shakespeare's cautionary sonnets to the fair youth may be taken to belong to the last year of their relationship and to the last year of the *Sonnets*, namely the summer and autumn of 1598. At this time it is likely that William Herbert's promiscuous living had courted disaster, a possibility which would explain his 'want of spirit' and 'melancholy' in the autumn of 1599.

Secondary relapses of untreated syphilis could easily occur 18 months after infection – the Oslo Study showed that they could occur up to 5 years later (Gjestland, 1955, pp.127, 142, 146) – and variable fever and headaches could be typical symptoms of a meningovascular syphilis in its early stages. Unbearable headaches accompanied the syphilitic infections of Schubert, Heine, Maupassant, Schopenhauer and Nietzsche, and they were also noted by William Clowes when writing about

'paines and aches in the head, shoulder blades, hips, thighes and ioints, which pains afflicting most in the night, and ceasing in the day time, a certaine heauines and painfull aking of the body after sleepe, as though they were broken asunder, sometimes a little feauer, and in some a lingring consumption or wasting of the bodie.' (Clowes, 1596, p.154)

'The paine of the Pockes is alwaies greater in the eueninges then in the morninges', adds Phillipp Hermann, 'and dooth encline to an Ague' (Hermann, 1590, p.4).

Yet another doctor, the London surgeon Joseph Binns (*floruit* 1633–63), testifies to the same symptoms in his syphilitic patients. 'My cousin Spooner's sister', he wrote in his casebook, 'consulted me for extreme pain in her head…it being all her head over & as much by day as night but somewhat worse in the night' (McCray Beier, 1987, p.93). Several days later she developed nodes on her forehead and pains in her shoulders, and Binns was able to diagnose her disease as that of syphilis and to prescribe a mercury flux.

## TOBACCO – AN 'INDIAN' WONDER DRUG FOR THE POX

William Herbert's recurrent 'ague' or 'tertian ague' – a loose Elizabethan term for bouts of fever – and the violent headaches attending his disease in the winter of 1599–1600 are suspicious, as is his use of tobacco in the treatment of his symptoms. Because syphilis was an 'Indian' disease, the English focused on the various herbs which the inhabitants of the New World used to cure the pox. Guaiac was the most famous of these herbal medicines, but tobacco came in second as an anti-syphilitic. This we know from an authority which is no less than the King of Scotland, James VI, later enthroned in England as King James I (*regnebat* 1603–25). A year after his coronation in London, he published a pamphlet entitled *A Counterblaste to Tobacco* (1604), in which he introduced the new American plant in the following way:

'Tobacco being a common herbe, which (though vnder diuers names) growes almost euery where, was first found out by some of the barbarous *Indians*, to be a Preseruatiue, or Antidot against the Pockes, a filthy disease, whereunto these barbarous people are (as all men know) very much subiect, what through the vncleanly and adust constitution of their bodies, and what through the intemperate heate of their Climat: so that as from them was first brought into Christendome, that most detestable disease, so from them likewise was brought this vse of *Tobacco*, as a stinking and vnsauourie Antidot, for so corrupted and execrable a Maladie, the stinking Suffumigation whereof they yet vse against that disease, making so one canker or venime to eate out another.' (James I, 1604, sig.Bi$^v$)

'It seemes a miracle to me, how a custome springing from so vile a ground, and brought in by a father so generally hated, should be welcomed vpon so slender a warrant. For if they that first put it in practise heere, had remembred for what respect it was vsed by them from whence it came, I am sure they would haue bene loath, to haue taken so farre the imputation of that disease vpon them as they did, by vsing the cure thereof.' (sig.B2$^{r-v}$)

King James goes on to satirize the alleged anti-syphilitic virtues of the tobacco plant, whose 'curative' effects he would rather prefer to ascribe to nature's own healing powers:

'For is it not a very great mistaking, to take *Non causam pro causa*, as they say in the Logicks? because peraduenture when a sicke man hath had his disease at the height, hee hath at that instant taken *Tobacco*, and afterward his disease taking the naturall course of declining, and consequently the patient of recouering his health, O then the *Tobacco* forsooth, was the worker of that miracle' (sig.C1ᵛ) ... 'But by the contrary, if a man smoke himselfe to death with it (and many haue done) O then some other disease must beare the blame for that fault. So doe olde harlots thanke their harlotrie for their many yeeres, that custome being healthfull (say they) *ad purgandos Renes*, but neuer haue minde how many die of the Pockes in the flower of their youth.' (sig.C2ʳ)

*A Counterblaste to Tobacco* finishes with King James's denunciation of the herb as an antidote and of smoking as 'A custome lothsome to the eye, hatefull to the Nose, harmefull to the braine, daungerous to the Lungs, and in the blacke stinking fume thereof, neerest resembling the horrible Stigian smoke of the pit that is bottome-lesse' (sig.D2ʳ).

A contemporary of King James testifies to the use of tobacco as an anti-syphilitic, not only after the disease has been contracted but also before a possible contraction of it. 'But the conceipt that is holden of Tobacco', Barnabe Rich observes in *The Irish Hubbub, or the English Hue and Crie,*

'how precious it is against the French pocks, may make some, that doe feele themselues to be distempered, to be the more inclining to it. Some other againe that be old fishmongers, and loues to follow the game, doe vse to fish those pooles, where they know the pocks are easily caught, doe therefore take Tobacco, to preuent perils.' (Rich, 1617, pp.41–2)*

## THE ABORTIVE BIRTH OF MARY FITTON'S SON

Whether William Herbert's tobacco cure or nature's own healing processes were responsible, the young nobleman's health appeared to have taken a turn for the better on February 26, 1600, when Rowland Whyte informs Robert Sidney that 'My Lord Harbert is well again; they all remove vpon Saturday to Wilton, to the Race' (Collins, vol.2, p.172). On March 22, 1600, Whyte tells Sidney the good news that William Herbert has gone up to Court, adding that 'I beleue he will proue a great Man in Court. He is very well beloued, and truly deserves it' (p.182).

Almost three months later, on June 16, 1600, a *grand fête* was held in London on the occasion of Anne Russell's marriage to Henry Herbert, son of the Earl of Worcester. Both William Herbert and Mary Fitton are known to have been present at the festivities, a fruit of which, perhaps, appeared some 8 months later when Sir Robert Cecil on February 6, 1601, wrote to Sir George Carey:

'We haue no newes but that there is a misfortune befallen Mistress Fitton, for she is proued with chyld, and the E. of Pembroke beinge examyned confesseth a ffact, but vtterly renounceth all marriage. I feare they will both dwell in the Tower awhyle, for the Queen hath vowed to send them thether.' (Gebauer, 1987, p.47)

On March 3, 1601, Tobie Matthew wrote to Dudley Carleton: 'The Earl of Pembroke is committed to the Fleet [Prison]; his cause [i.e., Mary Fitton] is delivered of a boy who is dead' (CSP, Dom. 1601–3, p.19).

The Herbert-Fitton scandal is the last in a considerable number of scandals at Queen Elizabeth's Court, involving such persons as Robert Dudley and Mrs.

---

*    cf. also pp.16–7.

Figure 39. A satirical poem of seven stanzas written by a sympathizer of the Earl of Essex, who had been executed in February of 1601, alludes to the contemporary Herbert-Fitton scandal:

> partie beard was aferd
> when they rann at the heard
> the Raine deer was imbost
> the white doe shee was loste
> pembrooke strooke her downe
> and tooke her from the clowne
> Lord for thy pittie. (Stopes, 1922, p.236)

Scholarly critics agree that the 'clown' with the 'party beard' in this poem alludes to Mary Fitton's aged and ridiculous suitor, Sir William Knollys (1547–1632), with his 'particoloured' beard streaked with grey. The model of Malvolio in Shakespeare's contemporary play *Twelfth Night* (1599–1600), Knollys had good reason to be 'afeared when they ran at the herd', or at the Queen's maids of honour, for on the occasion referred to, the Comptroller of Elizabeth I's household lost his 'white doe' to his younger rival – a stately, antlered 'reindeer', who, unfortunately, was 'imbost' or 'embossed'.

The expression 'embossed' has several connotations and may mean either 'foaming at the mouth' – like the slavering of a diseased or exhausted animal – or 'covered with boils or rounded swellings' – like the macular-papular syphilides of a secondary syphilitic eruption (Figure 16). In Elizabethan times, 'embossed' had a sinister connotation which Shakespeare makes use of both in *As You Like It*,

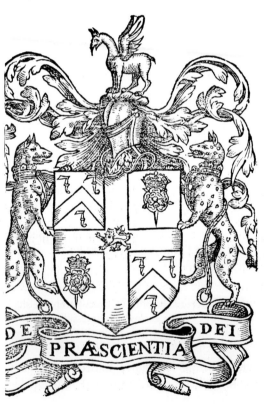

where he refers to the 'embossed sores' (2,7:67) of the syphilitic Jaques of Arden, and in *1 Henry IV*, where he alludes to Falstaff, the syphilitic, as an 'embossed rascal' (3,3:155). A second innuendo regarding syphilis is also found in the lampoon's opening stanza, in which it says of the Lord Chamberlain, Sir George Carey, second Lord Hunsdon (1547–1603), that 'quicksilver is in his head but his wit's dull as lead' (p.235). The courtier and nobleman referred to was known for his dissolute living and weak health and apparently died of syphilis in 1603.

The woodcut above depicts the coat of arms which was granted to the Barber-Surgeons' Company in 1569. This heraldic woodcut forms the frontispiece of William Clowes's 1579 treatise on syphilis, *A Short and Profitable Treatise Touching the Cure of the Morbus Gallicus by Unctions*. 'By God's foreknowledge,' reads the motto on the emblem, whose most interesting feature is the two embossed heraldic animals.

Cavendish; Walter Raleigh and Elizabeth Throgmorton; Robert Tyrwhitt and Bridget Manners; Southampton and Elizabeth Vernon; and Essex and Elizabeth Brydges, Mary Howard, Elizabeth Russell and Elizabeth Southwell. The young offenders were usually punished by the Queen by being sent for a short stay in the Tower or the Fleet, but they were normally forgiven and permitted to resume their place in the aristocratic hierarchy at Court. The young Earl of Pembroke proved an exception to this rule because his case varied in a number of critical ways. He had made a maid of honour pregnant and refused to marry her, and the young mother had given birth to a son who died shortly after delivery. Births at that time could be a very dangerous affair to both mother and child, but in Mary Fitton's case the mother survived while the child died. Mortality in neonates could be due to premature delivery, obstetric complications or infections in the newborn, sometimes passed on from the mother.

If Mary Fitton's son had been conceived on the night of the wedding of Anne Russell and Henry Herbert, his birth would have been a fortnight too early – hardly as early, however, as to warrant a premature delivery of a fatal nature. Of the two remaining possibilities, obstetric complications and infections in the newborn, the latter seems more likely. Sources indicate that William Herbert and Mary Fitton suffered illnesses at exactly the same time (see p.191), and in William Herbert's case the symptoms mimicked those of syphilis. Even if he had been infected as early as June 1598, his untreated syphilis would still be infectious two years after, in June 1600. Mary Fitton's illness in January and February of 1600 may have derived from William Herbert's unnamed disease, for it is likely that they entered into a sexual relationship with each other in the period 1599–1600. If Mary Fitton contracted syphilis during this period, she would have passed it on to her baby when she became pregnant in the summer of 1600. In that case congenital syphilis – a very common cause of stillbirths – would have caused the death of her baby, perhaps after premature delivery, in the beginning of March 1601.

William Clowes was one of the Queen's physicians, and it is feasible that he was consulted when Mary Fitton was taken into custody by Lady Hawkyns. He might also have diagnosed the death of Mary Fitton's newborn son as having been due to syphilis and might then have passed on his opinion to the Queen. If this hypothesis is correct, it would explain the Queen's extreme and unusual punishment of the Earl of Pembroke, who never again breathed freely while Elizabeth I was alive. In 1603, one of William Herbert's numerous poet friends, John Davies of Hereford, wrote to the young earl upon the coronation of James I shortly after Elizabeth's death:

> Pembrooke to Court (to which thou wert made strange)
> Goe, doe thine homage to thy Soveraigne,
> VVeepe, and reioyce, for this sadd-ioyfull Change;
> Then weepe for ioy, thou needst not teares to faine,
> Sith late thine Eies did nought els entertaine. (Davies, 1603, p.14)

# 10

# SHAKESPEARE'S UNCONSCIOUS IMAGERY

Around the turn of our century, Freud discovered that if he wanted to study his patients' secret thoughts and feelings – all that lies hidden beneath the surface of consciousness – he might do so by examining their dreams and free associations. Freud spoke of dreams as 'the royal road to the unconscious' (*via regia*) and established free associations as a parallel means of penetrating the hidden depths of the human mind. Freud also demonstrated that dreams and free associations rely heavily on the formation of *imagery (Bildersprache)* and that such spontaneously produced images may furnish an insight into the workings of the unconscious mind.

The modern study of the psychological significance of Shakespeare's imagery is perhaps the most rewarding aspect of Shakespearean scholarship in our time. With Shakespeare, the unconscious of the writer surfaces not only in the numerous dreams recorded in his plays but also in the author's free associations as expressed in his rich and varied imagery. This fascinating realm of Shakespeare's art was first opened up by Caroline Spurgeon in 1935 with her now famous *Shakespeare's Imagery and What It Tells Us*. In this pioneering study, Dr. Spurgeon demonstrates that Shakespeare's images connect up and have a consistency of their own, like vegetation under water, and that the study of this subworld may help to throw light on Shakespeare's unconscious mind.

Spurgeon defines an 'image' as any word or group of words conceived of as an analogical unit of thought or physical sensation. Thus, according to Spurgeon, every figure of speech such as a simile or metaphor might be conceived of as an 'image'. 'In the case of a poet', wrote Spurgeon, 'I suggest it is chiefly through his images that he, to some extent unconsciously, "gives himself away". He may be, and in Shakespeare's case is, almost entirely objective in his dramatic characters and their views and opinions, yet, like the man who under stress of emotion will show no sign of it in eye or face, but will reveal it in some muscular tension, the poet unwittingly lays bare his own innermost likes and dislikes, observations and interests, associations of thought, attitudes of mind and beliefs, in and through the images, the verbal pictures he draws to illuminate something quite different in the speech and thought of his characters. The imagery he instinctively uses is thus a revelation, largely unconscious, given at a moment of heightened feeling, of the furniture of his mind, the channels of his thought, the qualities of things, the objects and incidents he observes and remembers, and perhaps most significant of all, those which he does not observe or remember' (Spurgeon, 1935, p.4).

Writing in a time before the existence of computers, Caroline Spurgeon used index-cards to classify the various images occurring in Shakespeare's plays (some six thousand of which she collected). By means of this method she arrived at a number of interesting discoveries, two of which are notable in connection with this study. First, Dr. Spurgeon discovered the presence of recurrent, iterative or 'running' imagery in several of Shakespeare's plays. Like leitmotifs in a Wagnerian opera, a certain type of imagery tended to become insistent in a play, thus investing it with a certain atmosphere, mood or symbolic significance. 'By recurrent imagery', wrote Spurgeon,

> 'I mean the repetition of an idea or picture in the images used in any one play. Thus in *Romeo and Juliet* the dominating image is light with its background of darkness, while in *Hamlet* there hovers all through the play in both words and word pictures the conception of disease, especially of a hidden corruption infecting and destroying a wholesome body. This secondary or symbolic imagery within imagery is a marked characteristic of Shakespeare's art, indeed it is, perhaps, his most individual way of expressing his imaginative vision.' (p.213)

In addition to the recurrent imagery of Shakespeare's plays – their 'undersong' as she also called it (Spurgeon, 1931, p.4) – Spurgeon also studied a related aspect in the *statistical patterns* formed by the distribution of certain *image groups* in Shakespeare's works – yet another avenue into the poet's unconscious. Such distributions of specific image groups cannot, of course, be understood in terms of a deliberate and conscious process on the poet's part, but must be viewed as a spontaneous process unconsciously motivated and therefore tending to reveal certain aspects of and preoccupations of the poet's unconscious. Caroline Spurgeon, for instance, made a statistical chart of the number of images in Shakespeare's plays related to *'food, drink and cooking'* and also one illustrating the number of images concerned with *'sickness, disease and medicine'* (Figure 40). She found that these two image groups peaked in number during the period 1597/8–1601/2, where they were concentrated in the plays *2 Henry IV* (1597–8), *As You Like It* (1599–1600), *Hamlet* (1600–1), and *Troilus and Cressida* (1601–2). She also found that the distribution of such image groups reflected a qualitative as well as a quantitative factor (see further p.228).

To sum up, Caroline Spurgeon's study of the psychological significance of Shakespeare's imagery pointed out two royal roads for a study of the unconscious recesses of the poet's mind: *running symbolic imagery* and the *statistical distribution of certain image groups*, reflecting both quantitative and qualitative factors.

### SIR JOHN FALSTAFF: THE WORLD'S MOST FAMOUS SYPHILITIC

If one studies Caroline Spurgeon's chart in Figure 40, *2 Henry IV* (1597–8) shows a steep quantitative rise in the image group relating to 'sickness, disease and medicine' – imagery clustering around the figure of Falstaff. At the same time, this imagery reveals a *qualitative* change as well in that it is concerned with what Spurgeon calls 'foul disease' (1935, Chart VII), or with diseases related to lust and venery. Falstaff, the fat and dissolute knight, who is perhaps second only to Hamlet as

Shakespeare's most famous imaginative creation, makes his entry in the play in this striking fashion:

FAL.     Sirrah, you giant, what says the doctor to my water?

PAGE    He said, sir, the water itself was a good healthy water; but, for the party that owed it, he might have moe diseases than he knew for. (1,2:1–4)

Shortly afterwards, Falstaff points out two stages of life that have their own curses, which anticipate his own:

FAL.     A man can no more separate age and covetousness than 'a can part young limbs and lechery: but the gout galls the one, and the pox pinches the other…A pox of this gout! or a gout of this pox! for the one or the other plays the rogue with my great toe. 'Tis no matter if I do halt…A good wit will make use of anything; I will turn diseases to commodity. (1,2:229–32;244–7;249–50)

Falstaff's syphilitic illness is alluded to not only in his own humorous references to his aching bones and tabetic gait, but other characters in the plays refer to him as a 'whoremaster' (*1 Henry IV*, 2,4:463) and as a 'globe of sinful continents' (2,4:282). In the Boar's Head Tavern in Eastcheap he establishes his 'court' with the royal youth Prince Hal as his devoted friend and follower. 'Why, thou whoreson, impudent, embossed rascal', Prince Hal apostrophizes his 'sweet creature of bombast' (*1 Henry IV*,2,4:323), 'if there were anything in thy pocket but tavern reckonings, memorandums of bawdy-houses, and one poor pennyworth of sugar-candy to make thee long-winded, if thy pocket were enriched with any other injuries but these, I am a villain' (*1 Henry IV*,3,3:155–61). When Falstaff, after a drinking spree, asks the 'time of the day' of Hal, the latter explodes: 'What a devil hast thou to do with the time of the day? Unless hours were cups of sack, and minutes capons, and clocks the tongues of bawds, and dials the signs of leaping-houses, and the blessed sun himself a fair hot wench in flame-coloured taffeta, I see no reason why thou shouldst be so superfluous to demand the time of the day' (*1 Henry IV*,1,2:1;6–12).

When later Hal learns that Falstaff has been seen dining with a young woman called Doll Tearsheet at the Boar's Head Tavern, he wryly comments: 'This Doll Tearsheet should be some road' (*2 Henry IV*,2,2:159), to which his friend Poins answers: 'I warrant you, as common as the way between Saint Albans and London' (2,2:160–1). In what has been described as 'the finest tavern scene ever written',[*] Shakespeare at this point introduces the Hostess of the Boar's Head Tavern, Mistress Quickly, and the young prostitute Doll Tearsheet, two women who are both in love with Falstaff. Falstaff's association with Doll Tearsheet gives a graphic demonstration of the way in which the fat knight contracted his pox:

*Enter Falstaff singing.* 'When Arthur first in court' – Empty the jordan [chamber-pot]. [*Exit Francis*] – 'And was a worthy king' – How now, Mistress Doll?

HOST.   Sick of a calm, yea, good faith.

FAL.     So is all her sect; an they be once in a calm they are sick.

*    The Arden Shakespeare. *The Second Part of King Henry IV*, edited by A.R. Humphreys, London, 1966, p.62.

Figure 40. Caroline Spurgeon's Chart VII (1935): A Pictorial Statement of the Dominating Images in *Hamlet* and *Troilus and Cressida.* ('The chart was drawn up before Sir E.K. Chambers's book appeared, or I should have adhered to his dates' C.S.)

Reproduced by permission of Cambridge University Press.

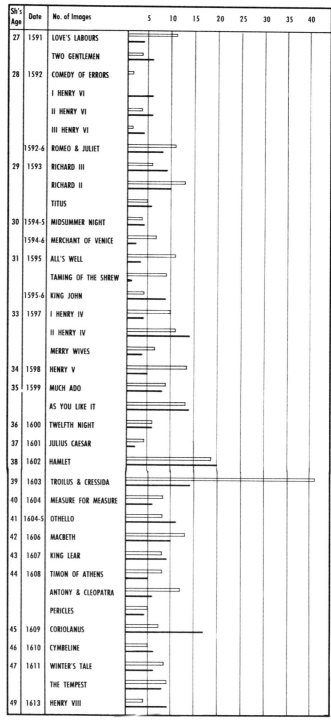

DOLL    A pox damn you, you muddy rascal, is that all the comfort you give me?

FAL.    You make fat rascals, Mistress Doll.

DOLL    I make them? Gluttony and diseases make them, I make them not.

FAL.    If the cook help to make the gluttony, you help to make the diseases, Doll. We catch of you, Doll, we catch of you; grant that, my poor virtue, grant that.

DOLL    Yea, joy, our chains and our jewels.

FAL.    'Your brooches, pearls, and ouches.' For to serve bravely is to come halting off, you know; to come off the breach, with his pike bent bravely; and to surgery bravely; to venture upon the charged chambers bravely –

DOLL    Hang yourself, you muddy conger, hang yourself! (2,4:33–53)

The quibbling of Falstaff's and Doll Tearsheet's amorous quarrel clearly centres on syphilis, its 'catching' nature and transmission through prostitutes, its hard chancres and macular-papular eruptions, and, finally, its debilitating symptoms and medical treatment. In his *Booke of Tumors* (1633), John Banister talks of 'the tumors of the yard, both inward and outward, as brooches of the French disease' (p.135), and in George Chapman's *The Widow's Tears* (1612) a 'diseased lord' has 'as many aches in's bones, as there are ouches in's skinne.' (Humphreys, 1966, p.66). Syphilitic 'gem' imagery also makes its appearance in *Love's Labour's Lost* (1594–5), in which Rosaline tells the Princess: 'O that your face were not so full of O's!' and receives the reply: 'A pox of that jest!' (5,2:45–6).

After their amorous quarrel at the Boar's Head Tavern, Falstaff and Doll Tearsheet begin to kiss and cuddle, while Hal and Poins enter the tavern disguised as drawers in order to observe 'Saturn and Venus this year in conjunction' (2,4:261):

FAL.    Thou dost give me flattering busses.

DOLL    By my troth, I kiss thee with a most constant heart.

FAL.    I am old, I am old.

DOLL    I love thee better than I love e'er a scurvy young boy of them all...

FAL.    Come, it grows late, we'll to bed...

DOLL    I'll canvass thee between a pair of sheets. (2,4:266–70;273;221)

For the rest of *2 Henry IV* nothing more is heard of Doll Tearsheet and Mistress Quickly until they reappear in the play's penultimate scene, where two beadles drag them along to the Clink, a prison for prostitutes, under the women's violent protests.

## A VENEREAL 'BURNING' IN WINDSOR FOREST

Prostitutes, the Clown jests in *The Comedy of Errors* (1592–3), 'appear to men like angels of light; light is an effect of fire, and fire will burn; ergo, light wenches will burn; come not near her' (4,3:53–5). Falstaff might have listened to this piece of advice to his own advantage, for at the end of *The Merry Wives of Windsor* (1597–8) the dissolute knight receives a powerful 'burning' under the oak of Herne the Hunter in Windsor Forest. Here, his punishment is meted out by Mrs. Ford and Mrs. Page, who decide that the promiscuous knight's behaviour toward them calls for a proper 'medicine' (3,3:178) to cure his 'dissolute disease' (3,3:177). Together with their husbands they dupe the old knight to appear at a nightly meeting in Windsor Forest, wearing a buck's head, and here they terrify the lecherous knight with a supernatural show in which he is assailed by a group of Windsor children disguised as fairies and hobgoblins. They 'pinch the unclean knight' (4,4:57) with burning tapers while singing:

> Fie on sinful fantasy,
> Fie on lust and luxury...
> Pinch him, fairies, mutually;
> Pinch him for his villainy;
> Pinch him, and burn him, and turn him about,
> Till candles and starlight and moonshine be out. (5,5:94–5;100–4)

After Falstaff has been burnt by the punitive symbols of his own 'wicked fire of lust' (2,1:65), the repentant knight finally promises to mend his ways while sighing: 'This is enough to be the decay of lust and late-walking through the realm' (5,5:144–6).

The epilogue of Falstaff's libidinal adventures strikes a rather sombre note as revealed in the sequel to *The First and Second Part of Henry IV* and *The Merry Wives of Windsor*. In *Henry V* (1598–9), Pistol turns up before the Boar's Head Tavern to inform the audience that he has married Mistress Quickly and thus become a host of the inn himself. During a quarrel with his friend Nym over the landlady, Pistol contemptuously advises his jealous friend to fetch a wife by going to the hospital:

PISTOL      O hound of Crete, think'st thou my spouse to get?
                 No; to the spital go,
                 And from the powdering tub of infamy
                 Fetch forth the lazar kite of Cressid's kind,
                 Doll Tearsheet she by name, and her espouse. (2,1:73–7)

Falstaff's prostitute girl friend is apparently under treatment for her 'lazar'-like disease in the barber-surgeon's infamous vessel, seeking cure in the mercurial 'fumes for the pox' (Figure 14). One is not surprised, therefore, to hear Pistol announce to his friends, at the end of *Henry V*, that young 'Doll is dead i'th' spital Of malady of France' (5,1:85–6).

At the same time it appears that Doll's old lover has also given up the spirit and left the stage. In a moving soliloquy, Mistress Quickly describes Falstaff's end in the Boar's Head Tavern, where she assures his cronies that the old knight is 'in Arthur's bosom' (2,3:9–10), since he has made a most Christian end. Nym and Falstaff's servant, however, express reservations on the latter point:

NYM     They say he cried out of [against] sack.

HOST.    Ay, that a' did.

BARD.    And of [against] women.

HOST.    Nay, that a' did not.

BOY      Yes, that a' did; and said they were devils incarnate.

HOST.   A' could never abide carnation; 'twas a colour he never liked.

BOY    A' said once, the devil would have him about women.

HOST.   A' did in some sort, indeed, handle women; but then he was rheumatic, and
        talked of the whore of Babylon. (2,3:28–40)

To all appearances, Shakespeare's merry old knight has died a misogynist and
entertained the conviction that Lucifer would take his soul as punishment for his
immoral dealings with women. On his deathbed, Falstaff appears to have received
his final bout of 'burning', his feverish ravings centering on the scarlet, archetypal
prostitute in the Bible – a replica of Doll Tearsheet who according to the fat knight
'is in hell already and burns poor souls' (*2 Henry IV*,2,4:335–6). Whatever the cause
of Falstaff's death and final 'burning', the lover of Doll Tearsheet and her crew
could only have escaped syphilitic infection short of a miracle – and the fat knight
was perhaps hardly the kind of man for whom heaven would have intervened.

## THE 'GOOSE CLUSTER'

While Falstaff is waiting under Herne's oak for his two women, he asks 'the
hot-blooded gods' (5,5:2) to assist him. In particular he calls on Jove or Jupiter who
transformed himself into a bull when attempting to rape Europa. 'You were also,
Jupiter', he goes on to apostrophize him, 'a swan for the *love* of Leda. O omnipotent
*love*, how near the god drew to the complexion of a *goose*! A *fault* done first in the
form of a *beast*: O Jove, a *beastly fault*! And then another *fault* in the semblance of a
*fowl*: think on't, Jove, a *foul fault*! When gods have *hot backs*, what shall poor men
do?' (5,5:6–12).

In this passage, the image of the goose is surrounded by a number of associations
(italicised) which center on 'love', 'beastly', 'foul', 'hot backs', and 'faults' – the last
word invested with the particular meaning of a 'foul' sexual sin. In his study of
*Shakespeare's Imagination* (1946), the English ornithologist and psychologist Edward
A. Armstrong demonstrated that in Shakespeare the image of the goose is always
accompanied by a satellite system of associations centering on 'lust', 'lechery',
'punishment' and 'disease'.

Armstrong was one of Caroline Spurgeon's followers, and the main object of his
studies was the associative processes of Shakespeare's imagination. In this field,
Caroline Spurgeon had made yet another pioneering venture with her discovery of
certain *associative linkages* or *'clusters' of associations* in Shakespeare's work. 'The
repeated evidence of clusters of certain associated ideas in the poet's mind', wrote
Spurgeon, 'is one of the most interesting of studies, and throws a curious light on
what I suppose the psycho-analyst would call "complexes"; that is, certain groups
of things and ideas – apparently entirely unrelated – which are linked together in
Shakespeare's subconscious mind, and some of which are undoubtedly the outcome
of an experience, a sight or emotion which has profoundly affected him' (1931,
p.13).

Spurgeon pointed out the presence of a 'dog cluster' in Shakespeare's plays and stated that 'this curious group of images is but one example of many such associated groups, which, when studied together, throw a distinct light on Shakespeare's likes and dislikes, physical sensations, experiences, and emotions, and sometimes on his deepest thought and feelings' (p.17).

Spurgeon demonstrated that whenever the idea of false friends or flatterers occurs in Shakespeare, there is a rather curious set of images which play round it. These are, a dog or spaniel, fawning and licking, candy, sugar or sweets, thawing or melting. So strong is the association of these ideas in Shakespeare's mind, that whenever he begins with one of these items – dog or sugar or melting – it almost invariably gives rise to the whole series. Spurgeon interpreted the 'dog cluster' in terms of a psychological 'complex' in Shakespeare which betrayed his deep personal disgust at 'feigned love and affection assumed for a selfish end' (1935, p.195): 'So there come to be linked in his mind two things he intensely dislikes, one in the physical everyday world, the other in the world of mind and emotions: the fawning cupboard love of dogs, their greed and gluttony, with its sticky and disagreeable consequences, and the other fawning of insincere friends, bowing and flattering for what they hope to get, and turning their backs when they think no more is coming to them' (1931, p.15). She thought it

> 'as certain as anything can be, short of direct proof, that he had been hurt, directly or indirectly, in this particular way. No one who reads his words carefully can doubt that he had either watched someone, whose friendship he prized, being deceived by fawning flatterers, or that he himself had suffered from a false friend or friends, who, for their own ends, had drawn out his love while remaining "themselves as stone".' [A quotation from Sonnet 94, with reference to the 'Unmovèd, cold' youth, who may have been the origin of this particular 'complex' in Shakespeare.] (1935, p.195)*

## ARMSTRONG'S AND WENTERSDORF'S 'GOOSE CLUSTER'

In *Shakespeare's Imagination*, Edward A. Armstrong pursued Spurgeon's method in order to explore what she had termed 'this habit in Shakespeare of returning under similar emotional stimulus to a similar picture or group of associated ideas' (Spurgeon, 1931, p.17). Armstrong succeeded in isolating a number of associative linkages such as a kite-bed-death-spirits-birds-food 'cluster'; a beetle-crow-mice-night-death-madness-fairies-cliff 'cluster'; a drone-weasel- (king-creature) -creeping-cat-mood-sucking-music 'cluster'; and the like. The most interesting 'cluster' discovered by Armstrong was the goose-lust-diseases-punishment 'cluster', which looked like the following:

---

\*    Dr. Spurgeon's discovery of the dog cluster and its chain of associations was anticipated at the end of the 18th century in a book by Walter Whiter (1758–1832) entitled *A Specimen of a Commentary on Shakespeare* (1794). Whiter's work summarized the researches done into the area of associations since antiquity, in which Aristotle had formulated the main laws of association. According to the Greek philosopher, these laws followed the laws of resemblance, contrast, and contiguity (in space and time), to which the English philosopher David Hume added the law of cause and effect.

| Context | Goose | Disease | Music | Bitterness | Seasoning | Restraint |
|---|---|---|---|---|---|---|
| 1 H. VI 1.3.53 | goose[53] | | | | | rope[33] |
| L.L.L. 1.1.97 | geese[97] | pain[73]<br>blind[76]<br>blinded[83] | sing[103] | | saucy[85] | |
| 3.1.98-123<br>4.3.75 | goose[98] etc.<br>goose[75] | | | liver-vein[74] | | bound, etc.[126] |
| Two Gent. 4.4.35 | geese[35] | blind[4] | | | | hanged[5]<br>hang[24]<br>stocks[33]<br>pillory[35] |
| R. & J. 2.4.75-90 | wild-goose[75]<br>goose[86, 90] | | | bitter sweeting[83] | saucy[53]<br>sauce[84] | ropery[153] |
| M.N.D. 3.2.20<br>5.1.235-38 | wild-geese[20]<br>goose[235, 238] | | | | | |
| M. of V. 5.1.105 | goose[105] | blind[112]<br>sick[124] | sing[102 104]<br>music[97]<br>musician[106] | | season[107]<br>season'd[107] | stockish[81] |
| 1 H. IV 2.4.152 | wild-geese[152] | plague[148] | sing[147] | | | stocks[130]<br>unhanged[144] |
| 3.1.232 | goose[232] | | sing[216, 223]<br>music[232]<br>musician[235] | | | hang[227]<br>penn'd[209] |
| 2 H. IV 1.2.196 | gooseberry[196] | | singing[213] | livers[198]<br>bitterness[198]<br>galls[199] | gravy[184] | |
| 5.1.79 | wild-geese[79] | diseases[85]<br>ache[93] | | | | |
| M.W. 3.4.41<br>5.1.27<br>5.5.9 | geese[41]<br>geese[27]<br>goose[9] | sickly[61] | tune[21] | gall'd[5] | | pen[41] |
| A.Y.L.I. 2.7.86 | wild-goose[86] | infected[60]<br>sores[67] | | | | |
| 3.4.48 | goose[48] | | | bitterness[3.5.3] | | |
| T. & C. 5.10.55 | goose[55] | aching[51]<br>diseases[57] | sing[42] | galled[55] | | |
| Ham. 2.2.359 | goose-quill[359] | | sing[363] | | | |
| Tw.N. 3.2.53 | goose-pen[53] | | | gall[52]<br>liver[66] | | hang[29]<br>-pen[53]<br>wainropes[64] |
| K.L. 2.2.89 | goose[89] | plague[87]<br>epileptic[87] | | lily-liver'd[18] | saucy[103] | cords[80] |
| 2.4.46 | wild-geese[46] | blind[49]<br>dolours[54] | | | saucily[41] | stocks[65] |
| Mac. 2.3.17 | goose[17] | | | | | hanged[5]<br>turning the key[2] |
| 5.3.12-13 | goose[12]<br>geese[13] | sick[19] | | lily-liver'd[15] | | |
| Cor. 1.1.176 | geese[176] | itch[168]<br>sick[182] | | | | hang[185] |
| 1.4.34 | geese[34] | contagion[30]<br>boils[31]<br>plagues[31]<br>infect[33]<br>agued[38] | | | | shut[47] |
| Temp. 2.2.135 | goose[135] | ague[139] | | | | |

Figure 41. Armstrong's 'goose cluster' (1946, p.65)

TABLE 1

| | BETRAY TRAITOR | REVOLT REBEL- LION | FALSE DECEIT- FUL | TRICKS COUNTER- FEIT | SWEARING PERJURY | VOWS OATHS |
|---|---|---|---|---|---|---|
| *1 Hen. VI*, I.iii | traitors proditor | conspirator | hypocrite | conveyance* | | |
| *T.G.V.* IV.iv | traitor | | false deceive | trick | perjury | vow, promise break oaths |
| *L.L.L.* I.i | mutiny | | falsely | | swear, sworn forsworn | oath(s) break troth |
| *L.L.L.* III.i | betray betrayed | | | | perjured | |
| *L.L.L.* IV.iii | betrayed traitors treason | | false hypocrisy | tricks cheat | perjury perjured forsworn | oaths, vows break vow break faith |
| *Romeo* II.iv | | | deceived | counterfeit | | |
| *Dream* III.ii | | conspired | false | counterfeit | swear swore | oath, vow, troth vows of faith |
| *Dream* V.i | | | deceiving | tricks | | promise |
| *Merch.* V.i | treason | stratagems | false deceived | | swear | vows of faith oath(s) |
| *1 Hen. IV*, II.iv | | | false deceiveth | trick, convey counterfeit | swearest | |
| *1 Hen. IV*, III.i | | | | | swear | oath(s) promises |
| *2 Hen. IV*, I.ii | | rebels rebellion | | trick | sworn | |
| *A.Y.L.* III.iv-v | | | false, falser dissembling | counterfeit | swear | oath(s) vows |
| *Twel.* III.i-ii | betray | | false | feigning policy | | oaths |
| *Ham.* II.ii | treason treacherous | rebellious | falsely deceived | tricked policy | | vow |
| *Wives* III.iii-v | betray traitor | | deceived dissembling | trick(s) conveyance | swears sworn | promise(d) |
| *Wives* V.v | | | deceit | | swearings | |
| *Troi.* V.x | traitors | | | | | |
| *Lear* II.ii | | rebel | | | | |
| *Lear* II.iv | | revolt | | tricks | | |
| *Macb* II.iii | treason treasonous | | false | counterfeit | swear | |
| *Macb.* V.iii-v | | revolts | false | | | faith-breach |
| *Cor.* I.i | mutinous | revolt rebellion | | | | promise |
| *Cor.* I.iv-ix | | | falsed-faced | | | vows promise-breaker |
| *Temp.* II.ii | perfidious | | | tricks | swear sworn | troth |

*conveyance*, 'trickery'

Source: Wentersdorf, 1972, pp.245–53

Figure 42. Wentersdorf's 'goose cluster'.

In 1972, Karl P. Wentersdorf developed the 'goose cluster' in its fullest form, adding to Armstrong's one table of associative linkages no less than 8 tables (above and on the following pages).

TABLE 2

| | GOOSE WILD-GOOSE | SAUCE SEASONING | TASTE RELISH | SWEET BITTER | GALL LIVER | PEN PAPER | BLACK WHITE |
|---|---|---|---|---|---|---|---|
| *1 Hen. VI*, I.iii | goose (line 53) | | | | | | |
| *T.G.V.* IV.iv | geese (37) | | sweet | bitterly | | paper | black |
| *L.L.L.* I.i. | geese (97) | saucy season | | sweet | | pen, ink paper | black-, white |
| *L.L.L.* III.i. | goose (98) | | | sweet sweetly | | | white |
| *L.L.L.* IV.iii | goose (75) | saucers* | taste | sweet bitter | liver-vein | pen, ink paper | black |
| *Romeo* II.iv | wild-goose, goose (75-91) | sauce saucy sharp | | sweetest bitter | | | black white |
| *Dream* III.ii | wild-geese (20) | salt | | sweet bitter | | | black white |
| *Dream* V.i | goose (235-40) | saucy | | sweet | | pen | black |
| *Merch.* V.i | goose (105) | season seasoned | | sweet(er) sweetly | | pen | |
| *1 Hen. IV*, II.iv | wild-geese (152) | sauce peppered | taste | sweet | livers | papers | black-, white |
| *1 Hen. IV*, III.i | goose (232) | pepper- | taste | sweet | | | |
| *2 Hen. IV*, I.ii | gooseberry (195) | saltness | relish smack | sweet bitterness | livers gall galls | | white |
| *A.Y.L.* III.iv-v | goose (48) | sauce | | sweet bitter bitterness | | inky | black cream |
| *Twel.* III.i-ii | goose-pen (ii.53) | | taste tastes | | gall liver | -pen, ink paper | |
| *Ham.* II.ii | goose-quills (359) | sallets savory | taste | sweet bitter | -livered gall | -quills | black white |
| *Wives* III.iii-v | geese (iv.41) | season pepper-box | | sweet | galled | pen | |
| *Wives* V.v | goose (9) | | | sweetheart | | | black |
| *Troi.* V.x | goose (55) | | | sweet | galled | | |
| *Lear* II.ii | goose (89) | saucy | | | -livered | | |
| *Lear* II.iv | wild-geese (46) | saucily sharp | taste | sweet | | | black |
| *Macb.* II.iii | goose (16) | | | | | | |
| *Macb.* V.iii-v | goose (12) geese (13) | | | sweet | -livered | | black cream-faced |
| *Cor.* I.i | geese (176) | | | | | | |
| *Cor.* I.iv-ix | geese (34) | sauced | | | | | |
| *Temp.* II.ii · | goose (135) | savor | taste | | | | black |

*saucers*, dishes for sauce or salt; here, for blood

TABLE 3

| | WHORES BAWDS | DISEASES PLAGUE | BLIND | PINCH PRICK | PAIN SUF-FERING | MEDICAL TREAT-MENT |
|---|---|---|---|---|---|---|
| *1 Hen. VI*, I.iii | whores | | | | pain | |
| *T.G.V.* IV.iv | | | blind blinded | pinches | suffered | starved |
| *L.L.L.* I.i | | sick bedrid | blind blinded lose eyes | pricks | pain painfully | fast physic |
| *L.L.L.* III.i | | French crown plague | purblind | | groans | salve purgation |
| *L.L.L.* IV.iii | whoreson light wenches | sick to death maladies, plagues | blind blinded | | groans pains | fasting, cures incision, salve |
| *Romeo* II.iv | whore, harlot bawdy | pox | blind | prick prick-song | groaning | |
| *Dream* III.ii | | -sick | | | | remedy medicine |
| *Dream* V.i | | | | | moans | surgeon recover** |
| *Merch.* V.i | | sick | blind | | pains | starved |
| *1 Hen. IV*, II.iv | whoreson harlotry | plague, dropsies bald crown | | | | starveling |
| *1 Hen. IV*, III.i | harlotry | distemperature | | pinched | | |
| *2 Hen. IV*, I.ii | whoreson stews | diseases, pox sick, gout | | pinches | | physician, sweat minister, remedy |
| *A.Y.L.* III.iv-v | | | | | hurt | fasting heal, relief |
| *Twel.* III.i-ii | Pandarus | corrupter | | | | |
| *Ham.* II.ii | whore, strumpet bawdy, drab | distemper | | | | |
| *Wives* III.iii-v | stewed* | sickly, disease distemper rotten | blind | | pains suffered | physician, pills bath, sweating medicine |
| *Wives* V.v | pander | corrupt corrupted | | pinch | suffered pain | balm remedy |
| *Troi.* V.x | bawds pander | plagues diseases | eyes half out | | aching groans | medicine starve, sweat |
| *Lear* II.ii | whoreson bawd, pander | plague, corrupter epileptic | | | | remedies |
| *Lear* II.iv | stewed* whore | sick, disease plague, boil corrupted | blind blinding | pinch | suffer dolors | |
| *Macb.* II.iii | | feverous | destroy sight | | pain | sweat physics |
| *Macb.* V.iii-v | | sick diseased | | prick | | minister, cure purge, physic |
| *Cor.* I.i | | sick itch, scabs | | | suffering | minister hunger |
| *Cor.* I.iv-ix | | infect, agued, con-tagion, murrain, boils, plague(s) feverous, fester | | | | sweat dieted balms |
| *Temp.* II.ii | | infections, ague, disease, plague, itch, scurvy, rotten | | pinch pricks | suffered | relief recover** |

*pun on *stew(s)*, 'brothel'          **recover, 'cure'

TABLE 4

| | LECHERY WILD LUST | FLESH BLOOD | HEAT PASSION | MAD MOON | HORNS CUCK-OLD | BURN FIRE | COLD ICE |
|---|---|---|---|---|---|---|---|
| *1 Hen. VI*, I.iii | | -blood | | | | | |
| *T.G.V.* IV.iv | | | passioning | | | | cold coldly |
| *L.L.L.* I.i | | flesh and blood | heat passion | | | fire | snow |
| *L.L.L.* III.i | wanton | flesh | passionate | | | fired | |
| *L.L.L.* IV.iii | wanton | flesh and blood | passion | mad moon | horns | fire fiery | |
| *Romeo* II.iv | lustier | flesh | | mad | | | |
| *Dream* III.ii | | | passion passionate | mad(ly) moon | | fiery | snow |
| *Dream* V.i | rage wildest rage | blood | hot passion | mad, moon frenzy lunatic | horns horned | burning fire | ice snow cool |
| *Merch.* V.i | wild, rage wanton | blood flesh | hot | mad moon | cuckolds | | |
| *1 Hen. IV*, II.iv | wild | flesh blood | hot passion | mad | cuckolds | fire | cold |
| *1 Hen. IV*, III.i | wanton rage | blood | hot passion | mad | | fiery fire | |
| *2 Hen. IV*, I.ii | lechery | blood | heat | | horn | | |
| *A.Y.L.* III.iv-v | lusty | bloody | | | | | ice |
| *Twel.* III.i-ii | wanton | blood | | | | fire | icicles |
| *Ham.* II.ii | lecherous rage | bleeding | hot passion(ate) | mad(ness) lunacy | | fire burning | |
| *Wives* III.iii-v | wild lecher | | hot heat | mad, -mad lunatic | cuckold horns horn-mad | fire | cold cool snowballs |
| *Wives* V.v | luxury, lust fornications | hot-blooded bloody | hot rut-time | moonshine | horns cuckold cuckoldly | fire burn flames | cold cool snow |
| *Troi.* V.x | rage | flesh | | frenzy's | | | cold |
| *Lear* II.ii | | flesh fleshment | passion | mad moon(shine) | | fire | snow colder |
| *Lear* II.iv | wantons, wild, lusty, rage | flesh, blood hot-blooded | hot passion | mad | adultress | burn fiery | cold |
| *Macb.* II.ii | lechery | blood | | | | bonfire | cold |
| *Macb.* V.iii-v | | flesh | | | | | |
| *Cor.* I.i | | blood | | moon | horns | fire | ice |
| *Cor.* I.iv-ix | | blood | | | | fires | |
| *Temp* II.ii | | | | mad(ness) mooncalf | | firing | |

TABLE 5

| | LAW JUDG- MENT | OBEY OBEDIENCE | PRISON CONFINE- MENT | BEATING WHIP- PING | DEATH HANGING | SUNDRY PUNISH- MENTS |
|---|---|---|---|---|---|---|
| *1 Hen. VI*, I.iii | law | | | beat rope | death | |
| *T.G.V.* IV.iv | judge judgment | | | whip | hang, hang-man, executed | stocks, stocked pillory |
| *L.L.L.* I.i | law, laws decree | | | | death | punishment |
| *L.L.L.* III.i | | | restrained immured, bound | whip | | |
| *L.L.L.* IV.iii | law(ful) decree justice | obey obedient | dungeons immured | whip whipping | hangs, Tyburn death execution | punishment losing tongue |
| *Romeo* II.iv | law | | constrains | ropery cords | | torments |
| *Dream* III.ii | judgment | | constraineth | whip with a rod | hang death | |
| *Dream* V.i | | | | | hanged death | |
| *Merch.* V.i | judge | | bound | | death | stockish |
| *1 Hen. IV*, II.iv | judge | | bound | beat cart | hang, hanging unhanged halter, death | nether-stocks strappado racks |
| *1 Hen. IV*, III.i | | | | | hang | |
| *2 Hen. IV*, I.ii | laws judgment | | imprisonment | | hang, hanged death | punish by the heels |
| *A.Y.L.* III.iv-v | | | | | executioner axe, death | |
| *Twel.* III.i-ii | judgment | obey | fetter | wainropes | hang | stockings |
| *Ham.* II.ii | law, judge judgments justly | obey obedience | prison prisoner dungeons | beaten whipping carters | death | rack |
| *Wives* III.iii-v | judge judgment | obey | | | hang death | punishment set quick in earth |
| *Wives* V.v | | disobedience | | swinged | hanged | arrested |
| *Troi.* V.x | | | | | death | |
| *Lear* II.ii | | | constrains restrained | beat cords | | punished |
| *Lear* II.iv | | obedience | turns the key restrained | beat | death | stocks, stocked nether-stocks |
| *Macb.* II.iii | | | turning the key | | hanged death | |
| *Macb.* V.iii-v | just | obedience | constrained | beat | hang death | |
| *Cor.* I.i | justice | | restrain(ed) chain up | | hang | |
| *Cor.* I.iv-ix | decrease | obeyed | pound up prisoner put in manacles | beat whip | hangmen death | |
| *Temp.* II.ii | | | | beat | hang death | torment |

TABLE 6

| | GOD HEAVEN | DEVIL HELL | PRAYER WORSHIP | SIN OFFENCE | FAULT GUILT | REPENTANCE CONFESSION | PAGAN DEITIES |
|---|---|---|---|---|---|---|---|
| *1 Hen. VI*, I.iii | God | devil | religion | sin | wrongs | | |
| *T.G.V.* IV.iv | god heaven(ly) | | worshipped | | fault | | Jove idolatry |
| *L.L.L.* I.i | God, god-heaven | | pray | | | confess penance | |
| *L.L.L.* III.i | heaven | | pray worship | | | | Cupid |
| *L.L.L.* IV.iii | God, gods heavens heavenly | hell devil | religion deity | sin offend offending | fault guilty | confess | Jove, Cupid Juno, Bacchus idolatry |
| *Romeo* II.iv | God heaven | devil | | sin | fault | shrift shrived | |
| *Dream* III.ii | gods heavens | devilish | prayers | offend | fault wrong | | Cupid |
| *Dream* V.i | God heaven | devils hell | | offend(ed) wicked | | repent confess | Jove Bacchanals |
| *Merch.* V.i | God heaven | | prays | | fault wrong | | |
| *1 Hen. IV*, II.iv | God heaven | devil | pray praying | sin, vice wicked | | | |
| *1 Hen. IV*, III.i | God heaven | devil hell | | | fault | | |
| *2 Hen. IV*, I.ii | God | ill-angel | pray worship | | | repents confess | |
| *A.Y.L.* III.iv-v | heaven | | worship religiously | offence | | | |
| *Twel.* III.i-ii | heavens | | | | guilt wrong | | Jove |
| *Ham.* II.ii | God, god heaven heavens | devil hell hellish | | sin | guilty | confession remorse remorseless | idol |
| *Wives* III.iii-v | heaven heavenly | devil hell | | sin, sins offended | faults wrong | confess remorse | |
| *Wives* V.v | god, gods heaven | devil hell | prayers irreligious | sin, sinful offence wicked | fault wrong guiltiness | | Jove Cupid Jupiter |
| *Troi.* V.x | gods | | | wicked | | | |
| *Lear* II.ii | heaven's | | | offence | fault | | |
| *Lear* II.iv | gods heaven heavens | | | offended offence wicked | wronged | confess | Jove Juno Jupiter |
| *Macb.* II.iii | God Heaven | devil hell | | | | repent | |
| *Macb.* V.iii-v | | devil | | | | | |
| *Cor.* I.i | gods heaven | | worshipful | sin, vice offence | fault | confess | |
| *Cor.* I.iv-ix | gods heaven | hell | | sin | | | Jupiter |
| *Temp.* II.ii | god heaven | devil devils | | | | | |

TABLE 7

| | TRADE MARKET | MONETARY TRANSACTIONS | MONEY PURSE | THIEF | ROB STEAL | TALE TAIL | SUIT ARGUMENT |
|---|---|---|---|---|---|---|---|
| *1 Hen. VI*, I.iii | | | purses | | | | |
| *T.G.V.* IV.iv | market-place offer(ed) | | purse | | steals stolen | | suit |
| *L.L.L.* I.i | | buy, profit purchased | | | | | |
| *L.L.L.* III.i | market bargain | buy, bought purchased sell, sold | penny pennyworth price | | | | argument |
| *L.L.L.* IV.iii | | buys sale, seller | -purses | thief, theft pickpurses | | | suit argument |
| *Romeo* II.iv | merchant offer(ed) | | penny | | | tale | argument |
| *Dream* III.ii | | buy, pay(s) paying | fee | thief | steal stolen | tales | argument |
| *Dream* V.i | | paying | | | | story | argument |
| *Merch.* V.i | | | fee | | steal stealing | | |
| *1 Hen. IV*, II.iv | trading | buy, spendest paid paid back | money purses pennyworth | thieves thief | stolest rob (bed) robbery | tale tailor | suits argument |
| *1 Hen. IV*, III.i | bargain | profited | | thief | steal rob | tailor | |
| *2 Hen. IV*, I.ii | offer | buy bought | money, purse pence, penny pounds | | robbery | | |
| *A.Y.L.* III.iv-v | markets offer | sell, bought sale-work | -purse | pickpurse | -stealer | | |
| *Twel.* III.i-ii | trade | | | | | | suit argument |
| *Ham.* II.ii | offer | profit | money fee | | | tale | argument |
| *Wives* III.iii-v | | | money, purse halfpenny | | stole | tailor longtail | suit |
| *Wives* V.v | | buys, sold paid, repay | money pounds | | | | |
| *Troi.* V.x | trade traders | | | | | tail | |
| *Lear* II.ii | trade | | pound | | pilfer-ings | tailor wagtail | suit |
| *Lear* II.iv | | | | | | tales | |
| *Macb.* II.iii | trade | | | | stole steal(ing) | tailor | argument |
| *Macb.* V.iii-v | | profit | | | | tale story | |
| *Cor.* I.i | | pays | price | | steal rob | tale | suitors arguing |
| *Cor.* I.iv-ix | market-place | buy, pay sell | doit drachme | theft | | | |
| *Temp.* II.ii | | pay, paid lay out | doit piece of silver | | rob | tailor | |

TABLE 8

| | DOG CUR | HUNT CHASE | MUSIC MUSICIAN | SING TUNE | PROCREATION PREGNANCY, BIRTH | CHILD INFANCY |
|---|---|---|---|---|---|---|
| *1 Hen. VI*, I.iii | | chase | | | | child's |
| *T.G.V.* IV.iv | dog, cur currish | | | | | infancy |
| *L.L.L.* I.i | | hunt hunteth | music minstrelsy | sing harmony | a-breeding, birth born, first-born | infants child |
| *L.L.L.* III.i | | hunt | | sing tune | with child | child |
| *L.L.L.* IV.iii | | hunting | musical minstrels | tune harmony | born, new-born engenders, with child | infant, child infancy |
| *Romeo*, II.iv | dog's | chase | | tuners sing, -song | conceive, great | |
| *Dream* III.ii | dog, cur hounds | | | | born, nativity | child childhood |
| *Dream* V.i | | | music | sing singer | bride-bed, nativity | issue, child children |
| *Merch.* V.i | | | music musician | sings harmony | conceive | |
| *1 Hen. IV*, II.iv | | | | sing | begets, misbegotten | |
| *1 Hen. IV*, III.i | | | musical musicians | sing, sung song | birth, born | |
| *2 Hen. IV*, I.ii | dog | hunt | | singing | pregnancy, born | |
| *A.Y.L.* III.iv-v | | | | | | children |
| *Twel.* III.i-ii | dogged | chase | music | | bred, pregnant | |
| *Ham.* II.ii | dog | hunts | | sing | breed, pregnant conceive, conception | baby, child children |
| *Wives* III.iii-v | dog bitch | | | | | child |
| *Wives* V.v | dogs | hunter hunting chased | | tune sing | birth | infancy |
| *Troi.* V.x | | | sweet notes | sing | | |
| *Lear* II.ii | dog dogs | | | | | |
| *Lear* II.iv | dogs | | | | young bones | child(hood) children |
| *Macb.* II.iii | | | | | new hatched | |
| *Macb.* V.iii-v | dogs | | | | born of woman | |
| *Cor.* I.i | dog curs | hunt | | | | |
| *Cor.* I.iv-ix | | chase | | | | progeny |
| *Temp.* II.ii | dog | | | sing tune | | |

## THE 'WINCHESTER GOOSE'

What was the conclusion that Armstrong and Wentersdorf drew from the 'goose cluster' and its strange chains of association? They both attempted to decipher the weird bird in the centre of the cluster, and they both arrived at the same conclusion. The key to the solution of the mystery proved to be the 'Winchester goose' of *1 Henry VI* (1,3:53) and the 'goose of Winchester' of *Troilus and Cressida* (5,10:55). To the satisfaction of the two scholars, the bird in both cases pointed in an unequivocal direction.

In the third scene of the opening of *Henry VI*, Shakespeare lays out the dissension between the two Lancastrian factions, one headed by Gloucester, the King's Protector, the other led by the Bishop of Winchester. Gloucester's supporters are called 'traitors' (1,3:15) by one Lieutenant Woodville, while Winchester is denounced by Gloucester as a conspirator against the authority of the King: 'Thou that contrived'st to murder our dead lord; *Thou that giv'st whores indulgences to sin*' (1,3:34–5). This reference is apparently to the Southwark stews which were under the control of the Bishop of Winchester, who lived near by in Winchester House and enjoyed revenues from extensive properties in the unsavoury Bankside district. One of these brothels even bore the sign of the Cardinal's Hat (see p.61). Gloucester boasts that he will manhandle the bishop – 'Under my feet I'll stamp thy cardinal's hat' (1,3:49) – and when Winchester threatens to make his opponent answer for such insolence before the Pope, Gloucester cries out: '*Winchester goose!* I cry, "A rope! a rope!"' Now beat them hence...Out scarlet hypocrite!' (1,3:53–4;56). In effect, Gloucester is calling Winchester a bawd, and his cry 'a rope!' is a sarcastic call for a humiliating punishment of the prelate usually reserved for bawds and harlots in the Clink.

The only other mentioning of the 'Winchester goose' in Shakespeare occurs at the end of *Troilus and Cressida* (5,10:55), where the symbolic bird appears in the epilogue spoken by Pandarus, the archetypal bawd with the pander's classic diseases, osteoscopic pain and primary optic atrophy. Here the Winchestrian goose is steeped in allusions to syphilis and prostitution, and the occasion is Troilus's curse of the pander who ruined his life by procuring Cressida for him, the play's faithless and promiscuous heroine.

TROILUS      Hence, broker-lackey! Ignomy and shame
             Pursue thy life, and live aye with thy name!

PANDARUS     A goodly medicine for my aching bones! O world, world, world!
             Thus is the poor agent despised. O traitors and bawds, how ear-
             nestly are you set awork, and how ill requited. Why should our en-
             deavour be so loved and the performance so loathed? What verse
             for it, what instance for it? – Let me see:

                 Full merrily the humble-bee doth sing
                 Till he hath lost his honey and his sting;
                 And being once subdued in armed tail,
                 Sweet honey and sweet notes together fail.

> Good traders in the flesh, set this in your painted cloths:
> As many as be here of Pandar's hall,
> Your eyes, half out, weep out at Pandar's fall;
> Or if you cannot weep, yet give some groans,
> Though not for me, yet for your aching bones.
> Brethren and sisters of the hold-door trade,
> Some two months hence my will shall here be made.
> It should be now, but that my fear is this:
> Some galled goose of Winchester would hiss.
> Till then I'll sweat and seek about for eases,
> And at that time bequeath you my diseases. (5,10:33–57)

## THE SYPHILITIC BIRD

The earliest appearance of the 'Winchester goose' yet found is in *The Resurrection of the Masse...by Hughe Hilarie(?)* (Strasbourg, 1554), which is a parody of the Catholic Mass, the Pope and the clergy, written by an exiled Protestant who is probably identical with John Bale. In a stanza where 'The Masse speaketh', the Masse lewdly claims that

> There is no disease in the countrie
> Whyther it be pockes or other sickenes
> But to heale it I haue habilitie.
>
>            (Hilarie, 1554, sig.A3. See also Garret, 1940, p.149)

In the poem, a member of the old clergy is shortly afterward seen to say that 'A Wynchester goose to heale is my gyse' (Hilarie, 1554, p.150) – an apparent reference to Stephen Gardiner who, at the time of the poem's publication was Bishop of Winchester and Queen Mary's Lord Chancellor (see p.78).

A later reference to the venereal bird is found in *The Nomenclator, or Remembrancer of Adrianus Junius* (1585), one of the first English dictionaries in Tudor times. The book defines a 'bubo', or hard chancre, as 'a sore in the grine or yard, which if it come by lecherie, it is called a Winchester goose, or a botch' (Junius, 1585, p.439).

A final reference to the promiscuous living and superstitious practices of the old clergy is found in Thomas Becon's *The Displaying of the Popish Mass*, which was not printed until 1637 but was written c. 1550. Here the author accuses priests of applying their masses to the 'driving away of devils, chasing away of agues, putting back of pestilences, curing of measled swine, healing of sick horses, helping of chickens of the pip, making whole of a Winchester goose' (Becon, 1844b, pp.283–4).

In Jacobean England, the 'Winchester goose' reappears in the works of John Taylor, Ben Jonson, and Thomas Dekker. In a satirical poem termed *Taylors Goose* (1621), the 'Water Poet' presents 'the true nature and profit of all Geese' (Taylor, 1630, p.104), which ultimately concludes with a description of the most odious specimen of all geese:

> Then ther's a Goose that breeds at *Winchester*,
> And of all Geese, my mind is least to her:
> For three or foure weekes after she is rost,

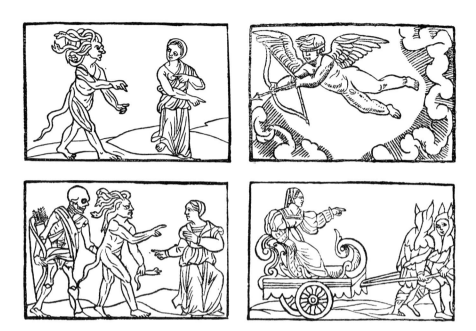

Figure 43. Montaiglon, 1874, emblema XXXIV, XXXV, XXXII/XL, and XLI. With *Troilus and Cressida*, Shakespeare wrote an unsavoury brothel drama in which human attachment is presented as 'hot blood, hot thoughts and hot deeds' (3,1:127–8). The statement is made by Pandarus, who also seems to think that 'love [is] a generation of vipers' (3,1:129), thus availing himself of serpents as symbolic expressions of poisonous love. Similar imagery surfaces in the woodcuts above from the Rabelaisian poem *The Triumph of the High and Mighty Dame Syphilis* (Lyons, 1539). Here the hot female figure of 'Voluptuousness' is approached by the Moirai and Erinyes of the Greek underworld who come to her with snakes, and are followed by Death carrying arrows – snakes and arrows symbolizing human sexuality in the poem. Later, while 'infecting Venus' (emblema XLVII) begins her triumphal procession through the country, enthroned in her chariot and drawn by ass-eared fools, Cupid shoots his poisoned arrows at loving couples, thus symbolizing the sinister tingeing of sexuality with disease in post-Columbian Europe.

*Troilus and Cressida* is a classic example of this trend, which is expressed in the play's merging of its two dominant image groups: 'sickness, disease and medicine' and 'food, drink and cooking'. Critics agree that the latter group is an expression of the sensual faculties of man, with particular emphasis on their libidinal aspect (Muir, 1982, p.29). The blending of the two image groups in the play's iterative or 'running' imagery therefore points to an unconscious, symbolic pattern which reveals the poet's preoccupation with libidinal appetite as related to disease and medicine.

Troilus and Hamlet are passionate and idealistic lovers who share the tragedy of believing that their beloved is a woman pure, only to discover in due time that they were actually whores (Cressida-Gertrude/Ophelia). The language used by the two heroes to describe their disillusioned view of love draws upon the goose cluster of images and shares Pandarus's view of human yearnings.

> She keepes her heat more hotter then a tost.
> She's seldome got or hatch'd with honesty,
> From Fornication and Adultery,
> From reaking Lust, foule Incest, beastly Rape,
> She hath her birth, her breeding, and her shape.
> Besides Whoremongers, Panders, Bawds & Pimpes,
> Whores, Harlots, Curtezans, and such base Impes,
> Luxurious, letcherous Goates, that hunt in Flockes,
> To catch the Glangore, Grinkums, or the Pockes,
> Thus is she got with pleasure, bred with paine.
> And scarce ere comes where honest men remaine.
> This Goose is worst of all, yet is most deare,
> And may be had (or heard of) any where.
> A Pander is the Cater to the Feast,
> A Bawde the Kitchin Clerke, to see her drest.
> A Whore the Cooke, that in a pockey heate,
> Can dresse a dish fit for the Deuill to eate.
> The hot whore-hunter for the Goose doth serue,
> The whil'st the Surgeon, and Physician carue.
> The Apothecary giues attendance still,
> For why the sauce lyes onely in his Bill.
> ...
>
> This Goose is no way to be tolerated,
> But of good men to be despisde and hated,
> For one of these, if it be let alone,
> Will eate the owner to the very bone. (p.105)

In Ben Jonson's poem *Execration against Vulcan* (1640), a work said to have been written on the occasion of the burning of his library, the author describes various historical instances of the ravages caused by Vulcan, the god of fire. In the middle of the poem, Jonson mentions the burning of the Globe in 1613 when sparks from a cannon fired during the performance of Shakespeare's play *Henry VIII* set its thatched roof on fire. Jonson's poem places the Globe in the middle of the Southwark stews on the unsavoury Bankside and also mentions the Puritans' gleeful slander that the theatre was 'some Relique of the Stewes' and therefore justly destroyed by 'a Sparkle of that fire'. 'But, O those Reeds!', Jonson apostrophizes Vulcan,

> thy meere disdaine of them,
> Made thee beget that cruell Stratagem,
> (Which, some are pleas'd to stile but thy madde pranck)
> Against the *Globe*, the Glory of the *Banke*.
> Which, though it were the Fort of the whole Parish,
> Flanck'd with a Ditch, and forc'd out of a Marish,
> I saw with two poore Chambers [volleys] taken in,
> And raz'd, e're thought could urge, This might have bin!
> See the worlds Ruines! nothing but the piles
> Left! and wit since to cover it with Tiles.
> The Brethren, they streight nois'd it out for Newes,

'Twas verily some Relique of the Stewes:
And this a Sparkle of that fire let loose
That was rak'd up in the *Winchestrian Goose*
Bred on the *Banck*, in time of Poperie,
When *Venus* there maintain'd the Misterie [craft].
But, others fell with that conceipt by the eares,
And cry'd, it was a threatning to the beares;
And that accursed ground, the *Parish-Garden*:
Nay, sigh'd a Sister, 'twas the Nun, *Kate Arden*,
Kindled the fire! But then, did one returne,
No Foole would his owne harvest spoile, or burne!
(Jonson, 1925–52, vol.8, pp.208–9)

Kate Arden was a famous 'nun', or prostitute, to whom Jonson also refers in his Epigramme 133:

Neuer did bottome more betray her burden;
The meate-boate of Beares colledge, *Paris-garden*,
Stunke not so ill; nor, when shee kist, *Kate Arden*. (p.87)

Jonson concludes his *Execration against Vulcan* by invoking Pandora, the mythical woman in whose box all the evils that afflict mankind were locked. His exchange of the letter 'p' for 'b' in his poem is a humorous attempt to specify one of the worst evils of his own time, presented as if Pandora herself had suffered from it:

Pox on thee, *Vulcan*, thy *Pandora's* pox,
And all the Evils that flew out of her box
Light on thee: Or if those plagues will not doo,
Thy Wives pox on thee, and *B[ess] B[roughton]s* too. (p.212)[*]

A final and, perhaps, most interesting reference to the 'Winchester goose' is found in Dekker's play *Westward Hoe* of 1604. Here the author gives an account of the way in which the bird had fluttered about most dangerously the year before when the Michaelmas law term had been moved from Westminster to Winchester because of the plague that was raging in London in 1603. The London season consisted in four law-terms called Michaelmas, Hilary, Easter, and Trinity. The law courts were held in Westminster, and it was during these sessions that the city was most crowded and the traffic greatest for thieves and whores. 'Every throng is sure of a pick-pocket', says Trapdore in Dekker's *The Roaring Girl* (1608), 'as sure as a whore is of the clients all Michaelmas term, and of the pox after the term' (3,3:28–30).

---

[*] Bess Broughton would have remained an obscure person lost to history if it had not been for John Aubrey, who has provided us with a full account of her life and career (ms. 6, f. 101 b). Bess, he tells us, came of an old family in Herefordshire, where her father 'lived at the Mannour-house at Canon-Peon'. She was seduced by the clerk of the parish, whom Audrey remembered in 1660 as 'a pittifull poor old weaver'. Bess's father locked her up in the turret of the house, but she got down by a rope, and set herself up in London as a whore. 'She was a most exquisite beautie, as finely shaped as nature could frame, and had a delicate Witt. She was soon taken notice of at London; and her price was very deare. a second Thais. Richard Earl of Dorset kept her...At last she grew common, and infamous, and had the Pox, of which she died. I remember thus much of an old song of those dayes which I have seen in a Collection, 'twas by way of Litanie, viz.,
 'From the Watch at Twelve a clock
 'And from Bess Broughtons buttond smock
  Libera nos Domine.' (Jonson, 1925–52, vol.8, p 81)

According to the passage quoted below from *Westward Hoe*, the law term's change of residence from Westminster to Winchester had given rise to an epidemic of syphilis which migrated from community to community, and from area to area. 'How came the goose to be put upon you, ha?', asks the Boy of the Italian merchant Justiniano, who appears in the disguise of a collier:

> '*Justiniano.* I'll tell thee, the term lying at Winchester in Henry the Third's days, and many French women coming out of the Isle of Wight thither (as it hath always been seen), though the Isle of Wight could not of long time neither endure foxes nor lawyers, yet it could brook the more dreadful cockatrice [whore]. There were many punks in the town (as you know, our term is their term), [and] your farmers that would spend but three pence on his ordinary [restaurant] would lavish half-a-crown on his lechery: and many men (calves as they were) would ride in a farmer's foul boots [fuck] before breakfast, the commonest sinner had more fluttering about her than a fresh punk hath when she comes to a town of garrison, or to a university. Captains, scholars, servingmen, jurors, clarks, townsmen, and the black-guard [the lowest order of domestics] used all to one ordinary, and most of them were called to a pitiful reckoning, for before two returns of Michaelmas, surgeons were full of business, the cure of most secrecy grew as common as lice in Ireland, or as scabs in France. One of my tribe, a collier, carried in his cart forty maimed soldiers to Salisbury, looking as pitifully as Dutchmen first made drunk, then carried to beheading. Every one that met him cried, 'ware the Goose, Collier, and from that day to this, there's a record to be seen at Croydon, how that pitiful waftage, which indeed was virtue in the collier that all that time would carry no coals [would put up with no affront], laid this imputation on all the posterity.' (3,3:8–31)

The words 'term' and 'returns' in the passage above refer to the returns of the Sheriff's reports upon any writs directed to them during Michaelmas Term, which lasted from October 10 to November 28 and which had eight returns. This periodic return explains a passage in Dekker's 'Epistle Dedicatory' to his *News from Gravesend* (1604), in which he alludes once more to the syphilitic epidemic of 1603–4 in London. '*O Winchester*', he cries out,

> 'much mutton hast thou to answer for, which thou hast made away…thy maid-seruants best know how, if they were cald to an account. It was happy for some, that 4. of the Returnes were cut off [those that had occurred in London before adjournment to Winchester], for if they had held together, many a one had neuer returned from thence his owne man. Oh beware! your *Winchester-Goose* is tenne times more dangerous to surfet vpon, than your *S. Nicholas* Shambles-Capon.' (Dekker, 1925, p.76)

In order to make his message perfectly clear, Dekker, at the end of his satirical epistle – written 'in the taile of the Plague' (p.66) during the Christmas season of 1603–4 – asserts that

> 'if thou hadst hirde a Chamber [in Winchester] (as would to heauen thou hadst) thou wouldst neuer haue gone to any Barbers in *London* whilst thou hadst liude, but haue bin trimd only there, for they are the true shauers, they haue the right Neapolitan polling.' (p.78)

A similar warning against the syphilitic bird was issued four years later by the anonymous author of a satirical tract entitled *The Penniles Parliament of Threed-bare*

*Poets* (1608). Here the 'Winchester goose' is spoken of as 'the pigeon', and the following bit of advice on how best to avoid it is given:

'Those who play fast and loose with women's apron-strings, may chance to make a journey for a Winchester pigeon; for prevention thereof, drink every morning a draught of *noli me tangere*, and by that means thou shalt be sure to escape the physician's purgatory.' (*The Harleian Miscellany*, London, 1808, vol.1, p.185)

### STRONG AND WEAK EMOTIONAL BONDS OF A CLUSTER

While Armstrong and Wentersdorf were not acquainted with many of the sources collected above, Armstrong knew of the Winchestrian Goose of Ben Jonson's *Execration against Vulcan* (Armstrong, 1946, p.62), and this made it possible for him to decipher the meaning of the symbolic bird found in the middle of Shakespeare's cluster. He concluded that the 'Winchester goose' must symbolize 'a person suffering from venereal disease' (p.62), a conclusion later agreed to by Wentersdorf in his equally pioneering work on the subject (Wentersdorf, 1972, pp.242–56).

Armstrong's decoding of connotations for the term was strongly supported by satellite elements of the cluster such as 'lechery, whores, procreation, trademarket, falsehood, diseases, suffering, sin, punishment and damnation'. The only modification necessary of the two scholars' interpretation of the symbolic bird is the term 'venereal disease' which must be viewed as a little too general. The associations to 'pox' and 'blindness', 'corruption' and 'plague' and the various medical treatments that are enumerated all show that the 'goose cluster' is clearly concerned with *syphilis*.

Armstrong's discoveries gave rise to a new literary discipline known as 'cluster criticism'. It proved a useful tool for determining the authenticity of passages attributed to Shakespeare by some scholars, but whose authorship was doubted by others. Coleridge, for instance, had raised doubts as to the authenticity of the Porter scene in *Macbeth* (2,3:1–40) because he felt that Shakespeare could never have written anything so coarse. Armstrong proved the authenticity of the passage by demonstrating the presence of all of the elements of the 'goose cluster', of which he found nearly 30 examples in the canon.

Apart from 'cluster criticism', Armstrong's conclusions were not revelatory. This was due to his ignorance of depth psychology, which prevented him from realizing the true importance of his discoveries. Armstrong's remarks on the difference between the 'drone-weasel cluster' and the 'goose cluster' throw his lack of psychological understanding into relief:

'Although the imagery [of the drone-weasel cluster] undoubtedly appertains to the Pride category and there are references to disagreeable moods the personal emotional content of the cluster is comparatively meagre. The contrary is true so far as the goose-disease linkage is concerned. The emotional bond is so evident that it needs no further emphasis. So persistent is the linkage, so fierce is the underlying loathing of venereal diseases that there cannot be the slightest doubt that Shakespeare was intimately acquainted with and revolted by these maladies and their dreadful sequelæ, such as blindness. More than this we cannot infer from the evidence.' (Armstrong, 1946, pp.167–8)

While this statement shows Armstrong's ability to distinguish between a weak and a strong emotional bond in an associative 'cluster' of images and ideas, it reveals at the same time his inability to draw conclusions from this difference. Obviously, Armstrong was not well acquainted with the work of the Swiss psychiatrist C.G. Jung who, forty years before Armstrong's studies on *Shakespeare's Imagination*, had conducted a series of important experiments in word associations. It was out of these experiments that Jung formulated his well-known concept of emotionally charged 'clusters' – the so-called 'complexes' – which soon became as important a theoretical formation of psychoanalysis as Freud's concept of dreams and the repressed unconscious.

## JUNG'S STUDIES IN WORD ASSOCIATION

Freud's early work on psychoanalysis at the beginning of our century had established dreams and free association as a method of penetrating the unconscious and uncovering the hidden strata of the human mind. While Freud was exploring the dynamic possibilities of such an approach in Vienna, Jung in Zürich was conducting a series of experiments in free association as another means of establishing direct contact with the unconscious.

Jung's experiments in word association consisted of a very simple procedure. The experimenter called out a word to the test-person, and the test-person immediately replied with the next association that came into his mind. The lag time between the stimulus word and the reply – the 'reaction-time' – was measured by a stop-watch and, after the experiment had been concluded, the test-person was asked to repeat, one by one, the answers to the stimulus words (the 'reproduction method'). One would expect all simple words to be followed by an equally short reaction-time, and all difficult or rare words to cause a more prolonged reaction-time. But Jung's experiments demonstrated that the reaction-times differed on this account far less than from other important reasons. Some very long reaction-times were produced unexpectedly by very simple stimulus words, while in the same case, there might be no delay in replying to quite unusual stimulus words. Furthermore, it turned out that the stimulus words which produced the prolonged reaction-time were also the words that produced incorrect reproduction. Finally, Jung found that 'critical' stimulus words had an effect on the replies to new stimulus words which followed immediately afterward and that this effect showed in prolonged reaction-times or incorrect reproduction (the so-called 'perseveration' phenomenon). Figure 44 illustrates an actual association experiment carried out by Jung with a young woman.

The shortest reaction-time occurs in connection with the ink–black linkage and the long–table linkage (1.2 sec.), while the longest reaction-time occurs in connection with the ship–wreck linkage (3.4 sec.), the swim–know linkage (3.8 sec.), the lake–water linkage (4.0 sec.) and the water–deep linkage (5.0 sec.). Significantly, these linkages are also the ones that produce the incorrect reproduction words *swim*, *steamer, blue, water*. By cautiously questioning the woman, Jung was informed that she had recently gone through a critical and painful period, during which she had seriously contemplated suicide by drowning herself (Jung, 1973, p.486).

Jung surmized that certain of this patient's stimulus words had struck a complex of ideas and images related to 'water', and that this associative 'cluster' of ideas and images was affectively toned by feelings of a painful and disagreeable nature. Like underwater vegetation, this affective mass of images and ideas appeared to possess a life and consistency of its own and had interfered with the reply so that its smooth passage towards conscious reproduction had been obstructed. 'Why cannot an idea which is closely associated with [such] a complex be reproduced "smoothly"?', Jung asked. The answer he found was that

| Stimulus-word | Reaction | Reaction-time sec. 1/10 | | Reproduction |
|---|---|---|---|---|
| head | hair | 1 | 4 | + |
| green | meadow | 1 | 6 | + |
| water | deep | 5 | | swim |
| stab | knife | 1 | 6 | + |
| long | table | 1 | 2 | + |
| ship | wreck | 3 | 4 | steamer |
| question | answer | 1 | 6 | + |
| wool | knit | 1 | 6 | + |
| insolent | gentle | 1 | 4 | + |
| lake | water | 4 | | blue |
| ill | well | 1 | 8 | + |
| ink | black | 1 | 2 | + |
| swim | know | 3 | 8 | water |

Figure 44. Jung's association experiment (1973, p.485).

'The prime reason for the obstruction is emotional inhibition. Complexes are mostly in a state of repression because they are concerned as a rule with the most intimate secrets which are anxiously guarded and which the subject either will not or cannot divulge.' (Jung, 1960, p.45)

Just as Jung's theory had explained the phenomena of prolonged reaction-time, incorrect reproduction and perseveration, it also explained the absence of such phenomena in the associative linkages ink–black, head–hair and long–table. For these images, their personal emotional bond was so weak or neutral that the reply encountered no obstruction on its way towards conscious reproduction. The opposite was true of the water–ship–wreckage linkage, whose strong emotional bond turned it into a complex. Jung cited Freud's contemporary theories of the *repression* of painful and disagreeable feelings, whose piling up in the unconscious accounted for a number of psychological disturbances such as neuroses and hysterical disorders.

Jung, concurring with Freud, stated that a repressed idea can be linked with an affect. In his association experiments Jung called this combination of a repressed idea and its affect a 'complex'. He defined 'affect' as Bleuler had, as a feeling, tone, mood, or emotion that is a 'driving force' seeking conscious expression. 'It was not difficult to see', concluded Jung, 'that while complexes owe their relative autonomy to their emotional nature, their expression is always dependent on a network of associations grouped round a centre charged with affect. The central emotion generally proved to be individually acquired, and therefore an exclusively personal matter' (Jacobi, 1959, p.ix). 'Every affective event becomes a complex', he repeated, 'the strongest feelings and impulses are connected with the strongest complexes. It is therefore not surprising that the majority of complexes are of an erotic-sexual nature, as also are most dreams and most of the hysterias' (Jung, 1960, p.67).

Jung envisaged the nucleus of the complex as a kind of psychological magnet. It has value in terms of the energy it can produce, and it automatically attracts associations to itself in proportion to its energy. The stronger the emotional or affective energy of the nucleus, the greater its associative range and differentiation (Figure 42, Tables 1–8). This characteristic explains the ability of the complex to carry on a totally separate existence in the background of the psyche, where it behaves like a state within the state. For this reason, Jung speaks of the independence or *autonomy* of the complex.

Freud and Jung arrived, by entirely different paths, at similar conclusions regarding the nature and effects of those psychic factors known as 'complexes'. It was this agreement that first, in 1902, called their attention to one another's work, and later, in 1907, brought the two psychologists together for a time. Today, the theory of the complex is one of the firmest and most well established foundations of depth psychology. Its value becomes clear if we apply the theory of the complex to the associative patterns of Shakespeare's 'image clusters'.

SHAKESPEARE'S 'IMAGE CLUSTERS'

According to Jung's definition, every complex consists primarily in a 'nuclear element' which is beyond the realm of the conscious will and therefore unconscious and uncontrollable; and secondarily, in a number of associations connected with that nuclear element and capable of being 'broadened' in direct proportion to the unconscious energy or autonomy of the complex. The third and final characteristic of the complex is the strong emotional or affective bond which connects its associations and turns them into a psychological magnet of great power.

The 'image clusters' in Shakespeare's works offer a variegated picture concerning associative range and differentiation and emotional or affective quality. The 'drone–weasel cluster' (Figure 45), on the one hand, presents a small associative range with little differentiation and a neutral affective quality. The opposite is true of the 'goose cluster' (Figure 46), which thus emerges as a *complex* in Shakespeare. In between these two 'clusters', we find the 'dog cluster' which has a wider associative range and differentiation and a much stronger affective quality than the 'drone–weasel cluster' – if not as strong as the 'goose cluster'. The 'dog cluster' is thus to be conceived of as a complex of a milder sort – the frustration and disappointment of a man who had experienced a betrayal of friendship and trust (see pp.203 and 242–7).

As to the strong emotional bond of the 'goose cluster', it may be argued that it is a natural feature once the connection has been established between 'goose' and syphilis. The revulsion and horror expressed by the 'goose cluster' reflects the Elizabethans' attitude towards the new venereal disease, and so Armstrong is probably right when he concludes that the strong emotional bond of the cluster expresses the fact 'that Shakespeare was intimately acquainted with and revolted by these maladies and their dreadful sequelæ, such as blindness. More than this we cannot infer from the evidence' (Armstrong, 1946, p.168).

Armstrong, however, ignores an important element of the 'goose cluster' which turns it into an idiosyncratic phenomenon and shows that its central emotion is individually acquired and therefore an exclusively personal matter. This is the element of *guilt* in the cluster, an emotion which Wentersdorf has isolated in his Tables 5 and 6. He lists each word pair relating to guilt in the cluster as follows: 'God–heaven, devil–hell, prayer–worship, sin–offence, fault–guilt, repentance–confession, pagan deities, law–judgement, obey–obedience, prison–confinement, beating–whipping, death–hanging, sundry punishments' (pp.209–10). Here the symbolic goose is brought before both the high Court of Heaven and the lower courts of mundane affairs and subjected to savage, even capital punishment. These features of the 'goose cluster' establish it as a complex in the Jungian sense of the word, just as its unique associative structure supports its idiosyncratic nature and turns it into a highly individual phenomenon, not found in any other writer of the Elizabethan or Jacobean period.*

Born in Shakespeare's debut-work *Henry VI* and powerfully erupting in *Love's Labour's Lost*, the 'goose cluster' grows to full maturity in the great tragedies and culminates in *Measure for Measure*, which contains a full-scale projection of all of the elements of the 'goose cluster'. The complex-like nature of the cluster is finally proved by the fact that it appears to lose its intensity in Shakespeare's last plays. Here the image suffers the depotentiation of a complex that has been raised to consciousness and assimilated emotionally by the author as a result of his own personal maturation and insight and due in no small degree to his creative writing.

---

* The closest approximation to Shakespeare's 'goose cluster' is found in the passage quoted above from Dekker's *Westward Hoe*, where the 'Winchester goose' is seen to constellate the same erotic, promiscuous and diseased elements as it does in Shakespeare's works. The 'goose' imagery in Dekker also includes the same economic element (prostitution) and the same elements of sexual infidelity and falsehood. While Dekker's 'goose cluster' thus constellates the first five items as does Shakespeare's 'goose cluster', depicted in Figure 46, it is weak in its representation of Shakespeare's sixth, seventh and eighth elements. The punitive, guilty and 'religious' aspects of the Shakespearean 'goose cluster' only appear in Dekkers's one reference each to 'repentant' (3,3:104), 'sinner' (3,3:18), 'confession' (3,3:45–6), and 'weeping' (3,3:77) and in his two references to 'pillory' (3,3:4–5). Dekker's works, also, include only one 'goose cluster', while Shakespeare presented almost 30 more examples. The works of John Taylor and Ben Jonson include a 'Winchester goose' resembling Dekker's cluster more than Shakespeare's in that they share a weak emotional bond and single appearance (see pp.214–7).

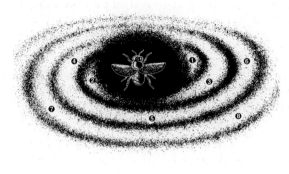

Figure 45. The drone cluster (drawing by René Terney).

1. drone, drone-like.
2. weasel.
3. king-creature: eagle, lion, whale, ape, dog-ape.
4. creeping, sneaking, snail, snail-slow.
5. cat, wild-cat, gib cat.
6. mood: spleen, melancholy, sad-eyed, surly, quarrelous, jangling.
7. sucking, sucks eggs, drink, swallow, play with mammets.
8. music: song, sing, lute, pipe, bagpipe, fife, drum, bells.

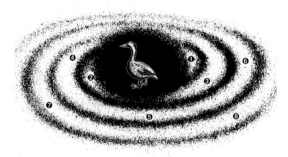

Figure 46. The goose cluster (drawing by René Terney).

1. goose, whores-bawds, diseases-plague, blind, pinch-prick, pain-suffering, medical treatment.
2. lechery-wild lust, flesh-blood, heat-passion, mad-moon, horns-cuckold, burn-fire, cold-ice.
3. dog-cur, hunt-chase, music-musician, sing-tune, procreation-pregnancy-birth, child-infancy.
4. trade-market, monetary trans-actions, money-purse, thief, rob-steal, tale-tail, suit-argument.
5. betray-traitor, revolt-rebellion, false-deceitful, tricks-counterfeit, swearing-perjury, vows-oaths.
6. sauce-seasoning, taste-relish, sweet-bitter, gall-liver, pen-paper, black-white.
7. law-judgement, obey-obedience, prison-confinement, beating-whipping, death-hanging, sundry punishments.
8. god-heaven, devil-hell, prayer-worship, sin-offence, fault-guilt, repentance-confession, pagan deities.

## JAQUES OF ARDEN: THE SYPHILITIC IN THE FOREST OF ARDEN

As noted above, Caroline Spurgeon's statistical chart in Figure 40 depicting the imagery of 'sickness, disease and medicine' shows a steep rise in *2 Henry IV* (1597–8), where it is connected with the emergence of Falstaff. Chronologically, the next play to show a similar concentration of imagery is *As You Like It* (1599–1600), in which 'sickness, disease and medicine' cluster around the figure of Jaques of Arden. Jaques is a strange character who is quite incongruous with the play's pastoral idyl and the enchanted Forest of Arden. In this fairy-tale world, a number of exiles live like Robin Hood and his Merry Men, and the romantic atmosphere of the forest is conducive to four young people's falling in love and marrying at the end of the play. Here the Duke is also united with his lost daughter in the forest and restored to his lost dukedom.

Through a large number of experiments, C.G. Jung discovered that most associative linkages are of a neutral emotional character (Figure 45), but that a few of them are strongly affectively toned (Figure 46). This latter group of associations is also characterized by such phenomena as prolonged reaction-time, incorrect reproduction, and perseveration. Jung's experiments in word association demonstrated a peculiarity of man's psychic makeup, namely the tendency of ideas to become associated round certain basic nuclei. These nuclei and their 'clusters' of associated ideas – which are held together by a particular emotional tone – were termed 'complexes' by Jung. He agreed with Freud that complexes are the products of psychic mechanisms of repression and that most complexes result from an attempt to evade the conflict between the primitive sexual urges of man and the moral and social constraints imposed on him by his surroundings. 'It may be permissible to point out once more', Jung wrote in 1905, 'that an overwhelming number of the complexes we have discovered in our subjects are erotic. In view of the great part played by love and sexuality in human life, this is not surprising' (Jung, 1973, p.137).

Complexes do not arise out of the blue since they are connected with an individual's most personal and painful experiences and conflicts. Shakespeare's 'goose cluster' is an example of such a conflict, and its network of associations grouped around its powerful nucleus is one that would almost certainly have disturbed the poet's reply to the stimulus word 'goose'. This symbolic bird's most powerful complex-characteristic is the emotion of guilt connected with the erotic ideas that are expressed by its clustering associations. A second characteristic is the fear of illness and punishment in connection with the promiscuous sexuality and unbridled lust which are a part of the same cluster. With its strong emotional bond of fear, guilt and revulsion, the 'goose cluster' denotes the moral and aesthetic conflict that one would expect in a married man living in the loftiest spheres of poetry and philosophy while not being unacquainted with the 'vice' that Clowes condemned so strongly in his fellow-citizens.

The moral qualms which went into the formation of Shakespeare's 'goose cluster' were succinctly formulated by Erasmus in his colloquy *A Problem* (1533): 'Figure out for yourself, then, how much bitterness is mingled with those pleasures, falsely so called, produced by shameless love, unlawful passion, excessive wining and dining – not to mention the worst of all: torments of conscience, enmity with God, expectation of eternal punishment. I ask you: which sort among these "pleasures" does not bring in its train a vast throng of external evils?' (Erasmus, 1965, p.543).

---

Shakespeare's romantic comedy is among his most glorious creations, and the happy atmosphere of *As You Like It* is only disturbed by Jaques of Arden, whose melancholy casts a gloom over the sun-lit setting of the play. Shakespeare's inclusion of this incongruous figure is a remarkable phenomenon for several reasons. The fact is that Shakespeare modelled his play relatively closely on Thomas Lodge's novel *Rosalynde, Euphues' Golden Legacie* (1590), whose plot and characters he adopted almost wholesale. Jaques of Arden is *not* found in Lodge's novel, and so a strong unconscious motivation accounts for his inclusion in *As You Like It*. Shakespeare did, of course, add two more figures to his play who are not found in Lodge's novel: the clown Touchstone and his country wench Audrey. However, the addition of these two characters was almost inevitable in a Shakespeare comedy from this period, where the Clown and his Wench are stock figures. Touchstone serves in part to ridicule pastoral love and its romantic follies and in part to participate in a comic *drame à trois* in which he courts Audrey and, with exaggerated threats, dismisses her former lover, the mild-mannered William. William, too, is an invention, as is the character Sir Oliver Martext, a foolish vicar who appears in the play with three short lines by which he marries Touchstone and Audrey.

While these additions are perhaps minor, Jaques of Arden is a major and significant addition for a number of reasons: (1) Jaques of Arden sustains the high quantitative level of the imagery of 'sickness, disease and medicine' established in *2 Henry IV* and is presented as a 'cousin' of Falstaff; (2) he resembles the venereal couple in *2 Henry IV* – Falstaff and Doll Tearsheet – in that he too brings about a qualitative change in the imagery toward images of 'lust', 'lechery', and 'foul disease'; (3) he is accompanied by the Shakespearean 'goose', as is Falstaff; (4) he is, in effect, a preliminary study of Prince Hamlet and shares not only Hamlet's profound melancholy, disillusioned spirits and mad foolery but also his vital interest in the theatre and the world of acting; (5) he sees the world as a diseased and corrupt place and professes a desire to 'Cleanse the foul body of the infected world' (2,7:60). In this, he anticipates Hamlet's world-view and the Prince's interpretation of his responsibility and purpose; (6) he provides the 'running imagery' of *Hamlet*, which Caroline Spurgeon indicates is governed by 'the conception of disease, especially of a hidden corruption infecting and destroying a wholesome body' (Spurgeon, 1935, p.213).

Heralding the 'mid-life crisis' of Shakespeare's 'black' tragedies, Jaques of Arden personifies a spirit of melancholy, frustration and bitterness which finds expression in his moving soliloquy on the seven ages of man (2,7:139–66). Jaques's imagery and point of view as expressed in one of Shakespeare's most famous monologues are interesting because they are those which would come naturally to a playwright, actor and stage-director. 'All the world's a stage' (2,7:139) echoes the *Totus mundus agit histrionem* motto of the Globe Theatre, which opened in the summer of 1599 – at the same time as *As You Like It* was written.

Jaques's statement represents an inversion of the view that the theatre is a mirror of life. In his soliloquy, life is seen as a mirror of the theatre – a view likely to be held by a dramatist such as Shakespeare whose whole life *was* the theatre. Jaques, we may infer, is a self-portrait of the poet, placed in a corner of his enchanting painting of Arden and its inhabitants. The fruits of that forest are so mellow that autumn, decomposition and withering are furthered by the mere course of time; and so Jaques sums up his awareness of the future in a passage which sounds touchingly personal:

> 'Tis but an hour ago since it was nine;
> And after one hour more it will be eleven;
> And so, from hour to hour, we ripe and ripe,
> And then, from hour to hour, we rot and rot;
> And thereby hangs a tale. (2,7:24–8)

Jaques's quotation of the clown Touchstone's wisdom concludes in a peal of laughter. 'When I did hear The motley fool thus moral on the time', Jaques tells the Duke, 'My lungs began to crow like chanticleer, That fools should be so deep-contemplative' (2,7:28–31). For almost three hundred years, critics and audiences have been unable to explain why Touchstone's philosophical commonplace could induce Jaques to 'laugh, sans intermission, An hour by his dial' (2,7:32–3) and to admire the subtlety of Touchstone's 'brain' (2,7:38) which

hath strange places crammed
With observation, the which he vents
In mangled forms. O that I were a fool!
I am ambitious for a motley coat. (2,7:40–3)

In his classic study of *Shakespeare's Pronunciation* (1953), Helge Kökeritz has managed to explain the ambiguous meaning of the Clown's wisdom and the reason for Jaques's boisterous laughter. The fact is that 'hour' and 'whore' were homonyms in Shakespeare's time, that is, they were pronounced in the same way as in *The tretece of the pokkis*, where the doctor orders a syphilitic patient into a hot chamber, 'and with this water hote make hym swete an hor in a stew' (Zimmermann, 1937, p.464).

The underlying meaning of Touchstone's bawdy moralizing and of Jaques's informed laughter are thus found within the sphere of the 'goose cluster': 'From whore to whore, we search and search, and then from whore to whore, we rot and rot, and thereby hangs a tail' (Kökeritz, 1953, pp.58–9). The diseased penis imagery concluding the passage comes about from the pun on *tale-tail* and on the slang meaning of *tail*, one of the bawdiest of Elizabethan jokes. The 'rotting' motif of the passage finds its final and most well-known expression in Jaques's soliloquy in the same scene on the seven ages of man. Here, an inexorable process of transformation is said to make mankind 'rot from hour to hour' until he is 'sans teeth, sans eyes, sans taste, sans everything' (2,7:165–6).

Significantly, Jaques's laughter at Touchstone's wisdom and his subsequent soliloquy form part of a conversation with the Duke (2,7:9–166) during which the Shakespearean 'goose' makes its first appearance in the play (2,7:86). (Its second appearance is in 3,5:40.) Here Duke Senior is seen to remind the railing satirist that anyone so well informed about the vices of the world must himself be a person of vices and someone who actually discharges his own filth upon the world when criticising it:

DUKE S.    Fie on thee! I can tell what thou wouldst do.

JAQ.       What, for a counter, would I do but good?

DUKE S.    Most mischievous foul sin, in chiding sin;
           For thou thyself hast been a libertine,
           As sensual as the brutish sting itself;
           And all th'embossed sores and headed evils
           That thou with license of free foot hast caught
           Wouldst thou disgorge into the general world. (2,7:62–9)

This passage, which comments upon Jaques's own character and career, recalls the background of the world of *Avisa* and the *Sonnets*. The choice of words in connection with the Duke's description of Jaques, the 'libertine', is telling: 'sores' appearing as 'bosses', or small protuberances (hard chancre), and 'evils' that have 'come to a head' (chancre sores enlarging and breaking in the centre, leaving a shallow ulcer) suggest syphilitic infection, 'caught' by the promiscuous living of a tavern-haunter and Bohemian when using his 'license of free foot'. Falstaff was also called a 'whoreson, impudent, *embossed* rascal', with nothing in his pockets but 'tavern-reckonings [and] memorandums of bawdy houses' (*1 Henry IV*, 3,3:155–8).

That venereal infection is on Shakespeare's mind here is supported by the passage immediately following in which Jaques defends his criticism of sinful man, adding that, in individual cases, 'if he be free, Why then my taxing *like a wild-goose flies*, Unclaimed of any man' (2,7:85–7).

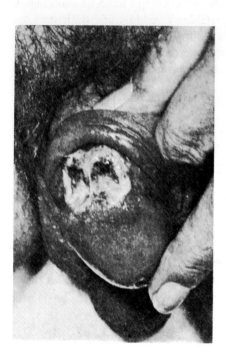

Figure 47. (Nielsen and Schmidt, 1985, fig.33) John C. Bucknill was the first medical writer to call attention to the syphilitic implications of the Duke's condemnation of Jaques of Arden: 'When Jaques expresses in medical form of thought and phrase his desire to reform the moral evils of the world', Bucknill wrote in *Shakespeare's Medical Knowledge* (1860), 'the class of disease to which the half-technical phrase of "cleansing the foul body" appears to refer to, is that which by its novelty and prevalence engrossed so much attention at that time. The reply of the Duke makes this certain' (p.108). The Duke's reference to 'embossed sores' suggests the primary lesion of syphilis, which occurs at the site of inoculation, usually the genitalia. It is marked by the appearance of a small, hard, painless swelling, and when it 'comes to a head' the chancre enlarges and often breaks in the centre, leaving a shallow, purulent ulcer which is rounded, regular and clearly defined in outline. It feels hard and indurated on palpation and has given rise to the term 'hard chancre'. The serous exudate of the ulcer contains numerous spirochetes and is very infectious.

## MEDICINE FOR A FOUL DISEASE

Caroline Spurgeon's demonstration of a steep quantitative rise in the imagery of 'sickness, disease and medicine' in *2 Henry IV, As You Like It, Hamlet* and *Troilus and Cressida* was accompanied by her parallel demonstration of a *qualitative* change of this imagery as follows:

> 'The early [sickness images] are chiefly of corrosive or balm applied to wounds, broken limbs and bruises or light references to plague and pestilence. Only in the later ones comes the feeling of horror and disgust at foul disease, and in *Hamlet* we are almost startled at the constant conception of a corrupt and hidden tumour or cancer which is the central imaginative symbol of the tragedy.' (Spurgeon, 1935, Chart VII)

Jaques's 'embossed sores, and headed evils' arising from his own 'Most mischievous foul sin' have some interesting associative ramifications in *2 Henry IV*, where the imagery of 'sickness, disease and medicine' is also found *outside* the Falstaff episodes. 'The time will come, that foul sin, gathering head, Shall break into corruption' (3,1:76–7), the King muses in his gloomy conversation with Warwick, who is asked to 'perceive the body of our kingdom, How foul it is, what rank diseases grow, And with what danger, near the heart of it' (3,1:38–40). 'It is but as a body yet distempered', Warwick reassures his monarch, 'Which to his former strength may be restored With good advice and little medicine' (3,1:41–3). 'We are all diseased', concurs the Archbishop of England, 'And with our surfeiting and wanton hours [pun on 'whores'] Have brought ourselves into a burning fever' (4,1:54–6). He goes on to envisage himself as 'a physician' (4,1:60) who must 'diet rank minds sick of happiness' (4,1:64). Another figure envisaging himself as both physician and patient is Jaques of Arden, who promises to 'Cleanse the foul body of the infected world, If they will patiently receive my *medicine*' (2,7:60–1).

In the plays of the period 1597/8–1601/2, the associative ramifications of the word 'medicine' present another interesting picture. 'If the rascal have not given me *medicines* to make me *love* him, I'll be hanged', says Falstaff in *1 Henry IV*. 'It could not be else: I have *drunk medicines*' (1,2:17–9). 'His *dissolute disease* will scarce obey this *medicine*' (3,3:177–8) observes Mrs. Page in *The Merry Wives of Windsor*, with reference to the same 'embossed rascal'. In *Much Ado About Nothing* (1598–9), Don John wonders that Conrade, his companion, 'goest about to apply a moral *medicine* to a mortifying *mischief*' (1,3:11–2). Another figure connected with 'medicine' is Pandarus of *Troilus and Cressida*, whose own 'Most mischievous foul sin' makes him cry out for 'A goodly *medicine* for my *aching bones*' (5,10:35). The last emergence of the word is in *Hamlet*, where the Danish prince is treacherously poisoned by the poisoner-king, the latter's 'treacherous instrument' being finally clutched by Hamlet's hand. 'Hamlet, thou art slain', Laertes cries at him,

> No *medicine* in the world can do thee good;
> In thee there is not half an hour's life.
> The *treacherous instrument* is in thy hand,
> Unbated and *envenomed*. The *foul practice*
> Hath turned itself on me. Lo, here I *lie*,
> Never to *rise* again. Thy mother's *poisoned*.
> *I can no more. The King, the King's to blame.* (5,2:319–21)

Jaques's vision of 'the foul body of the infected world', to be 'cleanse[d]...If they will patiently receive my medicine' is interpreted by the Duke as a *projection* on Jaques's part of his own life. In *Hamlet*, written the following year (1600), this projection is so strong and ubiquitous that it has influenced the 'running imagery' of the play, which Caroline Spurgeon pinpoints in the following way:

'In *Hamlet*, we find in the "sickness" images a feeling of horror, disgust and even helplessness not met before (save for a touch of the first two in Jacques' bitter moralising and the duke's answer, *A.Y.L.I.* 2. 7. 58–61, and 67–9); and the general sense of inward and unseen corruption, of the man helplessly succumbing to a deadly and "foul disease," which feeds "even on the pith of life" (4,1:19) is very strong. This is accompanied by the impression that for such terrible ill the remedy must be drastic, for "diseases desperate grown By desperate appliance are relieved, Or not at all" (4,3:9), and that anything short of this is but to "skin and film the ulcerous place, Whiles rank corruption, mining all within, Infects unseen" (3,4:147)...Anguish is not the dominating thought, but *rottenness*, disease, corruption, the result of *dirt;* the people are "muddied," "Thick and unwholesome in their thoughts and whispers" (4,5:82); and this corruption is, in the words of Claudius, "rank" and "smells to heaven," so that the state of things in Denmark which shocks, paralyses and finally overwhelms Hamlet, is as the foul tumour breaking inwardly and poisoning the whole body, while showing "no cause without Why the man dies" (4,4:28).' (Spurgeon, 1935, pp.133–4, 318)

# 11

# SHAKESPEARE'S MID-LIFE CRISIS

The works written by Shakespeare from c. 1600 to 1608 have puzzled critics and audiences alike. These works followed Shakespeare's so-called Comic Period (c. 1595–1601) in which romantic love and a sense of *joie de vivre* inform the comedies and the historical plays in which Falstaff appears. When Shakespeare was in his mid-thirties, however, he entered his so-called Tragic Period (c. 1601–1608), in which his protagonists are enveloped in a 'black' world of suffering, despair and death.

Modern depth psychology has observed that this sort of transformation of mood is a regular occurence for men and women in their thirties. Elliott Jaques coined the term 'mid-life crisis' for this period of transition and defined it as a time of anguish and depression arising out of an emotional awareness that time is running out and death will come (Jaques, 1965, pp.502–14). Jung termed this same stage of life *Lebenswende* and defined it as the onset of the second half of life in which an emotional awareness of the tragedy of personal death is accompanied by the sense of grief appropriate to it (Fabricius, 1976, pp.98–9).

When Hamlet speaks of 'the heart of my mystery' (3,2:356–7), he alludes to this inexplicable change in mood and outlook following his father's death, which makes him view the earth as 'a sterile promontory' (2,2:299) and 'Denmark [as] a prison' (2,2: 243). 'How weary, stale, flat, and unprofitable Seem to me all the uses of this world', he sighs, adding that it has become to him 'an unweeded garden That grows to seed; things rank and gross in nature Possess it merely. That it should come to this!' (1,2:133–7).

While the gloom and despair of Shakespeare's Tragic Period is thus to be explained as a predictable reaction to the poet's mid-life crisis, there are other features belonging to this period which deviate from the general pattern of this crisis and thus establish themselves as phenomena which are idiosyncratic to Shakespeare. The almost physical disgust for sex that is so prominent in *Hamlet* is not a standard feature of a mid-life crisis, neither is the strong misogyny which permeates the plays of Shakespeare's Tragic Period. Ernest Jones interprets these features as expressive of some 'bitter disappointment at the hands of the opposite sex', adding that 'his [Shakespeare's] way of responding was to compose a tragedy whose theme was the suffering of a tortured man who could not avenge his injured feelings…towards the faithless couple' (Jones, 1949, pp.114, 120).

We have advanced the thesis that the triangular drama and 'foul play' (1,2:256) described in *Hamlet*'s ghostly tale may reflect a real experience in the poet's life. The play depicts King Hamlet as a man betrayed by his wife, a 'most pernicious woman' (1,5:105), and as a man poisoned at the hand of a 'bawdy villain' (2,2:576), a man who has already 'whored' (5,2:64) and seduced the two men's common love object. These events may reflect similar 'foul play' as they happened to Shakespeare in a Bohemian setting, where the poet may have been infected with syphilis through a rival who had infected the unfaithful woman they shared (see p.46).

As demonstrated by Caroline Spurgeon, the occurrence of the 'sickness, disease and medicine' cluster of images reaches alarming heights in *Hamlet* – a drama in which love is perverted into lust, and sexuality into an act of treachery and deceit. This state of moral and physical corruption is epitomized in Marcellus's statement that 'Something is *rotten* in the state of Denmark' (1,4:90). Without warrant in his sources, Shakespeare has transformed his play into a poisonous drama which ends the lives of all parties involved. The poison coursing through the veins of the drama itself springs from a demonic centre – the Ghost's tale – whose patterns of association express a syphilitic symbolism, as we have attempted to demonstrate (see pp.43–5 and 50–1). Since Prince Hamlet is so completely absorbed by the Ghost and his commandment, Hamlet is finally brought to share the King's fate at the hands of the same treacherous and poisonous serpent which killed his father.

Significantly, the play's poisoner 'villain' (1,5:106) is seen as poisonous himself and is described by Hamlet as 'this *canker* of our nature' (5,2:69), and as 'a *mildewed* ear *Blasting* his wholesome brother' (3,4:64–5) (cf. pp.185–6). The 'running imagery' of the play centres on this consort of Gertrude, and constantly associates him with disease, just as the King speaks in metaphors of disease himself.

Perhaps the most fatal effect of the poisonous and villainous centre of *Hamlet* is the way in which the protagonist comes to view *all* women as treacherous creatures and evil prostitutes – even the fair and innocent Ophelia. Throughout the play, the melancholy Prince associates sexuality with 'an act' (3,4:40) that 'takes off the rose From the fair forehead of an innocent love, And sets a blister there' (3,4:42–4), thus availing himself of an obvious reference to syphilitic sores. Even the goddess of Fortune is made to conform to Hamlet's misogynist conception of woman, for Fortune is twice called a 'strumpet' (2,2:236;489). The bitter misogyny of Hamlet's exhortations to Ophelia and his treatment of her as if she were an inmate of a brothel (3,1:103–51) testify to the 'evil spirit' that has invaded him due to his ghostly vision.

Further imagery of prostitution, infection and disease appear in Hamlet's denunciation of Gertrude's adultery and of her shared responsibility for the poisoning of her consort. In the famous Closet scene, Hamlet presents the Queen with an ugly vision of the treacherous couple's 'making love…In the rank sweat of an enseamed [greasy] bed, Stewed in corruption' (3,4:92–4). Here, the stews, venereal disease and sexual disgust find one of their most forceful expressions. It is in conformity with Hamlet's revulsion for Gertrude's whorish behaviour that he says her 'reason panders will' (3,4:88) and that in her 'vice' (3,4:156) and 'trespass' (3,4:148) she is like one applying an ointment to a sore which will just cover up a foul, rotting 'ulcer' (3,4:149) that, nevertheless, eats away at her invisibly. 'Rank corruption, mining all within' while 'Infect[ing] unseen' (3,4:150–1) suggests that the same kind of poison which killed King Hamlet will spread everywhere.

Hamlet's metaphor clearly refers to the Renaissance practice of applying mercurial unctions to ulcerous and usually syphilitic sores. Hamlet also voices the observation and fear, shared by many doctors, that these ointments only healed the cutaneous lesions of syphilis, while the venereal disease itself spread invisibly and unchecked. Indeed, for precisely this reason, Villalobos and many early syphilographers maintained that mercurial unctions were ineffective against syphilis (Villalobos, 1870, p.117).

Hamlet's central metaphor – 'the foul body of the infected world' (As You Like It 2,7:60) – may thus be taken to have an intimate connection to another prominent feature of that play: Shakespeare's 'disgust at sexuality' (Sexualabneigung), as Freud termed it. 'This disgust surfaces with particular clarity in Hamlet's conversation with Ophelia', Freud observes in his well-known commentary on the play, 'a disgust that during the following years takes more and more possession of the poet's soul until it reaches its culminating expression in Timon of Athens. There can be no doubt that it is the poet's own psychological experience which confronts us in Hamlet' (Freud, 1953, p.265).

## 'TROILUS AND CRESSIDA': 'MY MIND IS NOW TURNED WHORE' (5,2:113)

The deep surge of bitterness, cynicism and misogyny in Hamlet (1600–1) continues in its companion piece Troilus and Cressida (1601–2), which was written shortly afterward. 'Did we not know it for other reasons', observes Caroline Spurgeon,

> 'we could be sure from the similarity and continuity of symbolism in the two plays that they were written near together, and at a time when the author was suffering from a disillusionment, revulsion and perturbation of nature, such as we feel nowhere else with the same intensity.' (Spurgeon, 1985, p.320)

In Troilus and Cressida, the 'sickness, disease and medicine' cluster of images reaches the same statistical high as it does in 2 Henry IV and As You Like It. In Troilus and Cressida, this cluster is concentrated in the brothel characters Thersites, Cressida and Pandarus. The last of these, Pandarus, is clearly a syphilitic (see pp.213–4), while the play's clown – 'a very filthy rogue' (5,4:29) named Thersites – may be characterized as a bawdy, syphilitic fool who wallows in repeated references to foul disease (2,1:1–13;27–9;2,3:18–21; 29–35; 73–7; 5,1:16–23; 65–6; 5,2:193–5). Thersites represents the 'undersong' of the play in that his 'spiteful execrations' (2,3:7) and 'comparisons with dirt' (1,3:194) express the play's 'running imagery', which fuses sexual appetite and punishment, lust and disease, lechery and rottenness. In similar fashion, Cressida emerges as the archetypal whore, to whom Shakespeare had previously referred as 'the lazar kite of Cressid's kind' in Henry V (2,1:76).

In Troilus and Cressida, once more a loving hero is betrayed by a 'most pernicious woman' and undone by a 'whoremasterly villain' (5,4:7), incarnate in part in Pandarus, and in part in the Greek commander Diomedes. As in Hamlet, the protagonist reacts with rage and jealousy, and, utterly disillusioned, comes to view his female idol as a 'false wench' (5,2:70).

In both tragedies, the character of love is poisonous and wounding. The 'serpent' that 'stings' the King in his orchard is resurrected in the 'generation of vipers' (3,1:129) that Pandarus presents to his clients as his gifts of 'love': 'Hot blood, hot thoughts, and hot deeds' (3,1:127–8). 'Gash', 'ulcer', 'knife' and 'balm' are the images recalled by Troilus for the way in which Cressida's love is experienced (1,1:53;61–3). Similarly, Hamlet and his father experience Gertrude's love as 'garbage' (1,5:57) and 'sty' (3,4:94), an 'ulcerous place' and 'rank corruption' (3,4:149–50).

The pervading atmosphere of the two plays is that of rottenness, disease, death and corruption. This is powerfully expressed in *Hamlet*'s final graveyard scene with its '*many pocky corses*' (5,1:160) and in *Troilus and Cressida*'s dead Greek who governs the play's final tableau: '*Most putrefied core, so fair without*' (5,8:1). The playwright's own 'goose quills' (*Ham.* 2,2:341) with which he wrote his most famous play and its companion piece trail many of the associations of the 'goose cluster' (Figure 46) – a fact which explains the remarkable similarity and continuity of symbolism in *Hamlet* and *Troilus and Cressida*. In addition to expressing the gloom of Shakespeare's mid-life crisis, the two plays depict the poet's bitterness at the faithlessness of women, just as they render his rage at adulterous couples, and his abysmal hatred of those like the 'lecherous, kindless villain' (*Ham.* 2,2:577) of *Hamlet* and *Troilus and Cressida* (Claudius–Pandarus–Diomedes) who poisoned the fountain of love.

### SHAKESPEARE'S 'WHORISH VISION' IN 'MEASURE FOR MEASURE' AND 'OTHELLO'

In *Troilus and Cressida*, one of the protagonists of Shakespeare's Greek drama says: 'My mind is now turned whore' (5,2:113). The 'whorish vision' governing *Hamlet* and *Troilus and Cressida* continues to project its energies in Shakespeare's two ensuing plays, *Measure for Measure* and *Othello* (1604–5). Shakespearean scholar Eric Partridge aptly calls these two dramas 'Shakespeare's most sexual, most bawdy plays' (Partridge, 1968, p.46). *Measure for Measure* (1604–5) is a remarkable literary creation in that it provides a *full-scale projection of all of the elements of the 'goose cluster'*.

In *Measure for Measure*, Shakespeare made the syphilitic shock of the Renaissance and the 'twin plague' of London 1603–4 (see pp.105–6 and 217–9) his principal subject. The play describes the relentless war waged by Puritan authorities against promiscuity and prostitution in a European metropolis poisoned by syphilis (see p.114). A dark comedy, full of bitter satire and cynicism, *Measure for Measure* presents sexuality as existing under the shadow of death and damnation, and features the protagonists of the play as sexual criminals who are sent to the block for adultery and fornication. Speaking of her brother's supposed beheading, Isabella says without sympathy: 'He did the thing for which he died' (5,1:447). The horror of sex in the play and its atmosphere of corruption and punishment thus turn this Shakespearean tragi-comedy into a dramatic version of the biblical dictum: 'The wages of sin is death' (*Rom.* 6:23).

In Shakespeare's companion piece *Othello* (1604–5), the 'goose cluster' projects its energies through the character of Iago, whose demonic vision of life as a place of lechery and lust, falseness and deceit, corruption and death, devil, hell and damnation is taken over wholesale by Othello. The Moor's transformation from a being living in a world of love and romance to one who sees only Iago's 'whorish vision' of the world thus reflects the poet's similar transition about the turn of the century from the world of his romantic comedies and chronicle plays to the world of his 'black' tragedies. The strange fascination of *Othello* is its juxtaposition of these worlds – one of supreme beauty, the other of supreme horror.

As Othello adopts Iago's 'whorish vision', the two men succeed in transforming the stage into a gigantic brothel, whose ugly climax is the scene in which Othello's 'horrible fancy' (4,2:26) makes him see Desdemona as a whore in a brothel and himself among her purchasers (4,2:20–96).

Caroline Spurgeon's examination of the recurrent imagery of *Othello* establishes theriomorphic imagery of a demonic nature as the play's 'undersong' or 'symbolic vision'. *Othello's* basic sense of 'foulness and dirt' (Spurgeon, 1935, p.161), as Spurgeon terms it, is expressed in yet another kind of dominant imagery which emerges as the olfactory counterpart of *Hamlet's* 'foul body of the infected world', first described by Jaques of Arden. 'The evil smell of sin is in *Othello* as constantly kept before us as are its foulness and dirt', Spurgeon suggests. 'The sickening smell of evil is the natural outcome of its being thought of as dirt and foul disease, and on the whole, perhaps, it is through this sense that Shakespeare most vividly pictures the horror of it' (p.161).

The association of evil smells with the world of prostitutes and brothels surfaces with particular force in *Measure for Measure* (3,2:25–8), where the Duke's Vienna smells as foully as Othello's Venice. In the final analysis, the two plays emerge as projections of the same unconscious complex, *Measure for Measure* and *Othello* assaulting the ears of the audience with the beating of the powerful wings of the Winchestrian Goose.

## SHAKESPEARE'S MISOGYNIST VISIONS IN 'KING LEAR' AND 'MACBETH'

While the word 'goose' itself does not appear in *Measure for Measure* and *Othello*, it emerges with great power in Shakespeare's ensuing plays *King Lear* (1605–6) and *Macbeth* (1605–6). In *Lear*, the 'goose cluster' surfaces twice in the play's second act (2,2:80 and 2,4:45), where its associative ramifications spread like a cancerous growth at the play's subliminal level to absorb two of Lear's daughters and to transform them into 'unnatural hags' (2,4:276). King Lear, whose 'hideous rashness' (1,1:150) the Earl of Kent refers to in ambiguous metaphors – 'Kill thy physician, and the fee bestow Upon the foul disease' (1,1:162–3) – compares his daughters to 'a disease that's in my flesh…a boil, A plague-sore, or embossed carbuncle, In my corrupted blood' (2,4:220–3). As the play unwinds, Lear's 'pelican daughters' (3,4:74) bring madness to the old king, whose misogyny culminates in the fourth act, where Lear who at around the age of eighty might be presumed past sexual obsession, works himself up into a fury on the devil in woman's flesh:

> Down from the waist they are Centaurs,
> Though women all above.
> But to the girdle do the gods inherit,
> Beneath is all the fiend's: there's hell, there's darkness,
> There is the sulphurous pit – burning, scalding,

> Stench, consumption; fie, fie, fie! pah, pah!
> Give me an ounce of civet, good apothecary,
> To sweeten my imagination. (4,6:123–30)

'Do thy worst, blind Cupid', Lear concludes, 'I'll not love' (4,6:136). 'Blind Cupid', incidentally, was not only an image of the little god of love but was also the sign of a brothel. '*Pick out mine eyes* with a ballad-maker's pen', says Benedick in *Much Ado About Nothing*, 'and hang me up at the door of a *brothel-house* for the sign of blind Cupid' (1,1:33–5). 'Do thy worst, *blind Cupid'*, has a further underlying meaning because Lear's words are addressed to Gloucester, the 'old lecher' (3,4:110) whose 'pleasant vices' (5,3:169) in 'The dark and vicious place…Cost him his eyes' (5,3:171–2).

Lear's final renunciation of love, then, is coloured both by his reference to 'blind Cupid' and by the fact that he is speaking with blind Gloucester. His reaction is interesting if viewed against the two men's experiences in love. As seen above, Edgar blatantly connects Gloucester's suffering with his adultery (5,3:169–72), just as Lear connects his 'pernicious daughters' (3,2:22) with an evil brought forth from his own 'flesh' (2,4:220). The association of procreation with blindness in Gloucester's case and of procreation with madness in Lear's case once more presents sexuality as a destructive force and female genitalia as a source of punishment and death. In Gloucester's case, it is referred to as 'The dark and vicious place' (5,3:171), and in Lear's case as 'hell', 'darkness', and 'the sulphurous pit' (4,6: 126–7).

On the heels of *King Lear* came yet another misogynist fantasy, *Macbeth*, where *Lear's* 'unnatural hags' (2,4:276) are resurrected in *Macbeth's* 'filthy hags' (5,1:115). Significantly, the tragedy is presided over by 'black Hecate' (3,2:41), the archetypal witch of mythology, and by Lady Macbeth, the archetypal witch of literary imagination. The play, in fact, opens with the witches' dance and reaches its dramatic climax in the witches' cave, 'at the pit of Acheron' (3,5:15), where the witches' cauldron 'Like a hell-broth boil[s] and bubble[s]' (4,1:19), its 'poison' (4,1:5) and 'venom' (4,1:8) to prepare Macbeth for his 'dismal and…fatal end' (3,5:21).

The poisonous mixture of Hecate's cauldron – spiced with 'Finger of birth-strangled babe Ditch-delivered by a drab' (4,1:30–1) – figures for the first time in *Hamlet*. In the play-within-the-play, the poisoning of King Hamlet is presented by the actor playing Claudius in this manner:

> LUCIANUS   Thoughts black, hands apt, drugs fit, and time agreeing;
> Confederate season, else no creature seeing;
> Thou mixture *rank*, of midnight weeds collected,
> With *Hecat's ban* thrice blasted, thrice *infected*,
> Thy natural magic and dire property
> On wholesome life usurps immediately.
> [*Pours the poison in his ears*]. (3,2:249–54)

The poison poured into Macbeth's ears is the witches' prophecy that he 'shalt be King' (1,3:50) – a venomous idea which works with particular effect when it is adopted by Macbeth's wife. The moment she ingests the witches' poison, Lady Macbeth is herself turned into a witch and 'fiend-like queen' (5,9:35). The scene depicting her transformation is one of the highlights of Shakespearean drama and is a culminating moment of the misogyny surrounding the poet's Tragic Period:

> The raven himself is hoarse
> That croaks the fatal entrance of Duncan
> Under my battlements. Come, you spirits
> That tend on mortal thoughts, unsex me here,
> And fill me, from the crown to the toe, top-full
> Of direst cruelty. Make thick my blood,
> Stop up th' access and passage to remorse,
> That no compunctious visitings of nature
> Shake my fell purpose nor keep peace between
> Th' effect and it. Come to my woman's breasts,
> And take my milk for gall, you murd'ring ministers,
> Wherever in your sightless substances
> You wait on nature's mischief. Come, thick night,
> And pall thee in the dunnest smoke of hell,
> That my keen knife see not the wound it makes,
> Nor heaven peep through the blanket of the dark
> To cry 'Hold, hold!' (1,5:38–54)

The first 'goose cluster' of *Macbeth* is found in connection with the Macbeths' castle at Inverness, which is guarded by a drunken Porter who compares himself to the 'porter of Hell Gate' (2,3:1–2). The 'goose' appearing in the Porter scene is surrounded by numerous classical elements of the cluster, its sexual elements blending with the equally important elements of equivocation, deceit, treachery, fear, horror, guilt, trial, punishment and damnation (2,3:1–40). This is a combination which has been cited by a number of critics as the theme and central idea of the play, which has been dubbed 'The great doom's image' (2,3:77).

The play's second 'goose cluster' is found in its final act (5,3:11–62), in which Macbeth realizes that his female demons have presented him with a 'poisoned chalice' (1,7:11) and in the process succeeded in effecting his mental ruin. Steeped in blood, Macbeth finds to his terror that his involvement with the 'secret, black, and midnight hags' (4,1:48) has only brought him the witches' crown and led him to his dismal end before Dunsinane Castle. The governing metaphor of his last speech is 'sickness, disease and medicine', which Caroline Spurgeon views as one of 'the chief symbolic ideas in the play' (Spurgeon, 1935, pp.331–2).

## THE TRAGEDY OF CORIOLANUS

A couple of years after *Macbeth*, Shakespeare wrote two Roman plays in which the bitterness, anger and frustration of his Tragic Period reach culminating heights with *The Tragedy of Coriolanus* (1607–8) and *The Life of Timon of Athens* (1607–8). Shakespeare took over the story of Coriolanus almost wholesale from the account of the life of Caius Marcius Coriolanus in the translation of Plutarch's *Parallel Lives* made by Sir Thomas North (1595). This wholesale adoption accounts for the protagonist's rather flat and stereotyped character, which makes him one of Shakespeare's weakest tragic heroes. While *Coriolanus* is still an interesting play, its interest lies in certain features which are not found in Plutarch and which therefore may be seen as expressing Shakespeare's own conception of the drama.

Foremost among these truly Shakespearean elements is the play's 'recurrent imagery' in which Shakespeare, according to Caroline Spurgeon, introduces the motif of 'sickness, disease and medicine' into his 'central theme' (Spurgeon, 1935, p.347), thereby establishing a connection between *Coriolanus, Hamlet* and *Troilus and Cressida*. 'The number of sickness images in *Hamlet*', observes Spurgeon, 'is greater than in any other play, and the number of them in Troilus is only surpassed (after *Hamlet*) by those in *Coriolanus*, where they arise out of the general dominating image of the body and its members' (Chart VII, see Figure 40).

The Roman hero of the play contributes greatly to its 'running imagery' because Coriolanus's own deep-seated anger and bitterness flow from him as a constant poison of invectives centring on foul disease and corruption, death and destruction. Significantly, the play's two 'goose clusters' are found in Coriolanus's two impassioned speeches, where he refers to the common people as 'measles, Which we disdain should *tetter* us, *yet sought The very way to catch them*' (3,1:77–9) – a reference to syphilis which was sometimes called 'the Measelles of the Indias' (see p.41). Coriolanus also sees the discontent of the people as self-made sores on the body, brought about by 'rubbing the poor itch' of their opinion, and so making themselves 'scabs' (1,1:163–4). 'All the contagion of the south light on you', he tells the cowardly soldiers, 'boils and plagues Plaster you o' er, that you may be abhorred Farther than seen, and one infect another Against the wind a mile! You souls of geese!' (1,4:30–4).

In addition to the play's 'running imagery', a second original motif introduced by Shakespeare is a strange feature of Coriolanus's electoral campaign, during which the first sign of a genuine, personal conflict appears in the Roman warrior. This almost unbearable conflict arises from the necessity of appearing naked to the public during his campaign for the office of consul, thereby revealing to curious and examining eyes the 'wounds' (2,2:138) and 'scars' (2,2:148) of his *skin*. While Plutarch's Coriolanus shows no reticence in showing his skin to the public, Shakespeare's hero appears to be held back by a strong 'skin-complex', possibly explained by the fact that ultimate horror in Shakespearean tragedy focuses on the skin. 'O horrible! O horrible! most horrible!', the poisoned King groaned in *Hamlet* as he described the way in which his 'smooth body' had been 'barked about, Most lazar-like, with vile and loathsome crust' (1,5:71–2;80).

As Kumar Sen demonstrates in his excellent analysis of the play, the public humiliation Coriolanus suffers when he is forced to show the lesions of his skin becomes the hinge on which the play turns (Kumar Sen, 1958, pp.334–5). In fact, Coriolanus's conflict proves of such magnitude that he appears both to submit to the ancient custom and in the end to manage to hide his skin from public view by a subtle manoeuver which calls down upon him the implacable wrath of the people and his own ultimate destruction. 'No man saw 'em' (2,3:163), the citizens grumble during Coriolanus's electoral campaign, with reference to Coriolanus's many 'wounds' (2,3:162). 'But this is something odd' (2,3: 82), a Third Citizen muses on the same occasion, once more reiterating the suspicion that 'if he show us his *wounds* and tell us his *deeds*, we are to put our *tongues* into those wounds and *speak for them*' (2,3:5–8).

The *double entendre* of the various references to Coriolanus's skin lesions also appears in the hero's own mentioning of them. 'I have some wounds upon me, and they smart To hear themselves remembered' (1,9:28–9), he confides to Cominius just before the election. And his old friend replies: 'Should they not, Well might they *fester* 'gainst ingratitude, And *tent* themselves with *death*' (1,9:29–31). 'Think Upon the *wounds* his body bears, which show Like *graves* i'th' holy churchyard' (3,3:49–51), Menenius later ruminates in similar telling manner.

To all appearances, Coriolanus's concern regarding his 'skin' and its 'wounds' and 'scars' received in the course of his many 'deeds' exhibits the features of a psychological complex. In an interesting way, the associations Shakespeare makes with the word 'skin' reveal the same developmental pattern as his images of 'sickness, disease and medicine'. While this latter group undergoes metamorphosis into horror and disgust at 'foul disease' after 1598, a similar movement may be discerned in the associative patterns in which the word 'skin' is embedded. The sexual and venereal character of Shakespearean associations to skin begin in *As You Like It* (4,2:10–19), and are followed by *Hamlet* (3,4:149–51), *Measure for Measure* (2,2:134–5), *All's Well that Ends Well* (2,2:20–6), *Lear* (3,4:6–9), *Othello* (5,2:4–6) and *The Tempest* (4,1:232–40).

The fusion of 'skin' imagery with the imagery of 'sickness, disease and medicine' in *Coriolanus* forms part of the same pattern developed in the earlier plays and helps to present the protagonist as a body spreading infection and disease throughout Rome. The tribune Sicinius denounces Coriolanus as 'this *viper* That would *depopulate* the city' (3,1:261–2) and further recommends total isolation of 'This *viperous* traitor' (3,1:284): 'It is a mind that shall remain a *poison* where it is, Not *poison* any further' (3,1:85–7). 'Pursue him to his *house*, and pluck him thence', continues the second tribune, Brutus, in similar ambiguous language, 'Lest his *infection*, being of *catching* nature, Spread further' (3,1:306–8). 'He's a *disease* that must be cut away' (3,1:292), Sicinius finally explodes, while Coriolanus's closest friend, Menenius Agrippa, attempts to defend him with the words: 'Oh, he's a *limb* that has but a *disease:* Mortal, to *cut it off;* to *cure* it, easy' (3,1:293–4). Menenius's attempts to negotiate between his friend and the plebeians earn him the rebuke of the tribune Brutus who tells him: 'Sir, those cold ways, That seem like prudent helps, are very poisonous Where the *disease* is *violent.* Lay hands upon him, And bear him to the rock' (3,1:218–21).

When Coriolanus manages to escape from the mob in the ensuing scuffle, he defects to join the Volscians, the enemies of Rome. However, here he is also treated as a viper and as a poisonous influence until finally he is killed as a traitor of the people by his many enemies. As the curtain descends on *Coriolanus*, the play's 'central theme of the body and sickness' (Spurgeon) materializes in a final dramatic and symbolic image of its hero bleeding to death from countless wounds.

Perhaps this ultimate fusion of the play's two image groups may be explained by an interesting dermatological aspect of the 'goose cluster'. As Ambrose King and Claude Nicol observe in their study of *Venereal Diseases* (1975):

'In the late latent stage of syphilis the scar of a primary lesion may sometimes be seen on the genital organs, and occasionally *Leucoderma...colli,* or 'collar of Venus,' is a residual depigmentation of the skin of the neck which is found not infrequently in dark-haired people who have suffered from secondary syphilis...Another occasional residual finding is 'macular atrophy,' presenting as small atrophic macules over the body surface at points where the original secondary papules were present.' (pp.41, 33–4)

## TIMON OF ATHENS

Shakespeare's second Roman play *Timon of Athens* (1607–8) was written at about the same time as *Coriolanus* and may be regarded as its companion piece. As demonstrated by G.W. Bentley, *Timon* is embedded in a web of syphilitic images and associations, and Timon, the final hero of Shakespeare's 'black' tragedies, brings to a head the plays' misogyny, sex-nausea and preoccupation with 'rottenness', the latter expression alluding both to physical and moral corruption (Bentley, 1989, pp.139–207). When the embittered and misanthropic Greek meets the prostitutes Timandra and Phrynia outside Athens, he tells them in fiery metaphors to use their occupation and their disease to destroy the city that has treated him so badly:

> Be whores still,
> And he whose pious breath seeks to convert you,
> Be strong in whore, allure him, burn him up;
> Let your close fire predominate his smoke,
> And be no turncoats...whore still;
> Paint till a horse may mire upon your face
> A pox of wrinkles! (4,3:141–45;149–51)

'Give them diseases', Timon advises Timandra as to how to take revenge on men,

> Make use of thy salt hours; season the slaves
> For tubs and baths; bring down rose-cheek'd youth
> To the tub-fast and the diet. (4,3:85–8)

Timon here of course refers to the common treatment of syphilis in Elizabethan times, and significantly his fiery address to the two courtezans culminates in one of the most vivid clinical pictures of the secondary and tertiary symptoms of syphilis written at the time:

> Consumptions sow
> In hollow bones of man; strike their sharp shins,
> And mar men's spurring. Crack the lawyer's voice,
> That he may never more false title plead,
> Nor sound his quillets shrilly. Hoar the flamen [priest],
> That scolds against the quality of flesh,
> And not believes himself. Down with the nose,
> Down with it flat, take the bridge quite away
> Of him that, his particular to foresee,
> Smells from the general weal. Make curled-pate ruffians bald,
> And let the unscarred braggarts of the war

Derive some pain from you. Plague all,
That your activity may defeat and quell
The source of all erection. (4,3:153–66)[*]

The pathology referred to would appear to be syphilitic osteitis; tabes with lightning pains and intractable leg ulcers; the raucous voice of laryngeal syphilis; the whitish or 'hoared' crusted lesions of the psoriasiform secondary syphilide; the flattened 'saddle nose' from a gumma of the bony bridge; and syphilitic alopecia. Impotence is not normally an effect of syphilis but may be a psychological side effect of contracting the disease. In Sir John Harington's epigram *Against an old Lecher*, the poet makes the following statement:

Since thy third curing of the French infection,
*Priapus* hath in thee found no erection:
Yet eat'st thou Ringoes, and Potato Rootes,
And Caueare, but it little bootes. (Harrington, 1930, p.244)

At the end of *Timon of Athens*, the protagonist arrives at the nadir of his depression, which he expresses symbolically by his desire to dig his grave on the beach and have the sea wash and dry his body until only the bones are left. The play represents the culmination of Shakespeare's Tragic Period and the extremity of his suffering, revealing a mind that has been transformed into a disillusioned misogynist and misanthrope – a nihilist without hope. In concluding our survey of this period of the poet's life and work, we shall attempt to illuminate Shakespeare's greatest nihilist and misogynist fantasy by a short examination of the psychological roots of misogyny – the most salient feature of the author's 'black' tragedies.

MISOGYNY IN MEN

If one disregards the cases in which misogyny appears as a concomitant of certain life styles such as homosexuality, misogyny in heterosexual men might reflect some traumatic experience at the hands of the opposite sex. In the 16th century, infection with syphilis could easily represent such an experience because of the incurable and often fatal nature of the disease. From later centuries we know of strong misogynist reactions in men who have been infected with syphilis. In a brilliant study entitled *The Horror of Life* (1980), Roger L. Williams has demonstrated the strong misogynist reactions of Charles Baudelaire, Jules de Goncourt, Guy de Maupassant and Alphonse Daudet – all men infected with syphilis at an early stage of their career.

Baudelaire recorded his misogynist views – especially in *Mon coeur mis à nu* – with unmistakable venom, regarding women as accomplices of the serpent that engineered the fall of man. 'The strange thing about woman', observed Baudelaire, 'her preordained fate, is that she is *simultaneously* the sin and the Hell that punishes it' (Williams, 1980, pp.19–20). In their novels *Charles Demailly* and *Manette Salomon*, Jules de Goncourt and his brother Edmond presented woman as a creature who achieves her domination of man by making herself an accomplice of that which is

---

[*]    The implications regarding syphilis of this passage have been noted by a number of medical observers, such as Smith, 1914, p.450. Packard, 1924, p.197. Wolfe, 1960, p.113. Rosebury, 1971, p.120. Simpson, 1959, pp. 251–2. Crosfill, 1957, pp.80–2.

basest in him, until the day arrives when a man is deprived of his talent and position, and his life ends in madness and tragedy (p.82–3). (As most will agree, this is very much the theme of *Macbeth*.)

Maupassant was a great lover of cats and once observed of 'the perfidious selfishness of their pleasure' that women were like cats: they open their arms and offer their lips, but as the man tastes the joy of their caresses, he realizes that he holds a perfidious cat, with claws and fangs, 'an enemy in love who will bite him when tired of his kisses' (p.222). Finally, Roger L. Williams demonstrates how Alphonse Daudet's view of woman corresponds with that of Baudelaire, the Goncourt brothers and Maupassant. Daudet conceives of woman as a creature instinctively false and bad for all men, especially those of superior talent. This is a logical concomitant to his sad appraisal of love as 'one of the inescapable sorrows of man' (p.283).

The most famous example in the 19th century of misogyny in a man infected with syphilis is, of course, the German philosopher Arthur Schopenhauer (1788–1860). At the age of 35 he contracted syphilis at Göttingen and underwent protracted mercury treatment, finally to die at the age of 72 of pneumonia. His misogyny appeared not only in his lifelong bachelorhood, but also in his philosophy, which denounces woman as the evil agent of procreation and generation. Iwan Bloch, who examined Schopenhauer's disease in an article published in 1906 (nos. 25, 26), concludes: 'Not until he had felt on his own body the whole tragedy of sensual pleasure, the demon of sexuality, and the "enmity" of love did he understand the full importance of the ascetic idea' (Bäumler, 1976, p.262).

In concluding our brief survey of famous misogynists in literature and philosophy, we should draw attention to the fact that even Shakespeare's humorous *bonvivant*, Sir John Falstaff, appears to have finished his life as an inveterate misogynist. On his deathbed he said of women that 'they were devils incarnate' (*Henry V*,2,3:32–3), and according to Mistress Quickly he finished his life with an ugly vision of 'the Whore of Babylon' (*Henry V*,2,3:39–40). Falstaff's view may be aptly explained by his own contraction of syphilis, such as later the two Hamlets may also have been expressing a hatred of women stemming from their contraction of the same disease.

THE SEXUAL 'CRIME' (120) OF THE 'SONNETS'

In concluding our chapters on Shakespeare, we shall now go on to explore whether the cluster 'sickness, disease and medicine' makes its appearence in Shakespeare's seemingly autobiographical *Sonnets*. This is indeed the case with Sonnets 34–37, which belong to a well-defined group comprising Sonnets 18–126. There is consensus among scholars that Shakespeare's *Sonnets* may be divided into three subgroups: (1) Sonnets 1–17 are an appeal to the fair youth to marry and beget children, an 'embassage' many critics believe to have been inspired by the noble youth's parents. With E.K. Chambers, we take these sonnets as Shakespeare's rendering of his commission from the Pembroke family to make William Herbert 'affect' Elizabeth Carey, the partner selected for him by the parents on both sides.

These negotiations took place in the late autumn of 1595, to which period Sonnets 1–17 may fittingly be assigned (see p.189).

(2) Sonnets 127–52 depict Shakespeare's infatuation with a dark lady, which we take to refer to the poet's love affair with Emilia Lanier, which probably began in 1594 (see p.182). The figure of Rosaline in *Love's Labour's Lost* (1594–5) and in *Romeo and Juliet* (1594–5) supports this date since she is obviously a portrait of the dark lady of the *Sonnets*. Further confirmation may be found in the sonneteering craze which is reflected so strongly in the two plays, which were written at the same time as the sonnets to the dark lady (Fabricius, 1989, pp.99–131).

(3) Sonnets 18–126 tell of Shakespeare's friendship with the fair youth and may be taken to cover the period 1595–98, or the 'Three winters…[and] three summers' described by Sonnet 104 (see p.183). It is in this group that we find in Sonnets 34–37, 67, 94–95, 111, and 118–20 the imagery of 'sickness, disease and medicine'.

Sonnet sequence 34–37 is conspicuous for its concentration of this imagery, which, significantly, is found in a sexual context more fully described by Sonnets 33–42. In this sequence, the fair youth has stolen the poet's mistress, and it appears that the two men have shared her favours for a while, each unknown to the other. When the poet learns the truth, he explains and forgives his friend's treachery (37–40) – 'Take all my loves, my love, yea take them all…Although thou steal me all my poverty' (40) – even if he cannot refrain from reproaching the 'straying youth' (41) for breaking a 'twofold truth' (41) and for not forbearing from occupying his 'seat' (41).

The *drame à trois* described by the sequence 33–42 is not necessarily the same as that described by Sonnet 144 to the dark lady, although they share the same fear of the medical consequences of triangular love. While Sonnet 144 broods over the possibility that the fair youth may be 'fired out' by the dark lady as a result of sexual intercourse, the traumatic event described by Sonnets 34–35 may allude to 'foul play' (*Ham.*1,2:256) in Shakespeare's own Bohemian world with its grave medical consequences, that is, an act of treachery by a rival who appears to have brought about the poet's infection through a common love object that has proved unfaithful (see p.46):

> Why didst thou promise such a beauteous day,
> And make me travel forth without my cloak,
> To let base clouds o'ertake me in my way,
> Hiding thy brav'ry in their rotten smoke?
> 'Tis not enough that through the cloud thou break,
> To dry the rain on my storm-beaten face,
> For no man well of such a salve can speak,
> That heals the wound, and cures not the disgrace.
> Nor can thy shame give physic to my grief;
> Though thou repent, yet I have still the loss.
> Th' offender's sorrow lends but weak relief
> To him that bears the strong offense's cross.
> Ah, but those tears are pearl which thy love sheeds,
> And they are rich and ransom all ill deeds. (34)

No more be grieved at that which thou hast done:
Roses have thorns, and silver fountains mud,
Clouds and eclipses stain both moon and sun,
And loathsome canker lives in sweetest bud.
All men make faults, and even I in this,
Authorizing thy trespass with compare,
Myself corrupting, salving thy amiss,
Excusing thy sins more than thy sins are;
For to thy sensual fault I bring in sense –
The adverse party is thy advocate –
And 'gainst myself a lawful plea commence.
Such civil war is in my love and hate
That I an accessory needs must be
To that sweet thief which sourly robs from me. (35)

The ensuing Sonnet 36 describes the poet's acceptance of both his friend's guilt as well as his own, although the Sonnet ends on a note of bitter resignation: 'So shall those *blots* that do with me remain, Without thy help, by me be borne alone' (36). The implications of the word 'blot' is borne out by Sonnet 95, which contains warning against syphilis to the fair youth, and its origin in his 'sins', 'canker', 'shame', 'sport' and 'vices' (95):

O, what a mansion have those *vices* got
Which for their habitation chose out thee,
Where beauty's veil doth cover every *blot*,
And all things turns to fair that eyes can see!
Take heed, dear heart, of this large privilege;
*The hardest knife ill-used doth lose his edge.* (95)

Our medical interpretation of sonnet sequences 34–37 and 40–42 solves the difficulties that commentators have had with the 'sickness, disease and medicine' imagery of Sonnet 37, in which the poet states that he has been 'made *lame* by Fortune's *dearest spite*' (37). In the 'sickness, disease and medicine' imagery of Sonnet 111 – '*willing patient...drink Potions...my strong infection...cure me*' (111) – 'Fortune' is presented as 'The *guilty* goddess of my *harmful deeds*' (111). Shakespeare's ailment was, perhaps, related to that resulting in Falstaff's halting gait and to the pains described by the subject of a contemporary popular ballad:

For I (sir) limping lame haue beene,
Sore bitten by the Scorpiuns keene,
In a bawdy house I vs'd to roare,
Till all my ioynts were pocky sore:
all this I haue endur'd
which vice procur'd
and since of health I am assur'd
I will doe what I can,
to hinder euery man
from that base course which once I ran. (*Roxburghe Ballads*, vol.1, p.478)

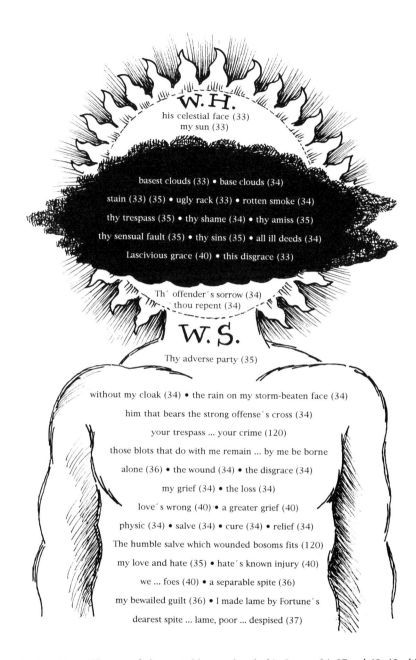

Figure 48. The fair youth's serious fault or moral lapse is described in Sonnets 34–37 and 40–42 which open with the symbolic sunrise of Sonnet 33, in which the youth is compared to the 'sun', at the same time as the poet attempts to justify 'the basest clouds' and 'ugly rack' that 'stain' the youth's 'celestial face'. The shared 'disgrace' occurs within a strong pattern of shared identity, the fair youth being perceived by the poet as an *alter ego* figure, or self representation. The drawing illustrates this psychological complex while rendering the associative patterns of the sexual 'crime' (120) committed by the fair youth as described in the above sonnet sequences. Seymour-Smith (1966, pp. 34–35) interprets Sonnets 33–36 as rendering a homosexual symbolism. Drawing by René Terney.

'Fortune's *dearest spite*' (37) is clearly meant to be the result of the sexual offense committed by the fair youth in Sonnets 34–36. Here it also results in a temporary estrangement or 'a separable *spite*' (36) between the two lovers. An echo of the same event may be heard in Sonnet 40 which laments the youth's seduction of the poet's love object while calling him '*Lascivious* grace, in whom all *ill* well shows. Kill me with *spites*; yet we must not be foes' (40). Another echo of the same seduction may be perceived in Sonnet 118, which, soaked in the imagery of 'sickness, disease and medicine', notes that '*Drugs poison him that so fell sick of you*' (118).

In Sonnet 120 the poet once more returns to the traumatic event of Sonnets 34–37 and 40–42, reminding the fair youth of how 'you were once *unkind*' (129) and 'how once I suffered in your *crime*' (120). Fittingly, the sonnet concludes with a sad reminiscence governed by imagery of 'sickness, disease and medicine':

> O, that our night of woe might have rememb'red
> My deepest sense how hard true sorrow hits,
> And soon to you, as you to me then, tend'red
> The humble salve which wounded bosoms fits!
> But that your trespass now becomes a fee;
> Mine ransoms yours, and yours must ransom me. (120)

This is possibly a standard exchange of apologies by two Bohemians or libertines, involved in amorous entanglements when 'trespassing' upon each other's property, for example by secretly sharing the same love object, as in Sonnets 144 and 34–42. 'Take all my loves, my love, yea take them all' (40) is another typical statement by a Bohemian when forced to acknowledge his defeat in love at the hands of an adored rival – the 'gentle thief' (40) and 'robber' of the same sonnet.

We have suggested a connection between the freewheeling life described in the *Sonnets* and their imagery of 'sickness, disease and medicine'. As demonstrated above, this specific image group undergoes a quantitative as well as qualitative change in the direction of horror and disgust at 'foul disease' with *2 Henry IV* (1597–8). This feature supports our medical interpretation of the sexual 'crime' (120) as committed in Sonnets 34–37 and 40–42 of the same period. The only topical allusion contained in the sonnets addressed to the fair youth that scholars have been able to agree on is the reference in Sonnet 66 to 'art made tongue-tied by authority' (66), which alludes to the Privy Council's closure of all the theatres of London on July 28, 1597, due to the scandalous performance of Nashe's and Jonson's play, the *Isle of Dogs*.

The 'beauteous day' (34) alluded to in Sonnet 34 is obviously one of summer, and this we take to belong to the last year of the poet's friendship with the fair youth, that is, 1598. Similarly we assume a connection between the estrangement described by Sonnets 33–42 and the unidentified disease contracted by William Herbert in June 1598 – most probably syphilis (see pp. 190–1). Thematically and chronologically, this hypothesis tallies with the two last poems of Shakespeare's *Sonnets* (153–54), which render the sad finale of the entire cycle. Steeped like the sonnet sequence 34–37 in imagery of 'sickness, disease and medicine', the final sonnets depict a frustrated and 'sick' (153) poet travelling to Bath to seek 'Against strange maladies a sovereign cure' (153). Describing himself as 'a sad distempered guest' (153) he further presents himself as 'my mistress' thrall' (154) and burnt by 'Cupid' (153) – his hope of a 'healthful remedy for men diseased' (154) proving to be 'a seething bath' (153), or the most common cure of syphilis (see pp.140–1).

A difficult and possibly odd play written by Shakespeare in the autumn of 1598 may help to shed further light on the enigmatic events described above. In *Much Ado About Nothing* (1598), the most interesting feature of the comedy is its 'amiable encounter…in the orchard' (3,3:146–7), where 'a liberal villain' (4.1:92) causes a young woman to be seduced and her lover 'poisoned' by this very act. Shakespeare's introduction of this subplot and its shocking denouement has puzzled critics and audiences because of its utter incongruity with the humorous main plot of the comedy. By an act of 'foul play' instigated by the villainous nobleman Don John, the protagonist of the play, Claudio, is presented with a love object whom he supposes faithful and chaste, only to discover later that she is actually 'a *contaminated stale*' (2,2:25) whose *'foul-tainted'* flesh' (4,1:143) belongs to that of an 'approved *wanton'* (4,1:44). Consumed with rage and jealousy, Claudio renounces his 'fair young Hero' (1,1:284) in front of the altar of their marriage ceremony and returns her to her father with the words: 'Give not this *rotten orange* to your friend' (4,1:31).

So powerful is this freely invented subplot that it later comes to fuel the main plots of *Hamlet, Troilus and Cressida, Othello, Cymbeline* and *The Winter's Tale* (Figure 49). Thus the traumatic event described by *Much Ado About Nothing* was possibly the same as that which was described by Shakespeare in sonnet sequence 33–42.

## THE MANNINGHAM ANECDOTE ABOUT SHAKESPEARE

In the final section of our chapters on Shakespeare's life and work, two more sources will be quoted to support our picture of Shakespeare as a Bohemian and a libertine. One is an anecdote from London, the other a piece of gossip from Oxford.

John Manningham (d. 1622) was a diarist and lawyer who lived in London during the first quarter of the 17th century. While a student at the Middle Temple he kept a diary for the period January 1602 to April 1603. The journal provides a number of interesting insights into early 17th-century London life, including an account of a performance of Shakespeare's *Twelfth Night* at the Middle Temple on February 2, 1602. On March 13, 1602, John Manningham records the following story as having been told him by Edward Curle, one of his fellow-students at the Middle Temple. The story deals with James Burbage (c. 1567–1619), the greatest actor of the day, and William Shakespeare:

> 'Upon a time when Burbage played Richard III, there was a citizen grew so far in liking with him that before she went from the play she appointed him to come that night unto her by the name of Richard the Third. Shakespeare, overhearing their conversation, went before, was entertained, and at his game ere Burbage came. Then message being brought that Richard the Third was at the door, Shakespeare caused return to be made that William the Conqueror was before Richard the Third. (Shakespeare's name William.)' (Chambers, 1930, vol.2, p.212)

John Manningham's diary was discovered by the Shakespearean scholar John Payne Collier (1789–1883), who was also a notorious forger, and in 1954 Sydney Race argued that the entry was a forgery inserted by Collier. But graphological evidence

Figure 49. 'Claudio…loved her so, that speaking of her foulness, Washed it with tears' (*Much Ado About Nothing*, 4,1:153–4). The drawing gives the common denominator of *Much Ado About Nothing, Hamlet, Troilus and Cressida, Othello, Cymbeline*, and *The Winter's Tale*. An idea so insistent in Shakespeare's dramatic imagination reveals a psychological complex, the structure of which may be outlined as follows: A woman whom the protagonist imagines 'pure' turns out to be a promiscuous woman, a prostitute in fact – 'whored' or 'bewhored' by a 'villain' who 'poisons' her and her lover while arousing the latter's abysmal hatred, jealousy and misogyny. Drawing by René Terney.

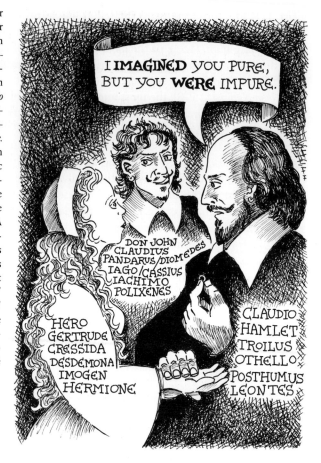

and recent microscopic and ultra-violet examination shows the entry to be genuine[*] and there is a contemporary allusion to the anecdote in *The Scourge of Folly* (c.1611) by John Davies of Hereford which also confirms its authenticity. In a poem addressed 'To our English Terence, Mr. Will. Shakespeare', John Davies alludes either to the anecdote or to the events it purports to narrate, in the following lines:

> Some say, good Will, (which I in sport do sing)
> *Hadst thou not played some kingly parts in sport,*
> Thou hadst been a companion for a king
> And been a king among the meaner sort.
>                                   (Chambers, 1930, vol.2, p.214)[**]

The meaning of the two last lines has defied interpretation for generations in spite of several scholarly efforts.

---

[*]   Manningham, 1976, p.328; Schoenbaum, 1975, p.152.
[**]  Modernized version; italics added.

THE ELIZABETHAN THEATRE: 'VENUS PALLACE AND SATHAN'S SYNAGOGUE'[*]

John Manningham's anecdote provides an interesting glimpse of the theatre milieu at Shakespeare's time, which in medical terms must be characterized as a dangerous one. The Puritans and other dissidents condemned not only the theatres as sources of sinful delight and moral corruption but as 'markets of bawdry' (Chambers, 1923, vol.4, p.218), that is, centres of prostitution.

> 'Satan hath not a more speedie way, and fitter schoole to work and teach his desire, to bring men and women into his snare of concupiscence and filthie lustes of wicked whoredome,' asserted a Gloucester minister, John Northbrooke, 'than those places, and playes, and theatres are; and therefore [it is] necessarie that those places, and players, shoulde be forbidden, and dissolued, and put downe by authoritie, as the brothell houses and stewes are.' (p.198)

In his treatise *The Schoole of Abuse* (1579), another Puritan extremist, Stephen Gosson, publicly accused the playhouse of being no more than an anteroom for the brothel (Chambers, 1923, vol.4, pp.203–4).[**] 'Pay thy two-pence to a player', one of Dekker's characters asserts in *Lanthorne and Candlelight* (1608), 'in his gallerie maist thou sitte by a Harlot'.[***] Not only were those persons associated with the theatre accused of encouraging 'Luxury and licentious ease' (Dekker, 1884–6, vol.2, p.53), but they were accused of partaking in it themselves. In Middleton's *A Mad World, My Masters* (1608), the Courtezan of the play witnesses an actor speaking the Prologue with such eloquence and charm that she cries out:

> 'A' my troth, an I were not married, I could find in my heart to fall in love with that player now, and send for him to a supper. I know some i' th' town that have done as much, and there took such a good conceit of their parts in th' two-penny room, that the actors have been found i' th' morning in a less compass than their stage, though 'twere ne'er so full of gentlemen.' (5,2:34–40)

A man on still more intimate terms with the world of the theatre was the popular actor Nathan Field (1587–1620), who in 1616 wrote a comedy called *Amends for Ladies*. In its tavern scene in the third act, a Drawer answers a 'roarer' named Whoore-bang who has just called for 'a whore':

> 'Why what d'ee thinke of me, am I an Infidell, a Turke, a Pagan, a Sarazin; I haue beene at *Bess Turnups*, and she sweares all the Gentlewomen went to see a play at the Fortune, and are not come in yet; and she beleeues they sup with the Players.'

To which another 'roarer' named Teare-chops replies: 'Damm-me, we must kill all those rogues, we shall neuer keepe a whore for them' (3,4:22–9).

The theatres, gardens, arenas and brothels on the Bankside formed what was popularly known as 'the Bears Colledge' because the education it offered was formidable. Not all members of the great metropolis, however, shared the enthusiasm of the common man for the various entertainments south of the Thames. Skeptics saw a connection between brothels and theatres which was more than one of geographical contiguity. When John Dryden (1631–1700), late in the 17th century, wrote his Prologue to Thomas Southerne's (1659–1746) *The Disappointment*, he

---

[*]   Philip Stubbes: *The Anatomie of Abuses* (1583), quoted by Chambers, 1923, vol.4, p.223.
[**]   cf. also pp.223–4.
[***]  Dekker, 1884–6, vol.3, pp.216–7. See also Gurr, 1987, p.128.

alluded to a state of affairs that had already been widely commented on in the Elizabethan period.

> The Playhouse is their place of Traffic, where
> nightly they sit to sell their rotten Ware.
> Tho' done in silence and Withoute a Cryer
> yet hee that bids the most is still the Buyer:
> for while he nibbles at her am'rous Trap
> she gets the Mony: he gets the Clap.
>
> (Burford, 1973, p.188)

## THE OXFORD GOSSIP ABOUT MISTRESS DAVENANT

London, Oxford and Stratford are the three main sources of information about Shakespeare, and the Oxford tradition is concerned exclusively with the rumour that the later Poet Laureate, Sir William Davenant (1606–68), was the natural son of Shakespeare and that this rumour had confirmation from Davenant himself when his tongue had been loosened by alcohol. The result of local tradition, the Oxford rumour was first put in print by William Rufus Chetwood in *A General History of the Stage* (1749), in which he gave the information that 'Sir William Davenant was by many, suppos'd the natural Son of Shakespeare' (Chambers, 1930, vol.2, p.285).

Of the other and earlier sources quoted by E.K. Chambers, the oldest and best-known account of William Shakespeare's 'relationship' with William Davenant derives from the English antiquarian and writer John Aubrey (1626–97). Aubrey's information is from 1681 and his three informants appear to have been the well-known Restoration actor William Beeston (c. 1606–82), the son of Christopher Beeston (d. 1638), Shakespeare's colleague; William Davenant's brother, the Reverend Robert Davenant; and the poet and satirist Samuel Butler (1612–80). In the following transcription, the passages in square brackets have been scored out by an unknown hand:

'Sr William Davenant Knight Poet Laureate was borne in —— street in the City of Oxford, at the Crowne Taverne (*In margin*, 'V.A.W. Antiq:Oxon:'). His father was John Davenant a Vintner there, a very grave and discreet Citizen: his mother was a very beautifull woman, & of a very good witt and of conversation extremely agreable...Mr William Shakespeare was wont to goe into Warwickshire once a yeare, and did commonly in his journey lye at this house in Oxon: where he was exceedingly respected. [I have heard parson Robert Davenant say that Mr W. Shakespeare here gave him a hundred kisses.] Now Sr. Wm would sometimes when he was pleasant over a glasse of wine with his most intimate friends e.g. Sam: Butler (author of Hudibras) &c. say, that it seemed to him that he writt with the very spirit that did Shakespeare, and was seemed contentended enough to be thought his Son: he would tell them the story as above. [in which way his mother had a very light report, whereby she was called a whore.].' (Chambers, 1930, vol.2, p.254. cf. also p.258)

The story of William Shakespeare's paternity of William Davenant circulated in Oxford in the form of a humorous anecdote which has been handed down in several versions. The best one of these reads as follows: 'One day going from school, a grave doctor in divinity met him [William Davenant] and asked him: "Child, whither art thou going in such haste?" To which the child replied: "O Sir, my godfather is come to town, and I am going to ask his blessing." To which the doctor said: "Hold child, you must not take the name of God in vain'" (pp.269–70. Cf also pp.271–2, 277, 284. Modernized spelling).

Chambers and most scholars refer Shakespeare's paternity of William Davenant to 'The Shakespeare-Mythos'. But the legend may be true. Chronology shows *Antony and Cleopatra* (1606–7) to be contemporaneous with the birth of William Davenant, and Shakespeare's rumoured affair with the boy's beautiful and charming mother provides an apt explanation of his remarkable departure in this play from the gloomy atmosphere of the 'black' tragedies. *Antony and Cleopatra* blazes like a fire in the night and presents the audience with one of the most magnificent love affairs the world has ever known. In Shakespeare's Eastern romance, the depressed and misogynist worlds of the author's Tragic Period are momentarily alleviated by a fresh outburst of sexual passion and by a heavenly sense of libidinal fulfilment and elevation. Antony himself touches on this glorious aspect of the play's royal love when he tells Cleopatra that if she would put a bourn to the measure of his love, she must 'needs find out new heaven, new earth' (1,1:17).

The woman who inspired *Antony and Cleopatra* was hardly the 52-year-old Anne Hathaway at Stratford who, according to tradition, was wont to receive her husband's visit 'once a yeare' (Chambers, 1930, vol.2, p.253). The muse to set Shakespeare's imagination on fire for the wonders of *Antony and Cleopatra* is rather to be sought elsewhere and this, possibly, in Oxford during the years 1606–7 when the play was written and when William Davenant was born on March 3, 1606.

In addition to chronology, there is the genetic evidence in favour of 'The Davenant Hypothesis'. The man who was ostensibly an innkeeper's son from Oxford did, in fact, become one of the most famous poets and playwrights of the 17th century, in addition to proving himself a successful theatre manager and producer. His first play, *The Tragedy of Albovine, King of the Lombards* (1629), was followed by many plays and masques at court. He stood high in royal favour and, in 1638, after the death of Ben Jonson, he was awarded a pension and the quasi-official title of 'Poet Laureate'. At his death in 1668, he was buried in Westminster Abbey in the Poets' Corner.

The tradition that Shakespeare was Davenant's 'godfather' may explain the latter's first name, *William*. Tradition also has it that William Davenant possessed an 'amicable letter' written to Shakespeare by James I (Chambers, 1930, vol.2, p.280).

There is finally the remarkable fact that Shakespeare's only portrait (Figure 35) was not in the possession of his family after his death. *It was owned by Sir William Davenant.* From him it passed on to the Duke of Buckingham and Chandos, and in 1848 it was sold among the other effects of the Chandos estate. It was then bought by the Earl of Ellesmere, who subsequently presented it to the nation. These scraps of information suggest that Shakespeare himself might have regarded William Davenant as more than a godson and looked upon him as a son – a substitute for Hamnet, his only son, whom the poet had lost in 1596 at the tender age of eleven.

Figure 50. Father and son? Engraving of William Shakespeare in the Folio edition of his collected works, 1623 by Martin Droeshout after the portrait of the poet by John Taylor c. 1608 (Figure 35); and engraving of William Davenant in the Folio edition of his collected works, 1673 by William Faithorne after a lost painting by John Greenhill. Davenant's nose bridge has been eaten away by syphilitic infection, a deformity which in the majority of cases is due to congenital syphilis. In Davenant's case, however, his 'saddle nose' appears to have been acquired later in life. John Aubrey in his *Brief Lives* says of Davenant that 'He gott a terrible clap of a Black handsome wench that lay in Axeyard, Westminster, whom he thought on when he speakes of Dalga in Gondibert, which cost him his Nose, with which unlucky mischance many witts were too cruelly bold' (1950, p.86). Davenant's syphilitic infection was complicated by poisoning from mercury, which was used clumsily at this time in the treatment of syphilis. In a poem *To Doctor Cademan, Physitian to the Queen* (Davenant, 1673, pp.234–5), a man whose widow Davenant was one day to marry, the poet thanked him 'For setting now my condemn'd body free, From that no God, but Devil Mercurie' (p.234). In another poem addressed to his friend and maecenas Endymion Porter, Davenant vowed never again to practice 'vice', 'Lest by a fiery surfeit I be led, Once more to grow devout in a strange bed' (p.218).

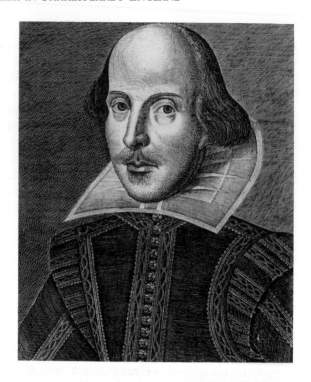

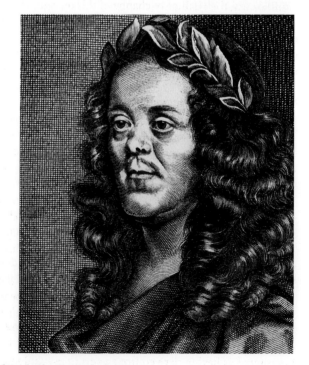

CONCLUSION

We have quoted *Willobie His Avisa, Shakespeare's Sonnets,* John Manningham's London anecdote about the poet, and the Oxford gossip about his paternity of William Davenant as evidence of Shakespeare's Bohemian tendencies and freewheeling life. In Elizabethan and Stuart London such a pattern of behaviour was extremely dangerous, and there is evidence that other leading members of literary and dramatic Bohemia in the capital contracted syphilis – Robert Greene, Thomas Nashe and George Peele among them.

Our hypothesis that Shakespeare might have contracted syphilis as well rests on internal evidence. Several features at the unconscious level of the poet's work point to Shakespeare's preoccupation with venereal diseases and their consequences. The quantitative and qualitative change of the statistical distribution of 'sickness, disease and medicine' imagery during the years 1597/98 – 1601/2 reveals a heightened awareness of and concern regarding 'foul disease'. Falstaff, the hero of *2 Henry IV* (1597–8), is a syphilitic libertine, and a second supposedly self-portrait in Jaques of Arden of *As You Like It* (1599–1600) answers to the same description.

The 'sickness, disease and medicine' imagery clustering around the two dramatic figures culminates in *Hamlet* (1600–1), where the hero's absorption by his ghostly vision is so complete that one may speak of an identity between the two Hamlets, father and son. The dramatic and symbolic centre of the play is King Hamlet's poisoning, which expresses a strong syphilitic symbolism, at the same time that it propels the imagery of 'sickness, disease and medicine' to skyscraper heights. Significantly, the qualitative change of this imagery is in the direction of 'horror and disgust at foul disease' (Spurgeon). Another unconscious aspect of Shakespeare's work – its running or symbolic imagery – supports this change in that the running imagery of *Hamlet* expresses Hamlet's symbolic vision of 'the foul body of the infected world', first envisaged by Jaques of Arden, Hamlet's forerunner.

The poisonous *drame à trois* in *Hamlet* is interpreted as reflecting a parallel drama in the poet's life which we have connected with the sexual 'crime' of the *Sonnets.* This is interpreted as rendering the poet's venereal infection by an unfaithful female love object who had herself been infected by the fair youth, who is the third party in the triangular drama. This 'fair youth' we have identified as William Herbert, whose known illnesses in 1598–1600 were probably of a syphilitic nature.

The traumatic aspect of love in the sonnets addressed to the fair youth is projected in the triangular dramas of *Hamlet* and *Troilus and Cressida,* whose running symbolic imagery describes the fateful connection between 'sickness, disease and medicine' and lust, jealousy and amorous betrayal. This complex of ideas explains why Shakespeare's two plays have come to express 'a disillusionment, revulsion and perturbation of nature, such as we feel nowhere else with the same intensity' (Spurgeon). Our interpretation of the dramatic core of the two plays further explains the disgust at sexuality and the misogyny of Shakespeare's Tragic Period.

A final unconscious phenomenon of Shakespeare's work is the 'goose cluster', which was first discovered by Edward Armstrong in 1946. The chain of associations of this image cluster has proved to be of a strongly idiosyncratic nature and is interpreted as having derived from a strong psychological complex in Shakespeare, expressive of the moral qualms and medical fears of a married man governed by 'All frailties that besiege all kinds of blood' (109) and recklessly obeying the motions of his 'sportive blood' (121).

# 12

# THE DANGEROUS INFIRMITY OF BURNING

In approaching the conclusion of this study, we shall mention one of the greatest difficulties for the assessment of the prevalence and severity of syphilis during the 16th and 17th centuries – in addition to the doctors' lack of diagnostic tools (above all the Wassermann test) and the public's suppression of the 'shamefull disease called the French Pockes' (see pp. 24–32).

This final difficulty is connected with the so-called 'unitarian' concept of syphilis and gonorrhea. The indiscriminate use of the words 'clap' and 'pox' in the 16th and 17th centuries reflects the confusion between gonorrhea and syphilis which was a prevalent feature of the time. Which physician started the heresy is a moot point, but by 1530 two leading venereologists, Jean de Béthencourt and Paracelsus, appear to have accepted the unitarian concept. In his treatise on the French disease, *Von der Frantzösischen Kranckheit Drei Bücher* (Nuremberg, 1530), Paracelsus presents syphilis and gonorrhea as part and parcel of the same disease. He prescribes a mercurial treatment for the syphilitic 'French blisters' (*französischen geschwer*), the origin of which he sees in the urethra when afflicted by 'French discharge and matter' (*französischen flüssen und materien*) (Paracelsus, 1922–33, vol.7, pp.123–4).

Paracelsus was later supported by Ambroise Paré (1510–90), another medical genius of the 16th century, and the two authorities were largely responsible for spreading the heresy, which in the 17th century was represented by the celebrated English physician Thomas Sydenham (1624–89), and in the 18th century by the great French physician and syphilographer Jean Astruc (1684–1766).

In Shakespeare's England the confusion between syphilis and gonorrhea appears in Marston's *The Dutch Courtesan* (1605), where young Freevill asserts that 'a strumpet is a serpigo, venom'd gonorrhy to man' (2,1:130–1), serpigo being a general term for creeping or spreading skin diseases and thus referring to syphilis and not to gonorrhea. Similarly, John Hester in *The Pearle of Practise* (1594) devotes a whole chapter to the description 'Of the Gonorrhæa, or running of the raynes, and the cure'. 'This disease', he asserts,

'is a corruption, caused of the superfluous vse of women, that are infected therewith: for such men as haue knowledge of them, they receiue the said corruption which afterward commeth forth of the yard, with great payne and difficultie in making water; and moreouer in the night, when that part is erected, it causeth great torment: which for fifteen or twentie dayes, causeth extreme payne. This is the beginning of the French pocks, a fit sawce for that sweet sinne of *Lecherie*. It bringeth most commonly payne in the interiour partes, or payne in the raynes, armes, and legges: in somuch that in fine, it commeth to that fowle disease. For such as haue this *Gonorrhœa*, neuer suspecting or fearing the afterclaps, suffer their disease, to grow on further and further till their cure will very hardly or neuer be accomplished. Therefore I wish euery man, to seeke helpe in time, least by letting it passe; in the end, it turne to his destruction.' (p.59)

Though John Hester can be seen as a Paracelsian iatrochemist operating on the fringes of medical science, the surgeons of the establishment held no more progressive views on the unitarian concept of the clap and the pox. In *An Easie, Certain and Perfect Method to Cure and Prevent the Spanish Sicknes* (1596), the Scottish surgeon Peter Lowe takes great pains to describe the gonorrheal symptoms that usually precede a syphilitic infection. 'Of those which goe before', he says,

'which we call precedents or forriders, is vlcers and cankors of diuers fashions in the yeard, burning of vrine, Chaudepisses, Carnosities, Pulluines, and such like. Yet sometimes any of these may happen without the sicknes [syphilis]. Those that followe, bee pustules and vlcers throughout all the bodie, cheefely in the secret parts, and also in the forehead, and diuers other parts of the head, in the emunctories, in the mouth, throat, and fundament, falling of hayre, dolors, and nodosities of the ioynts.' (sig.E1ᵛ)

Like Hester, Peter Lowe is aware of the dangerous 'afterclaps' of untreated gonorrhea and the 'destruction' that may follow in its wake. 'Accidents doe also happen sometimes by carnosities in the yeard', he writes, 'hindering the vrine to passe, so that oft commeth death, if suddaine order be not taken' (sig.E4ʳ). Urethral stricture and severe prostatitis caused insufferable pains and were not an uncommon way of meeting death. 'The strangury hath vndone me', is one of the translation examples provided in William Horman's *Vulgaria*, the best-known Latin-English dictionary used in Tudor grammar schools (Horman, 1926, p.59). Not surprisingly, the treatment of gleets and strictures was a lucrative business, and the surgeons of the time made large fortunes from the passing of catheters.

Technical advances also took place in surgical methods of relieving urinary obstruction. An advanced method of catherization was presented in 1588 by John Read, who advised his colleagues to use 'a fine tender Mallow stalke, or a smallage or Parseley stalke' (fol.74ʳ), instead of the more dangerous and painful metal syringe used by John Arderne. 'By these few notes and instructions', he piously concludes his chapter on gonorrhea,

'any skilfull Chirurgian may be able to iudge and discerne a carbuncle: and be also sufficiently instructed, by the might and power of GOD to cure the same. Who as he is wont to punish mankinde with innumerable diseases, to the ende to abate his pride, and to make him to know himselfe, so is he also accustomed to helpe and succor those, who flie vnto him for comfort, and doe trust in his mercy.' (fol.79ᵛ-80ʳ)

THE VENEREAL COCKTAIL: GONORRHEA, SYPHILIS AND LEPROSY

It is easy today to see how in an age of great promiscuity a person contracting both gonorrhea and syphilis during one intercourse would consider them to be one disease. The victim's only knowledge that he was ill would be the burning of gonorrhea after a few days and a syphilitic chancre after a few weeks. Physicians themselves thought that gonorrhea was caused by an ulcer inside the urethra which led to a discharge of pus, while syphilis produced an ulcer which appeared on the epidermis as a chancre. The confusion between gonorrhea and syphilis explains the tendency of the writers of the time to regard 'clap' as the early stage and syphilis as the later stage of 'the pox'. This view is incorporated in Alexander Pope's *The Satires of Dr. John Donne*, in which he speaks of 'Time that at last matures a clap to pox' (Pope, 1871–89, vol.3, p.429: Satire II, line 47). Humoral pathology also supported the unitarian concept by providing a ready explanation for gonorrhea as a kind of running off of the impurities of syphilis.

The unitarian concept was finally tested and 'proved' by John Hunter (1728–93), the famous 18th-century surgeon, who after a self-inoculation experiment thought that he had demonstrated the unity of the two diseases, commonly referred to as 'the venereal'. In the year 1767, Hunter made two punctures with a lancet, one on his foreskin, one on his glans. Into these punctures he rubbed 'the matter of a gonorrhoea'. Unhappily the case was one of mixed infection, and Hunter developed a chancre and the syphilis from which it is possible he died.

On top of this confusion between the two great venereal diseases of the time came the identification of gonorrhea and syphilis with *leprosy*. Part of the confusion was due to the fact that the papular lesions of syphilis often simulate the nodular lesions of leprosy. 'The fyrst kyndes of the french pockes', asserted Andrew Boord, 'be skabbes & pimples lyke to leprosyte' (1547, fol.1xxxvii[r]). In addition, syphilis and leprosy were both highly contagious, were transmitted sexually, had hereditary features, and responded to mercurial treatment – all of which fit the medieval concept of leprosy.

Diagnosis of the new venereal disease thus presented a difficult task to Renaissance physicians, and right down to modern times gonorrhea, leprosy and syphilis were confused by medical observers, who allowed such wholly different diseases to go undifferentiated. In the middle of the 19th century, a German doctor even maintained the origin of syphilis from leprosy (Simon, 1857–8, *passim*). In the 16th century, the first doctor to advance this view was Johannes Manardus of Ferrara (1462–1536), who in his treatise *De morbo Gallico* (Ferrara, 1525) stated that the new venereal disease was the successor of leprosy, had been evoked out of it, and had even been caught from the leprous by contagion. According to the Italian doctor, the disease had made its first appearance in Europe at Valencia, Spain, out of a case of leprosy (Creighton, 1891, pp.429–30).

In John Hester's translation of Phillipp Hermann's book *An Excellent Treatise Teaching How to Cure the French Pockes* (1590), it is stated that 'the Leprosie and this disease [syphilis] are so neere of kinne, that they are Cozen-germanes to each other' (Hermann, 1590, p.1). In his *Epistle Dedicatorie* 'To the worshipfull the Maister Wardens, and generall Assistants of the fraternitie of Chirurgions in London', Hester further speaks of the recent knowledge obtained of 'this filthy disease', but says parenthetically that 'I know some auer it to be *Lepram Arabum*...and therefore as this latter age of ours sustaineth the scourge thereof, a iust whyp of our lycentiousnes, so let it, (if there be any to be had) carry the credite of the cure [by quicksilver and guaiac], as some rewarde to some mens industries' (Hermann, 1590, *Epistle Dedicatorie*).

A final example of the confusion between leprosy and the two great venereal diseases of the Renaissance is Simon Fish's diatribe of 1529 against the Romish priests, where the three diseases are presented by the author as merely points on a continuum of one disease. He describes the priests as libertines

> 'that catche the pokkes of one woman, and bere theym to an other; that be brent wyth one woman, and bere it to an other; that catche the lepry of one woman, and bere it to an other; ye, some one of theym shall bost emong his felawes, that he hath medled with an hundredth wymen.' (see p.63)

## 'BURNING' BY SYPHILIS AND GONORRHEA

The most famous example of the confusion between syphilis and gonorrhea is the 'burning' metaphor that was used by the writers of the time, both lay and medical. One of the earliest examples of this 'fiery' blurring of the boundary between syphilis and gonorrhea is found in Andrew Boord's *Breviary of Helthe* from 1547, in which the author devotes his 376th chapter to 'a womans secret member the which is the gate or the dore of the matryx or bely, and there may brede many diseases as vlcers, skabbes, apostumes, fyssures, fystles, festures, the pockes, and burnynge of an harlot' (fol.cxxxviiii$^v$). 'Yf a man be burnt with an harlot', Boord further explains,

> 'and do medle with an other woman within a day, he shal burne the woman that he doth medle with al. Yf one be burnt let them washe theyr secret [parts] ii or iii tymes with whyte wyne, or els with secke and water. And yf the matter haue contynewed longe, go to some expert Chierurgion to haue helpe or els the gutt wyll burne and fall out of the bely.' (fol.xv$^v$)

The best early example of the confusion between syphilis and gonorrhea as it was expressed through the use of the 'burning' metaphor is the work of John Bale, the Protestant controversialist, bishop and dramatist. In rendering the relevant passages, we shall at the same time present the reader with an interesting glimpse of one of the leading figures of the Marian Restoration.

In *The Vocacyon of Johan Bale to the Bishoprick of Ossorie in Irelande* (1553), Bale gives an account of his persecution in Catholic Ireland by both the clergy and the general public alike. 'May I not be glad, that I am in sorowes for the Gospell', he consoles himself,

> 'and not pranked up in pompe and pleasures, lyke the wanton babes of this worlde? As at this daye is lecherouse Weston, which is more practised in the arte of breche burninge, than all the whores of the stues to the great infamye of his virginall ordre.' (Bale, 1810, p.439)

Dr. Hugh Weston (1505?–58) was one of the most prominent clergymen in England under the reign of Queen Mary, and in 1553 he was installed as Dean of Westminster as part of the monarch's Catholic Restoration. During this same period, anti-Catholic John Bale attacked the celibacy of the clergy as one of the pillars of whoredom. 'God sayth, it is not good for man to be alone, without an helpe, which is a wife in mariage', Bale asserted, with reference to the Popish priests then in power, adding that

Figure 51. One of the first pictorial records testifying to the confusion between syphilis and leprosy is a German flyleaf published c. 1497 in Vienna and containing a prayer for averting the new venereal plague. 'This prayer is good and protects against the blisters of the so-called French disease', it says. 'It was found in a delapidated monastery in France called Maliers in a stone column engraved with the year 104 [A.D.]; here this plague is called Job's blisters. Whoever carries this prayer on him or reads it aloud will be safe against the blisters' (Sudhoff, 1912, Tafel XXI).

Just as victims of AIDS in 1991 got their patron saint with San Luigi of Gonzaga, the Catholic Church provided the victims of syphilis with a patron saint in St. Job, together with Lazarus a famous leper of the Bible. This happened to

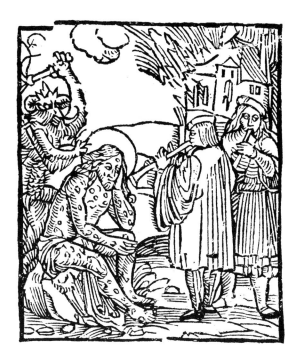

the annoyance of the Protestant reformers in England, who attacked the syphilitics' worship of St. Job as yet another example of the idolatry of the Old Church. 'If God punish the world with an evil pock', grumbled William Tyndale (c. 1490–1536), 'they immediately paint a block and call it Job, to heal the disease, instead of warning the people to mend their living' (Tyndale, 1850, p.105). 'The papists also bring in many gods, but covertly and privily', seconded his fellow partisan Roger Hutchinson (d. 1555). 'They teach the people to pray unto saints: to St. Luke for the ox, to Job for the pox, to Rocke for the pestilence' (Hutchinson, 1842, p.171. Cf also Bale, 1849, p.498 and Becon, 1884a, p.536).

In the 16th century when leprosy was disappearing or had already disappeared from Europe due to the rigorous quarantine measures of the late Middle Ages (see p.72), most allusions to leprosy were, in fact, synonymous with references to syphilis. This may be demonstrated by a wealth of examples from Elizabethan and Jacobean literature. Robert Greene describes the pox as 'loathsome leprosie' (see p.109) and as 'the infection of leprosie' (Greene, 1881–6, vol.8, p.290). Ben Jonson talks of the 'loath'd and leprous face' of the syphilized figure of Vice (*Cynthias Reuelle* 1,5:53), while Philip Massinger and Thomas Nabbes describe the disease as 'loathsome leprosie' (*The Guardian* 3,6:45) and 'foule leprosie' (*Tottenham Court* 5,6), respectively. In John Donne's elegy *The Perfume*, he writes that 'the seely [innocent] Amorous sucks his death By drawing in a leprous harlots breath,' an obvious allusion to syphilis (Donne, 1965, p.8). In *The Metamorphosis of Ajax*, Sir John Harington mentions 'Naaman the Syrian, that would disdaine to wash in Jordan, though it would cure him of the Leprosie, or the pox' (Harington, 1962, p.221).

Several of Shakespeare's associations to leprosy move within the same sphere: Doll Tearsheet is called a '*lazar* kite of Cressid's kind' (see p.233), just as three references to leprosy in *Timon of Athens* appear in a context of prostitution and foul disease (4,1:23–30; 4,3:34–45;362–7). The '*lazar-like*' skin symptoms of the poisoned King in *Hamlet*, which are produced by 'The *leperous* distilment' coursing through his blood, are therefore strong indications of syphilitic poisoning.

'They saye contrariously that it is more than good; for it is holy religiouse, and prest-like, to have no wives of their owne, whatsoever they have of other mennis, besides buggery boyes. I trowe Doctour Weston will saye none other at this daye; what though not longe ago he brent a beggar in S. Botolphe's parishe without Bishopsgate, gevinge her no wurse than he had received afore of that religiouse occupienge.' (p.462)

The probability that Weston's 'arte of brech burninge' or 'brenning' – elsewhere termed his 'botches & breche burninges' (see p.159) – is meant as a reference to syphilis is made certain by Bale's sarcastic report of the dean's role at the funeral of Edward VI in 1553. The painful scene described by Bale affords him an opportunity to highlight the hyprocrisy of the clergymen advanced to power by Bloody Mary after the boy-king's funeral.

'At the funerall masse of king Edward the VI (which he neuer by his life desyred but abhorred)', Bale begins his account,

'one Walker a syngyng man and chaplayne of the court, was deacon, which mindyng after the gospel, as the maner is in the popishe ceremony, to haue insensed the Quene, was forbidden to do it by doctoure Weston, because he hadde marryed a wife. Shamest thou not (sayth the sayde Weston) to do thys offyce, the hauing a wyfe, as thou hast? I tell thee, the Quene wyl not be insensed of suche a one as thou arte. And so wyth vyolence, he toke the sensers out of hys handes, and wyth that swete smoke perfumed the Quene, he beyng the same tyme sore bytten wyth a Wynchester gose, and not yet al healed therof. If Mary Hugsal of Oxford, hys olde famylyer, or hys prouyder good wife person eyther els Christyane Tompson the wydow whom he sealed wyth hys hot yron in the nether partes had bene there present to haue holden the shyppe, or geuen him the frankensence, the pageaunt hadde bene in the very ryght course. Loo, sir, these are the minysters of holy churches suffrages nowe a dayes.' (Bale, 1561, fol.68$^r$-69$^v$)

As demonstrated in an earlier chapter, a 'Winchester goose' was an Elizabethan slang expression for either a syphilitic prostitute, a person infected with the pox, or a syphilitic sore (see pp.214–9). According to John Bale, the 'Wynchester gose' which had 'bytten' Hugh Weston was also responsible for 'brenning' a woman in London, to whom the promiscuous clergyman had passed on his venereal infection.

William Bullein's *Bulwarke of Defence* (1562) provides a final 16th-century example of the ambiguous use of the word 'burning' or 'brenning'. In the treatise, the allegorical figure of Sickness demands of Health what he should do with 'a shamefull disease, called the Frenche Pockes', and Health answers him: 'I [would] not, that any should fishe for this disease, or be to[o] bolde when he is bitten, to thinke hereby to be helped: but rather eschue the cause of this infirmitie, and filthy, rotten, burning of harlottes' (Bullein, 1562, *The Booke of Compoundes*, fol.xlvii$^r$).

Later sources reflect the same confusion between the two great venereal diseases of the time. In Massinger's *The Emperour of the East* (1632), an Emperick and a Chirurgion attempt to cure the gout of a nobleman named Paulinus. 'An excellent receipt', says the surgeon sarcastically to the empiric after the latter has presented the patient with a wonder 'balsamum' (4,3:80) containing a number of ingredients, among them sassafras and guaiac.

| CHIRURGION | But does your Lordship<br>Know what it is good for? |
|---|---|
| PAULINUS | I would be instructed. |
| CHIRURGION | For the gonorrhea, or if you will hear it<br>In a plainer phrase, the pox. |
| EMPIRICK | If it cure his Lordship<br>Of that by the way, I hope Sir 'tis the better;<br>My medicine serues for all things, and the pox, Sir,<br>Though falsely nam'd the Sciatica, or goute,<br>Is the more Catholic sicknesse. |
| PAULINUS | Hence with the rascal! (4,3:83–90) |

One reason for the surgeon's sarcastic comment on the empiric's wonder medicine may be that guaiac by the last quarter of the 16th century appears to have lost much of its popularity. Although Clowes mentions it, he strictly favours mercury inunctions. And in 1596, Peter Lowe concludes:

> 'Among the foure wayes to heale this disease, I esteeme this [guaiacum wood] to be the most weake & most uncertaine, the which opinion is confirmed by all those that have written and practiced in this matter.' (Lowe, 1596, sig.C3ʳ)

## THE 'BURNING' CLAP OR POX

While the unitarian concept of gonorrhea and syphilis makes it difficult to distinguish which is which, it is clear from the context of Elizabethan and Jacobean sources that 'burning' in a great number of cases refers to syphilis. 'The country Gull, with *Punks* was so bepay'd, That he must needs seeke out for Surgeons ayde', Samuel Rowlands notes of a syphilitic named Humphrey in *A Paire of Spy-Knaues* (1619):

> A burning griefe did ouertake at last,
> And he must sweat to thinke on what was past,
> Take vp his Chamber and a while lye in.
> Oh Pockey griefe to thinke where he had bin!
> (Rowlands, 1880, vol.2, p.10)

On discovering his foul infection, Humphrey goes to see the woman who had shared his night's encounter and meets her with the words: 'Thou damned Whore hast giuen the Pox to me'. 'I giue the Pox?' laughs the girl,

> 'Tis false, I ne're gaue any:
> I sold the Pox, thou bought'st it with thy penny:
> We made a bargaine, I had thy French gold,
> And thou my French disease, full bought and sold. (p.10)

The prostitute's clever reply presents a slight variation on Doll Tearsheet's reply to Falstaff that he merely 'caught' the valuables that she had been given – 'our chains and our jewels…[our] brooches, pearles, and ouches' (*2 Henry IV*, 2,4:47–8). By these items Falstaff's prostitute girl clearly means the 'brooches of the French disease', as John Banister calls the cutaneous jewelry of the syphilitic skin lesions (Banister, 1633, p.135). In the same scene, Falstaffs tells his syphilitic girlfriend that 'you help to make the diseases, Doll; we catch of you, Doll' (2,4:44–5), later observing that 'she's in hell already, and burns poor souls' (2,4:335–6) – the fat knight himself being among her scorched victims (pp.198–200).

Another 'burnt' couple shows up in Rowlands's satirical poem *A Whole Crew of Kind Gossips, All Met to Be Merry* (1609), in which a frustrated wife complains of her 'lewd' husband that

> Ther's not a Whore in *London* nor about,
> But he hath all the haunts to find her out.
> He knowes the Pandars that can fit his turne,
> And Bauds that helpe good fellowes to the burne:
> Taffity Queanes, and fine light silken Whores,
> That haue the gift of pox in their owne pores.
>
> (Rowlands, 1880, vol.2, p.18)

In Fletcher's *Women Pleased* (c.1620), the 'burning' of venereal disease breaks into full flame when three gallants are asked by Penurio if 'not you three [are] going to be sinful?'

PENURIO  I have found your faces,
And see whore written in your eyes…
Have a care Gentlemen,
'Tis a sore age, very sore age, lewd age,
And women now are like old Knights adventures,
Full of inchanted flames, and dangerous.

2. GENT.  Where the most danger is, there's the most honor.

PENURIO  I grant ye, honor most consists in sufferance,
And by that rule you three should be most honorable.

3. GENT.  A subtle Rogue: but canst thou tell Penurio
Where we may light upon –

PENURIO  A learned Surgeon?

3. GENT.  Pox take ye fool; I mean good
wholsome wenches. (3,2:269)

## LUCIFER – THE 'BURNING' DEVIL

The fire of venereal disease blazes brightly in Middleton's *No Wit, no Help Like a Woman's* (1657), in which Sir George Lambstone in the play's allegorical Apotheosis appears 'in the character of Fire' (4,2:68). 'The wicked fire of lust Does now spread heat through water, air, and dust', he begins his Lear-like monologue,

> I that was wont in elder times to pass
> For a bright angel – so they call'd me then –
> Now so corrupted with the upstart fires
> Of avarice, luxury, and inconstant heats,
> Struck from the bloods of cunning clap-faln daughters,
> Night-walking wives, but, most, libidinous widows,
> That I, that purify even gold itself,

Have the contemptible dross thrown in my face,
And my bright name walk common in disgrace.
How am I us'd a' late, that I'm so handled, –
Thrust into alleys, hospitals, and tubs!...
These are the fires a' late my brightness darks,
And fills the world so full of beggarly sparks. (4,2:66–78;94–5)

'By my faith, monsieur Fire, you're a hot whoreson!' (4,2:97), Lady Goldenfleece comments succinctly.

A still more impressive incarnation of 'Fire' appears in the same author's *The Blacke Booke* (1604), in which Lucifer himself ascends from hell to speak a 'Prologue to his own Play', staged on the rails of the Earth. Here Lucifer tells the audience that he will join the members of the theatrical world and 'burn' the sexual parts of all those men and women who are

Pawn'd to luxurious and adulterous merit.
Yea, that's the sin, and now it takes her turn,
For which the world shall like a strumpet burn;
And for an instance to fire false embraces,
I make the world burn now in secret places:
I haunt invisible corners as a spy,
And in adulterous circles there rise I;
There am I conjur'd up through hot desire,
And where hell rises, there must needs be fire.
(Middleton, 1885–6, vol.8, pp.7–8)

Lucifer also turns up in one of Shakespeare's earliest plays in the context of promiscuity and prostitution, 'burning' and venereal disease. In *The Comedy of Errors* (1592–3), Antipholus of Syracuse and his servant Dromio come across a prostitute in the dark and dangerous streets of Ephesus. The alluring woman is met by the two men as a devilish temptation to be avoided at all costs, Dromio jestingly identifying 'light' wenches with Lucifer himself:

SYR. ANT.   Satan avoid, I charge thee tempt me not.

SYR. DRO.   Master, is this mistress Satan?

SYR. ANT.   It is the devil.

SYR. DRO.   Nay, she is worse, she is the devil's dam: and here she comes in the habit of a light wench, and thereof comes that the wenches say 'god damn me,' that's as much as to say, 'God make me a light wench.' It is written, they appear to men like angels of light; light is an effect of fire, and fire will burn; ergo, light wenches will burn; come not near her. (4,3:46–55)

Falstaff might have listened to this advice to his own good advantage.[*]

---

[*] Among Elizabethan and Jacobean authors, 'hell' was a popular comparison to the burning effects of gonorrhea and *ulcus molle* and the tormenting pains of syphilis. Sometimes these sufferings were also understood to prefigure the fate of the sexually sinful in hell. 'The world is become a Brothell house of sinne', Barnabe Rich fumed in *The Honestie of This Age* (1614). 'I tell thee, thou Adulterer, I speake it to thy face, that besides the poxe, and many other loathsome diseases that are incident to whore-maisters whilst they liue in this world, thy hot burning fire of lust will bring thee to the hot burning fire of hell' (Rich, 1614, pp.17, 53). In Dekker's

THE BURNING DEVIL TAKEN TO COURT

The burning devil of venereal disease appears not only in the dramatic and poetic works of the time but also in its court records. Like a number of present-day Americans, many men and women of Shakespeare's England discovered that the true fury of hell is not a lover scorned but a lover who contracts venereal disease from his or her sexual partner. There is evidence than many Elizabethans reacted to the growing venereal plague in the same way that modern Americans react to the epidemic of AIDS. The surge of litigation in regard to both diseases is largely based on the claim that one partner did not inform the other about his or her infection, and that the sexually transmitted disease subjected the infected partner to a painful and sometimes debilitating condition.

In two pioneering studies of the 1970s, F.G. Emmison and G.R. Quaife presented a wealth of entirely new material on the permissiveness of Elizabethan and Jacobean society. Emmison's *Elizabethan Life: Morals and the Church Courts* (1973) examines some 100,000 entries in the Elizabethan court books of the two Essex Archdeaconries. The Archdeacons' Courts (popularly known as the 'Bawdy Courts') dealt with offences such as absence from church, usury and a variety of other aberrations. Moral offences fill half of Dr. Emmison's book, and well over 10,000 members of the two adult generations of the Elizabethan period were charged with pre-marital intercourse, 'incontinence' in various forms, bastardy, or graver offences. 'Bridal pregnancy' was largely condoned because betrothal was regarded as quasi-marriage – like Shakespeare's. The court books throw fresh light on the growing scourge of venereal disease because a number of entries refer to prostitution, to men charged with 'burning' women, or vice versa, men and women presented because they were venereally infected, cases in which both parties were charged, unusual cases, and, finally, cases referring to 'surgeons'.

In the 1560s, for example, one man was prosecuted for the 'harbouring of harlots for a privy gain', and a wife was accused of being 'a keeper of common harlots and hath one now in her house which [who] is burned' (Emmison, 1973, p.21). In the same decade a woman sued another for 'calling her whore which burnt men' (1564). Two years later, the unnamed wife of the vicar of North Shoebury [Robert Hawks] was presented 'because she did burn William Steven of North Shoebury half a year past' (p.33). A certain Joan Gallowaie of Havering, 'in the extremity of sickness [childbirth]', named no less than five men, 'but she did falsely accuse them all' except for one who 'did burn her very pitifully' (1578) (p.34). A dire tragedy occurred when a 'Feering' wife was accused of 'committing fornication with Enoch Greve, who drowned himself, being so burned that he could not abide the pains' (1590) (p.35).

---

*Newes from Hell* (1606), the Devil is happy to describe his kingdom in terms that would be easily recognizable to an inhabitant of London. 'The *Vniuersall Region*', Lucifers asserts, 'is built altogether vpon Stoues and *Hotte-houses*, you cannot set foote into it, but you haue a *Fieri facias* seru'de vpon you: for like the Glass-house *Furnace* in Blacke-friers, the bonefiers that are kept there, neuer goe out; insomuch that all the Inhabitants are almost broylde like *Carbonadoes* with the sweating sicknes, but the best is (or rather the worst) none of them die on't. And such daungerous hot shottes are all the women there, that whosoeuer meddles with any of them is sure to be burnt' (Dekker, 1884–6, vol.2, pp.97–8). The association between prostitution and the kingdom of hell went back beyond Elizabethan times to the medieval morality drama, and even to the sermon.

Figure 52. An interesting variation upon the theme of this chapter is presented by the engraving from George Wither's *A Collection of Emblems, Ancient and Modern* (1635, Book 1, illustration XXVII, p.27). The picture shows two gentlemen duelling in front of a whore, while the accompanying verse launches a fierce attack on prostitution and promiscuity. The poet warns whoremongers that pursuit of loose women such as 'Hellen' of Troy will make them share the fate of 'burning' Troy, destroyed on the altar of lust and promiscuity, jealousy and rage. The engraving gives a rare picture of an English brothel.

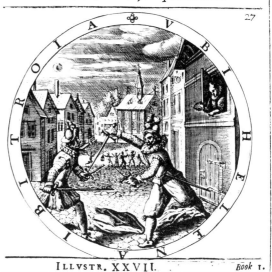

*Where* Hellen *is, there, will be* Warre;
*For,* Death *and* Lust, *Companions are.*

27

TROIA·VBI·HELENA·IBI

ILLVSTR. XXVII.    *Book* 1.

Heir foolish Guise, I never could affect,
 Who dare, for any cause, the *Stewes* frequent:
 And, thither, where I justly might suspect
A *Strumpet* liv'd, as yet, I never went.
For, when (as *Fooles* pretend) they goe to seeke
Experience, where more *Ill* then *Good*, they see;
They venture for their *Knowledge, Adam-*like;
And, such as his, will their *Atchievements* bee.
 Let, therefore, those that would loose *Trulls* detest,
Converse with none, but those that modest are;
For, they that can of *Whoredome* make a Iest,
Will entertaine it, ere they be aware.
*Chast Company,* and *Chast-Discourse,* doth make
The Minde more pleased with it, ev'ry day;
And, *Frequent viewes of Wantonnesse,* will take
The Sense and Hatred, of the *Vice* away.
 Some, I have knowne, by *Harlots* Wiles undone,
Who, but *to see their Fashions,* first pretended;
And, they that went *for Company,* alone,
By suddaine Quarrells, there, their Dayes have ended.
For, in the Lodgings of a *Lustfull-Woman,*
Immodest *Impudence* hath still her Being;
There, *Furie, Fraud,* and *Cruelties* are common:
And, there, is *Want,* and *Shame,* and *Disagreeing.*
Ev'n *Beauty,* of it selfe, stirres loose Desires,
Occasioning both *Iealousies,* and *Feares*;
It kindleth in the Brest, concealed *Fires,*
Which burne the Heart, before the *Flame* appeares:
 And, ev'ry day, experienced are wee;
 That, there, where *Hellen* is, *Troyes* Fate will bee.
                    E 2                          *No*

A certain John Grieve of Coggeshall was presented in 1588 because 'he is a surgeon and useth to heal those that be burned with committing fornication'. Another case was brought against a widow named Agnes Newman for 'keeping a harlot in her house, and being a common surgeon to common strumpets and such as be burnt, and keeping their counsel' (1580) (p.36).

One reference to the 'pox' notes its transmission through three individuals. This was the case against the wife of Andrew Knightbridge of Rayleigh, 'suspected of adultery with one Edward Leggatt of Hockley, who hath given her the pocks, and so she had given them to her husband' (1596) (p.35).

G.R. Quaife's examination of similar material in *Wanton Wenches and Wayward Wives* (1979) reveals the same picture. Quaife's source is the depositions presented between 1601 and 1660 to the ecclesiastical 'bawdy court' in Somerset, The Consistory Court of Bath and Wells. Quaife quotes a man who was presented because 'his pudenda were burned by means he had lived incontinently with some one woman or another'. Another man complained of a neighbour's wife that he 'had the carnal knowledge of her body and was burned by her'. In a similar situation in Axbridge, the infected man went to the husband and told him 'that he was a cuckold and that she was a whore and that he had the carnal knowledge of her body in Wrides Ditch...and that she burned him...or else he would have done the same again' (Quaife, 1979, p.186).

Numerous men in Quaife's material report that the woman had burnt them after intercourse. 'The pox frightened many men', Quaife concludes and instances a Sutton Mallet husbandman who, on contracting the disease and experiencing the symptoms of the primary stage, thought he was dying. He went to the local curate and confessed that 'he had received hurt by knowledge of a woman in his privy parts and said if he might have help it should be a warning for him as long as he lived' (p.186).

Community reaction seems to have been a desire to isolate the carrier and effect a medical cure. When one village discovered that a husband, after frequenting a travelling tinker woman, had given the disease to his wife, they forced him to flee. This action saved the village from further contamination, but it did little for the infected woman, who was 'left with a loathsome disease' (p.186). Quaife also mentions a man who showed some consideration for the health of his friends and neighbours after having been dangerously ill for three weeks. On discovering that 'it was the French pox', he asked them 'not to accompany or drink with him' (pp.186–7).

Quaife's sources suggest that medical treatment was readily available in the larger towns of the county, where quacks and surgeons had a regular business. A Wiltshire man built up a reputation throughout Eastern Somerset to the extent that a trip to Shaftesbury by a village male set the tongues a-wagging. Many men confessed, as did a Taunton husbandman, that 'he had an occasion to use a chirurgeon saying that his shaft or privities were much swelled' due to carnal intercourse. Another man who could not resist the allurements of a diseased married slut admitted to 'his lewd life with her, whereof he lay sick nine or ten weeks and was grievously tormented thereof, until he was much eased by the physician that discovered his disease unto him' (p.187).

Figure 53. A second emblem from George Wither's *A Collection of Emblems, Ancient and Modern* (1635, Book 4, illustration XIX, p.227) shows Cupid with his poisoned arrows and three loving couples beneath him, which by their 'willfull ignorance' of the dangers of promiscuity run the risk of 'dy[ing]…in an hospital'.

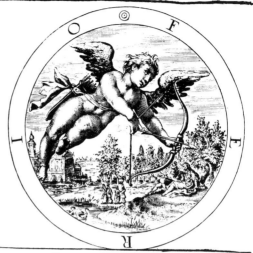

Be wary, whofoe're thou be,
For, from Loves arrow as none are free.

ILLVSTR. XIX.          *Book.4.*

Ood Folkes, take heede; for, here's a wanton *Wagge*,
Who, having *Bowes* and *Arrowes*, makes his bragg
That, he hath fome unhappy trick to play;
And, vowes to fhoot at all he meets to day.
Pray be not careleffe; for, the *Boy* is blinde,
And, fometimes ftrikes, where moft he feemeth kinde.
This rambling *Archer* fpares not one, nor other:
Yea, otherwhile, the *Monkey* fhoots his Mother.
    Though you be little *Children*, come not neere;
For, I remember (though't be many a yeare
Now gone and paft,) that, when I was a *Lad*,
My Heart, a pricke, by this young Wanton had,
That, pain'd me feven yeares after: nor had I
The grace (thus warn'd) to fcape his waggery;
But many times, ev'n fince I was a man,
He fhot me, oftner then I tell you can:
And, if I had not bene the ftronger-hearted,
I, for my over-daring, might have fmarted.
    You laugh now, as if this were nothing fo;
But, if you meet this *Blinkard* with his Bow,
You may, unleffe you take the better care,
Receive a *wound*, before you be aware.
I feare him not; for, I have learned how
To keepe my heart-ftrings from his Arrowes now:
And, fo might you, and fo might ev'ry one
That vaine *Occafions*, truely feekes to fhunn.
But, if you fleight my Counfells, you may chance
To blame at laft, your willfull ignorance:
    For, fome, who thought, at firft, his wounds but fmall
    Have dyed by them, in an *Hofpitall*.
                    H b 2                    *On*

While Quaife concludes that 'the reference of the court records was primarily to syphilis and in a few cases to gonorrhoea' (p.186), Emmison concludes that 'the prosecutions recorded in the Essex court books relate almost wholly to gonorrhoea except perhaps the single case of "pocks"' (Emmison, 1973, p.32). These contradictory conclusions reflect the difficulties researchers have had with the term 'burning', and with the ambiguity inherent in regarding syphilis and gonorrhea to be the same disease.

The use of the term 'burning' presented above from the literature of the 16th and 17th centuries and the additional material collected by Gordon Williams in his article *An Elizabethan Disease* (Williams, 1971, pp.48–50) show that the majority of the uses of the term appear in a definitely syphilitic context. Still, the diagnostic twilight of the two great venereal diseases and the looseness of their common epithet make it difficult to discern the source of the many 'burnings' described by Elizabethan and Jacobean authors. For all this, Emmison's conclusion seems reasonable enough in a certain type of case: urethral stricture and severe prostatitis could explain the terrible suffering of many of the patients described in his sources. The torments of these patients might in turn serve to modify Chauncey D. Leake's complacent statement on gonorrhea in his preface (1945) to William Clowes's 1596 treatise on the *morbus gallicus*:

> 'There was no need for Clowes to differentiate between the venereal plague [syphilis] and gonorrhea. Gonorrhea, the gleet or clap, was prevalent enough, but no one seemed to pay much attention to it. It was not considered to be much more serious than a "cold" and probably was just about as common. The really serious venereal plague in Clowes's time was syphilis. It produced severe symptoms and often caused death.' (pp.xix–xx)

## SYPHILIS AND SLANDER IN 16TH CENTURY ENGLAND

An interesting aspect of the cases tried at the ecclesiastical courts is presented in this final section because of the light these cases shed on our subject. One of the offences in English society that was strictly under the jurisdiction of the ecclesiastical courts was that of defamation and slander. The word 'defamation' was a technical term in church law and its use indicates that in Elizabethan times it was felt that to give someone an evil reputation was considered to be a serious enough crime to put a man on trial.

Saying that someone was a 'heretic and one of the new learning', for example, or calling him an adulterer would be considered slanderous, and a person tried and found guilty of defamation and slander in an ecclesiastical court would, depending on the severity of his crime, receive one of two punishments: either he would have to perform some kind of public atonement, or he would be excommunicated (Holdsworth, 1903, vol.8, p.348).

In *A History of English Law* (1903), Sir William Holdsworth has demonstrated that many cases of defamation and slander began to appear in the common law courts under Elizabeth I. This forced the courts to distinguish carefully the defamatory words which would be actionable in the common law courts from those which were actionable only in the ecclesiastical courts. If one called another person a 'thief' or 'traitor', the offence was punishable in the common law courts. If, on the other hand, one called another person 'heretic and one of the new learning', or an 'adulterer', the offence was 'merely spiritual', and no punishment was possible under common law. If the offence charged was punishable under both common and ecclesiastical law, the plaintiff could bring his action in either jurisdiction.

This presupposed that words imputing a criminal offence was actionable, while words imputing gross acts of immorality were not actionable, because such acts were only recognized by the ecclesiastical courts (p.348).

During the Renaissance, the question of syphilis became associated with that of defamation and slander. If a person accused someone of having a contagious disease such as leprosy, the plague, or syphilis, the accused person could, presuming he was healthy, bring an action of slander against his detractor. This was so because the imputation of having contracted syphilis was actionable, on the grounds that a person suffering from a contagious disease could legally be excluded from society and could suffer economic loss and social damage thereby (p.347).

There were, however, two factors mitigating the severity of the punishment meted out to slanderers under the law. In the first place, the words imputing gross acts of immorality were not actionable *per se* because they fell within the jurisdiction of the ecclesiastical courts. In the second place, the common law courts could apply the concept of *in mitiori sensu*, that is that words would be considered defamatory only if no other meaning could be read into them. Thus to say of a man that he was full of the pox was not actionable because that might mean merely smallpox, an infectious disease that did not require the removal of the afflicted person from society (pp.354–5).

Despite the complex legal and moral ramifications of these problems, it is interesting to note that, according to Holdsworth, the accusation of having contracted syphilis was much the most common in these legal reports (p.349).[*] Evidence from the annals of jurisdiction thus indicates that syphilis was a widespread disease among the English population, and that it was a feared one because of its moral, social and economic consequences.

---

[*] See also Sharpe, 1980, pp.1–36. For the central importance of slander of a syphilitic kind in Shakepeare's *Measure for Measure*, see Bentley, 1989, pp.101–34.

# 13

# CONCLUSION

1. Our starting point was Lawrence Stone's statement that 'the ubiquity of gonor-rhoea and the rarity of syphilis seems to have been an established feature of England at least by the late sixteenth century' (p.xi). On the basis of the sources examined in this study, this statement may be repudiated. In the first place, Stone's assertion is based on an erroneous conception of the two venereal diseases. In the course of the passage just quoted, he writes that 'the treatment [of gonorrhea] was almost as dangerous as the disease, since the most reliable cure was the ingestion of mercury, itself a dangerous poison, the other remedy being strict diet and sweating in a sweating-tub' (Stone, 1977, p.599).

As demonstrated in the study presented here, the 'mercury cure' was the common treatment for syphilis rather than gonorrhea. However, doctors of the age did not distinguish between the two venereal diseases since they were regarded as part and parcel of the same disease. Stone is clearly unaware of this 'unitarian' conception of syphilis and gonorrhea since he makes a distinction between them and then goes on to conclude – without quoting his sources – that gonorrhea was a common disease by the late 16th century, whereas syphilis was a rare one.

2. In all fairness, any assessment of the prevalence and severity of syphilis during the period 1495–1650 is difficult to make for at least four reasons. In the first place, doctors of the age were without our modern knowledge of syphilis and methods of diagnosis, foremost of which is the Wassermann test. In the second place, syphilis in its late stages simulates almost every disease known to man. Sir William Osler called syphilis the 'Great Imitator,' and added: 'Know syphilis and the whole of medicine is opened unto you' (Parran, 1937, p.15).

Third, the unitarian concept of syphilis and gonorrhea presents a diagnostic twilight which makes it impossible to discern the source of the many 'burnings' described by the authors of the time, both lay and medical. In the fourth place, syphilis was surrounded by an air of secrecy and shame so that any attempt at computing statistical records for the 'foul disease' is bound to fail – as John Graunt found out to his great annoyance (pp.29–30).

Even if these difficulties are taken into consideration, the sources examined in this study suggest that syphilis in Tudor and Stuart England was a 'common and ordinary…disease' according to Fuller (p.79), a 'too frequent Maladie' according to Graunt (p.30), and an infection 'as catching as the plague, though not all so general' according to Dekker (p.166). 'We seldom take physic [medicine] without it', asserts one of Middleton's characters, 'the pox is as natural now as an ague in the springtime' (p.110). And one of Greene's characters completes this statement by his assertion that 'the Poxe...is so surely now rooted in England, that by Syth it may better be called *A Morbus Anglicus* then *Gallicus*' (p.109).

The various books on syphilis published in the 16th century and the numerous references to the disease in the medical and lay writings of the time leave the impression that syphilis was spreading unimpeded among the population and that it was a matter of grave concern (pp.67–82 and 106–24). The prevalence of syphilis, particularly in London, must have been high (pp.107–8) – a fact which may have influenced William Clowes's apocalyptic vision of the 'foul disease' as a sickness that 'daylye spreadeth it selfe throughout all England and ouerfloweth as I thinke the whole world' (p.112).

3. A key indicator of the possible prevalence of syphilis during the 16th and 17th centuries is the extent of prostitution in the country. Sources indicate that prostitution was widespread in London and that the political and economic centre of the kingdom could also be regarded as a centre for prostitution as well. This was due in part to investments in the flesh trade made by the nobility, merchants, entertainment moguls and the numerous landlords of the capital (pp.118–21, 128–31 and 144–5). Jacobean City Comedy supports this picture of the English capital in its numerous references to brothels, pox, barber-surgeons, and medical treatments for venereal disease (pp.165–73).

4. In the provinces, sources indicate that prostitution was growing rapidly during the period due to the high degree of migration and the rapidly increasing number of alehouses. Factors contributing to the growth of prostitution in both the countryside and in London were a high unemployment rate and the widespread poverty of Tudor and Stuart England – partly caused by the population explosion of the period (pp.84–103).

5. Another indication of the spread of syphilis in England is the increase in political measures undertaken by the authorities to stem the disease. The temporary closure in 1506 of the Bankside brothels of London was the first official reaction to syphilis in England, and this measure was followed forty years later by the permanent closure of the stews of the capital – a move which dealt licensed prostitution its final death-blow.

A legislative act carried out a century later by the Puritan Government under Oliver Cromwell reflects the pressure for control of syphilis which had been at work over the previous decades. In the extremely harsh 1650 Commonwealth Act 'for the suppressing of the abhominable and crying sins of incest, adultery and fornication wherewith this land is much defiled and Almighty God highly displeased', the death penalty was introduced for incest and adultery. Fornication, a much less serious crime, brought the offender three months gaol and a good behaviour bond for a further year. Brothel-keepers were to be whipped, set in the pillory 'and there marked with a hot iron in the forehead with a B'. According to the same law, a second conviction brought death (Cobbett, 1810, vol.3 (1808), pp.1346–7).

These draconian measures reflect the Puritans' desperate efforts to root out an evil that in their eyes had corrupted the nation, physically and morally, for more than a century and a half.

6. If there is a connection between microbes and morals, as Theodor Rosebury maintains, there may even be a connection between the spread of syphilis and the growth of Puritanism in the 16th and 17th centuries. In a study entitled *Syphilis, Puritanism and Witch Hunts* (1989), sociologist Stanislav Andreski argues that syphilis played a crucial role both in the rise of Puritanism and in the 'purification' of the Catholic Church during the Counter Reformation. Andreski views Puritanism as an adaptive reaction which permitted the preservation of healthy genetic lines and the growth of population despite the debilitating impact of the new venereal disease. 'People of stern morals', he concludes, 'who avoided fornication and adultery and who chose as spouses persons of similar conduct, had a much better chance of a long life and of producing a large and healthy progeny, whereas libertines died young and left a few sickly descendants' (Andreski, 1989, p.15).

7. Sources examined in this study indicate that syphilis had a profound impact on the history of Western civilisation during the Renaissance. In the medical field, the disease furthered the growth of modern medicine, just as it confronted the existing health services with a new challenge at a time when the old one, leprosy, had almost been solved. In England there is evidence that the disease put strong demands on medical resources such as the lazarhouses of the country and the hospitals of London (pp.71–2 and 107–8). Probably the incorporation of the barbers and surgeons into the Barber-Surgeons' Company in 1540 reflects the same stress on the economy made by syphilis by showing the attempt of these practitioners to establish their ascendancy with respect to all venereal disease and thereby to cash in on a growing market for treatment.

8. The emergence of Paracelsian medicine and chemotherapy in the later decades of the 16th century is another indication of the spread of syphilis and of the barber-surgeons' attempts to cure it by new methods of treatment.

9. A final indication of the growing threat of syphilis to the population is the numerous warnings from the ecclesiastical establishment against promiscuity and whoredom (pp.17–20, 77–82 and 110–1) and the similar warnings made by social critics of the period, envisaging the physical and moral corruption of the nation and the undermining of its social and political structure (pp.101–3, 106–21 and 152–4). Referring to the practitioners of prostitution, one of these critics asserts that they 'are the decay of the forwardest Gentlemen and best wits...the verie causes of all the plagues that happen to this flourishing common wealth. They are the destruction of so manie Gentlemen in England. By them many Lordships come to ruine' (p.117).

10. Our examination of the various high-risk groups for the contraction of syphilis confirms this statement. In addition to sailors, soldiers, vagabonds and apprentices (pp.1–7, 88–100 and 147–8), sources indicate that numerous members of the nobility, particularly those serving at the Court of London, belonged to a high-risk group, as did the student population of the Universities and members of the Inns of Court of London – both establishments composed of members of the nobility and of the gentry (pp.148–60). Another section of the intelligentsia which

must be characterized as a high-risk group were the members of literary and dramatic Bohemia in the capital (pp.160–3).

11. Among notable members of the groups mentioned above, there is reason to believe that syphilis was contracted by the first Duke of Buckingham, the second Earl of Essex, the third Earl of Pembroke, Robert Greene, Thomas Nashe, George Peele, and William Davenant (pp.156–7, 184–95, 242–7 and 252). Circumstantial evidence examined on pp.175–254 further suggests that even William Shakespeare may have fallen a victim to syphilis – a disease which could well have contributed to his deep understanding of human suffering and despair.

12. In the final analysis, we concur with William Clowes, a notable witness of the period, that syphilis was 'a sicknes very lothsome, odious, troublesome, and daungerous' (p.112) and that it had a serious impact on the medical, social, economic, political, religious and cultural spheres of the English nation in the 16th and 17th centuries.

# BIBLIOGRAPHY

Acosta, J. de (1880) *The Natural & Moral History of the Indies*. Reprint 1880 of the English translated edition of Edward Grimstone (1604). London: Hakluyt Society.

Anderson, K. (1933) *The Treatment of Vagrancy and the Relief of the Poor and Destitute in the Tudor Period*. London University: History Theses 1901–70. Social History no. 2886. Jacobs, 1933.

André, B. (1858) *Annales Henrici VII. Historia Regis Henrici Septimi a Bernardo Andrea Tholosate conscripta* (edited by James Gairdner). Chronicles and Memorials of Great Britain and Ireland during the Middle Ages, no. 10. London.

Andreski, S. (1990) *Syphilis, Puritanism and Witch Hunts*. New York: St Martin's Press.

Appelboom, T. *et al.* (1986) 'Can a Diagnosis Be Made in Retrospect? The Case of Desiderius Erasmus.' *The Journal of Rheumatology, 13*, no.6, 1181–4.

Armstrong, E.A. (1946) *Shakespeare's Imagination: A Study of the Psychology of Association and Inspiration*. London: Lindsay Drummond.

Ashton, R. (1983) 'Popular Entertainment and Social Control in Later Elizabethan and Early Stuart London.' *London Journal, 9*, no.1, 3–19.

A. T. (1596) *A Rich Store-House or Treasury for the Diseased...Now Set Foorth for the Great Benefit and Comfort of the Poorer Sort of People That Are Not of Abilitie to Go to the Physitions*. London.

Aubrey, J. (1950) *Aubrey's Brief Lives* (edited by Oliver Lawson Dick). London: Secker and Warburg.

Aydelotte, F. (1967) *Elizabethan Rogues and Vagabonds*. London: Barnes and Noble.

Bacon, F. (1857–74) *The Works of Francis Bacon* (edited by J. Spedding, R.L. Ellis and D.D. Heath) vols. 1–14. London: Longman.

Bald, R.C. (1970) *John Donne: A Life*. Oxford: Clarendon Press.

Bale, J. (1561) *A Declaration of Edmonde Bonners Articles*.

Bale, J. (1810) *The Vocacyon of Johan Bale to the Bishoprick of Ossorie in Irelande* (1553). The Harleian Miscellany. London, vol. 6.

Bale, J. (1849) 'The Image of Both Churches.' *Select Works of John Bale* (edited by H. Christmas). The Parker Society. Cambridge, vol. 36.

Banister, J. (1575) *A Needfull, New and Necessarie Treatise of Chyrurgerie*. Reprint 1971 in The English Experience, no. 300. London.

Banister, J. (1633) *The Workes of That Famous Chyrurgian, Mr. John Banester. Booke of Tumors*. London.

Bannatyne, G. (1770) *Ancient Scottish Poems Published from the MS of George Bannatyne, 1568*. Edinburgh.

Barnard Jr., D.S. (1970) *Hollands Leaguer by Nicholas Goodman*. A critical edition by Dean Stanton Barnard Jr. The Hague-Paris: Mouton.

Barret, N.R. (1973) 'King Henry the Eighth.' *Annals of the Royal College of Surgeons in England, 52*, no.4, 216–33.

Bäumler, E. (1976) *Amors vergifteter Pfeile. Kulturgeschichte einer verschwiegene Krankheit*. Hamburg: Hoffmann und Campe.

Beaumont, F. and Fletcher, J. (1905–12) *The Works of Francis Beaumont and John Fletcher,* vols. 1–10 (edited by A. Glower and A.R. Waller). Cambridge: The University Press.

Beaumont, F. (1967) *The Knight of the Burning Pestle* (edited by John Doebler). Regents Renaissance Drama Series, BB 223. Lincoln: University of Nebraska Press.

Beckett, W. (1718) 'An Attempt to Prove the Antiquity of the Venereal Disease.' *Philosophical Transactions,* vol.30, 839–47. London.

Becon, T. (1843) *Early Works, Being the Treatises Published in the Reign of Henry VIII* (edited by John Ayre). The Parker Society, vol.9. Cambridge.

Becon, T. (1844a) *Catechism with Other Pieces Written by Him in the Reign of Edward VI* (edited by John Ayre). The Parker Society, vol.13. Cambridge.

Becon, T. (1844b) *Prayers and Other Pieces of Thomas Becon* (edited by John Ayre). The Parker Society, vol.17. Cambridge.

Beier, A.L. and Finlay, R. (eds) (1986) *London 1500–1700: the Making of the Metropolis.* London: Longman.

Bell, W.G. (1924) *The Great Plague in London in 1665.* London: John Lane.

Bentley, G.W. (1989) *Shakespeare and the New Disease: The Dramatic Function of Syphilis in Troilus and Cressida, Measure for Measure, and Timon of Athens.* New York: Peter Lang.

Béthencourt, J. de (1527) *Nova penitentialis qvadragesima, nec non purgatorium in Morbum Gallicum sive Venereum.* Paris.

Blanckaert, S. (1685) *Venus Belegert en Ontset.* Amsterdam.

Bloch, I. (1901–11) *Der Ursprung der Syphilis, 1–2 Abteilung.* Jena: G. Fisher.

Bloch, I. (1906) 'Schopenhauers Syphilis-Krankheit im Jahre 1823.' *Medizinische Klinik,* nos.25 and 26.

Boord, A. (1547) *The Breviary of Helthe, for All Maner of Syckenesses and Diseases the Whiche May Be in Man, or Woman Doth Follow.* Reprint 1971 in The English Experience, no.362. London.

Boord, A. (1870) *Andrew Borde's Introduction of Knowledge and Dyetary of Helth* (edited by F.J. Furnivall). Early English Text Society. Extra Series, no. 10.

Booth, S. (ed) (1977) *Shakespeare's Sonnets.* New Haven and London: Yale University Press.

Bradley, H. (1920) '"Cursed Hebenon" (or "Hebona").' *Modern Language Review, 15,* 85–7.

Brathwaite, R. (1887) *A Strappado for the Divell* (1615) (edited by J.W. Ebsworth). Boston: Robert Roberts.

Breton, N. (1879) *The Works in Verse and Prose of Nicholas Breton,* vols. 1–2 (edited by A.B. Grosart). Edinburgh: Chertsey Worthies' Library.

Brewster, P.G. (1958) 'A Note on the "Winchester Goose" and Kindred Topics.' *Journal of the History of Medical and Allied Sciences, 13,* 483–91.

Brinklow, H. (1874) *Henry Brinklow's Complaynt of Roderyck Mors* (edited by J.M. Cowper). Early English Text Society. Extra Series, no. 22.

Brinkman, A.A.A.M. (1982) *De Alchemist in de Prentkunst.* Amsterdam: Rodopi.

Browne, P. (1756) *The Civil and Natural History of Jamaica.* London.

Bucknill, J.C. (1860) *Shakespeare's Medical Knowledge.* London: Longman & Co.

Bullein, W. (1562) *Bulleins Bulwarke of Defence againste All Sicknes, Sornes, and Woundes.* Reprint 1971 in The English Experience, no.350. London.

Bullein, W. (1888) *A Dialogue against the Feuer Pestilence by William Bullein* (edited by M.W. and A.H. Bullen). Early English Text Society. Extra Series, no. 52.

Burckhard, J. (1717) *Ulrichi de Hutten ad B. Pirckheymer…epistola.* Wolfenbüttel.

Burford, E.J. (1973) *Queen of the Bawds.* London: Neville Spearman.

Burford, E.J. (1976) *Bawds and Lodgings.* London: Peter Owen.

Burford, E.J. (1990) *London, the Synfulle Citie.* London: Robert Hale.

Butler, C. (1936) *Syphilis sive Morbus Humanus.* New York: Science Press Printing Co.

Camden, C.C. (1975) *The Elizabethan Woman.* New York: Paul P. Appel Pub..

Camden, W. (1610) *Britain, or a Chorographicall Description of the Most Flourishing Kingdomes, England, Scotland and Ireland...Written First in Latin by William Camden...Translated Newly into English by Philemon Holland.* London.

Campbell, L.B. (1938–46) *The Mirror for Magistrates (1559). Parts Added to The Mirror for Magistrates by J. Higgins and T. Blenerhasset (1574),* vols. 1–2 (edited by L.B. Campbell). Cambridge: The University Press.

Campbell, O.J. and Quinn, E.G. (1966) *A Shakespeare Encyclopaedia.* London: Methuen & Co.

Cassel, J. (1987) *The Secret Plague: Venereal Disease in Canada 1838–1939.* Toronto: University of Toronto Press.

Cellini, B. (1771) *The Life of Benvenuto Cellini,* vols. 1–2 (translated by T. Nugent). London.

Chalfant, F.C. (1978) *Ben Jonson's London.* Athens, Ga: University of Georgia Press.

Chambers, E.K. (1923) *The Elizabethan Stage,* vols. 1–4. Oxford: Clarendon Press.

Chambers, E.K. (1930) *William Shakespeare: A Study of Facts and Problems,* vols. 1–2. Oxford: Clarendon Press.

Chambers, E.K. (1944) *Shakespearean Gleanings.* Oxford: The University Press.

Chambers, J.D. (1972) *Population, Economy and Society in Pre-Industrial England.* Oxford: Oxford University Press.

Chettle, H. (1923) *Kind-Harts Dreame Conteigning Five Apparitions with Their Invectives against Abuses Reigning.* The Bodley Head Quartos, vol.4. London.

Clark, P. and Slack, P. (1976) *English Towns in Transition.* London: Oxford University Press.

Clark, P. (1983) *The English Alehouse: A Social History 1200–1830.* London: Longman.

Clowes, W. (1579) *A Short and Profitable Treatise Touching the Cure of the Disease Called Morbus Gallicus by Unctions.* Reprint 1972 in The English Experience, no. 443. London.

Clowes, W. (1579a) *Epistle to the Frendly Reader.*

Clowes, W. (1585) *A Briefe and Necessarie Treatise...Newly Corrected and Augmented.* London.

Clowes, W. (1596) *A Profitable and Necessarie Booke of Observations, for All Those That are Burned with Flame of Gun Powder, &...Last of All Adioined a Short Treatise for the Cure of Lues Venerea by Unction.* London. Reprint 1945 with introductions general and medical by De Witt T. Starnes and Chauncey D. Leake. New York.

Clowes, W. (1596) *A Briefe and Necessary Treatise, Touching the Cure of the Disease Now Usually Called Lues Venerea, by Unctions and Other Approoued Waies of Curing.* Included in the above title (Clowes, 1596), where it is printed on pp.145–229.

Cobbett, W. (ed) (1810) *Cobbett's Parliamentary History of England,* vols. 1–36. London, 1806–20.

Cock, W. (1924) 'An Early Prescription in English.' *The British Medical Journal,* May 17, 869–70.

Cole, H.N. (1952) 'Erasmus and His Diseases.' *Journal of the American Medical Association,* 148, 529–31.

Collins, A. (ed) (1746) *Letters and Memorials of State in the Reigns of Queen Mary, Queen Elizabeth, King James, King Charles I, Part of the Reign of Charles II and Oliver's Usurpation,* vols. 1–2. London. (Also called 'Sidney Papers').

Comrie, J.D. (1932) *History of Scottish Medicine,* vols. 1–2. The Wellcome Historical Medical Museum. London.

Copeman, P.W.M. and Copeman, W.S.C. (1969–70) 'Dermatology in Tudor and Early Stuart England.' *British Journal of Dermatology,* 1969, *81,* 303–11; 1970, *82,* 78–88; 1970, *82,* 182–91.

Coryat, T. (1905) *Coryat's Crudities,* vols. 1–2. Glasgow: James MacLehose and Sons.

Cotgrave, R. (1611) *A Dictionarie of the French and English Tongves.* London.

Cotta, J. (1612) *A Short Discoverie of the Unobserved Dangers of Severall Sorts of Ignorant and Unconsiderate Practisers of Physicke in England.* London.

Cranley, T. (1635) *Amanda, or the Reformed Whore.* London.

Creighton, C. (1891) *A History of Epidemics in Britain.* London. Second edition: London, 1965.

Crossfill, J.W.L. (1954–7) 'Classified Medical References in the Works of Shakespeare.' *Journal of the Royal Naval Medical Service,* 1954, *40,* 12–29 and 139–49; 1955, *41,* 35–53 and 149–67; 1956, *42,* 22–36 and 166–75; 1957, *43,* 76–88.

Crowley, R. (1872) *The Select Works of Robert Crowley* (edited by J.M. Cowper). Early English Text Society, Extra Series, no.15.

CSP, DOM. (1869) *Calendar of State Papers, Domestic. 1598–1601,* vol.5 (edited by E. Green). London.

CSP, DOM. (1870) *Calendar of State Papers, Domestic. 1601–1603,* vol.6 (edited by E. Green). London.

Davenant, W. (1673) *The Works of William Davenant.* London.

Davies, J., of Hereford (1878) *The Complete Works of John Davies of Hereford,* vols. 1–2 (edited by A.B. Grosart). London: Chertsey Worthies' Library.

Dee, J. (1842) *The Diary of Dr John Dee* (edited by J.O. Halliwell). The Camden Society, *19,* 14–7. London.

Dekker, T. (1612) *O per se O or A New Cryer of Lanthorne and Candlelight.* London.

Dekker, T. (1620) *Villanies Discovered by Lanthorne and Candlelight, and the Help of a New Cryer called O Per se O.* London.

Dekker, T. (1630) *The Honest Whore.* London.

Dekker, T. (1631) *Penny-Wise, Pound-Foolish.* London.

Dekker, T. (1638) *English Villanies Seven Severall Times Prest to Death.* London.

Dekker, T. (1884–6) *The Non-Dramatic Works of Thomas Dekker* (edited by A.B. Grosart), vols. 1–5. London: The Huth Library.

Dekker, T. (1925) *The Plague Pamphlets of Thomas Dekker* (edited by F.P. Wilson). Oxford: Clarendon Press.

Delicado, F. (1529) *El modo de adoperare el legno de India occidentale.* Venezia.

Dennie, C.C. (1962) *A History of Syphilis.* Springfield: C.C. Thomas.

Dohi, K. (1923) *Beiträge zur Geschichte der Syphilis.* Tokyo: Verlag von Nankodo.

Donne, J. (1965) *The Elegies and the Songs and Sonnets* (edited by H. Gardner). Oxford: Oxford University Press.

Donne, J. (1980) *Paradoxes and Problems* (edited by H. Peters). Oxford: Oxford University Press.

Dürer, A. (1963) *The Complete Woodcuts of Albrecht Dürer* (edited by W. Kurth). New York: Dover Publications.

Earle, J. (1633) *Microcosmographie.* London.

Edward, Lord Herbert of Cherbury (1649) *The Life and Raigne of King Henry the Eighth.* London.

Elyot, T. (1880) *The Boke Named the Governour* (1531), vols. 1–2 (edited by H.H.S. Croft). London: Kegan Paul and Co.

Emmison, F.G. (1970) *Elizabethan Life: Disorder.* Essex County Council. Chelmsford.

Emmison, F.G. (1973) *Elizabethan Life: Morals and the Church Courts.* Essex County Council. Chelmsford.

Erasmus, R. (1965) *The Colloquies of Erasmus* (translated by C.R. Thompson). Chicago and London: University of Chicago Press.

Erasmus, R. (1968), *Erasmus and Fisher. Their Correspondence 1511–1524* (edited by J. Rouschausse). Paris.

Erasmus, R. (1974–82) *Collected Works of Erasmus: The Correspondence of Erasmus. Letters, vols. 1–6.* Toronto: University of Toronto Press.

Fabricius, J. (1976) *Alchemy: The Medieval Alchemists and Their Royal Art.* Copenhagen. Reprint: The Aquarian Press. Wellingborough, 1989.

Fabricius, J. (1989) *Shakespeare's Hidden World: A Study of His Unconscious.* Copenhagen: Munksgaard.

Fabyan, R. (1938) *The Great Chronicle of London* (edited by A.H. Thomas and I.D. Thornley). London.

Farmer, J.S. (ed) (1906) *Six Anonymous Plays, second series.* London. Privately printed.

Fildes, V. (1988) 'The English Wet-Nurse and Her Role in Infant Care 1538–1800.' *Medical History, 32*, 142–73.

Finlay, R. (1981) *Population and Metropolis: The Demography of London 1580–1650.* Cambridge: Cambridge University Press.

Fish, S. (1871) *Simon Fish A Supplicacyon for the Beggers* (edited by F.J. Furnivall). Early English Text Society. Extra Series, no. 13.

Fisher, J. (1876) *John Fisher The English Works* (edited by J.E.B. Mayor). Early English Text Society. Extra Series, no. 27.

Florio, J. (1591) *Florios Second Frutes.* London.

Forbes, T.R. (1971) *Chronicle from Aldgate. Life and Death in Shakespeare's London.* New Haven and London: Yale University Press.

Ford, J. (1869) *The Dramatic Works of John Ford,* vols. 1–3 (edited by W. Gifford). London.

Foster, D.W. (1989) *Elegy by W.S.: A Study in Attribution.* Newark, London and Toronto: University of Delaware Press.

Fracastoro, G. (1930) *De contagione et contagiosis morbis* (translated and with notes by W.C. Wright). New York: G.P. Putnam's Sons.

Fracastoro, G. (1988) *Lehrgedicht über die Syphilis* (edited and translated by G. Wöhrle). Bamberg: Stefan Wendel Verlag.

Freud, S. (1953) *The Interpretation of Dreams.* The Standard Edition of the Complete Psychological Works of Sigmund Freud (translated and edited by James Strachey) vol.4/5. London: Hogarth Press.

Fuchs, C.H. (1843) *Die ältesten Schriftsteller über die Lustseuche in Deutschland, von 1495 bis 1510.* Göttingen.

Fuchs, C.H. (1853) 'Francesco Delicado über den Guajac. Ein Beitrag zur älteren Bibliographie und Geschichte der Syphilis.' *Janus, Neue Folge, 2,* 193–204. Gotha.

Fuller, T. (1655) *The Church History of Britain from the Birth of Jesus Christ until the Year MDCXLVIII.* London.

Fuller, T. (1938) *The Holy and the Profane State,* vols. 1–2 (edited by M. Graf Walten). New York: Columbia University Press.

Furnivall, F.J. (ed) (1868–72) *Ballads from Manuscripts* (edited by F.L. Furnivall). London: The Ballad Society.

Gale, T. (1563a) *An Antidotarie Conteyning Hidde and Secrete Medicines Simple and Compounde.* London.

Gale, T. (1563b) *Certain Workes of Chirurgerie.* Reprint 1971 in The English Experience, no. 420. London.

Garret, C. (1940) '"The Resurreccion of the Masse" by Hugh Hilarie – or John Bale (?).' Transactions of the Bibliographical Society. New Series, *21*, no.2. 149.

Gebauer, A. (1987) *Von Macht und Mäzenatentum. Leben und Werk William Herberts, des dritten Earls vom Pembroke*. Heidelberger Forschungen, 28. Heft, 1987. Heidelberg: Carl Winter Universitätsverlag.

Girtanner, C. (1788–9) *Abhandlung über die venerische Krankheit*, vols. 1–3. Göttingen.

Gjestland, T. (1955) *The Oslo Study of Untreated Syphilis*. Oslo.

Goethe, J.W. (1949) *Gedichte* (edited by Emil Steiger). Stuttgart: Manesse Verlag.

Gosson, S. (1595) *Quippes for the Upstarte Newfangled Gentlewoman*. London.

Graunt, J. (1662) *Natural and Political Observations Made upon the Bills of Mortality*. London.

Greene, R. (1881–6) *The Life and Complete Works in Prose and Verse of Robert Greene MA*, vols. 1–15 (edited by A.B. Grosart). London: The Huth Library.

Greene, R. (1905) *The Plays and Poems of Robert Greene* (edited by J. Churton Collins), vols.1–2. Oxford: Clarendon Press.

Greene, R. (1966a) *Greenes Groatsworth of Witte, Bought with a Million of Repentance (1592)*, in Elizabethan and Jacobean Quartos, no.5 (edited by G.B. Harrison). Edinburgh: The University Press.

Greene, R. (1966b) *The Repentance of Robert Greene Maister of Artes (1592)*, in Elizabethan and Jacobean Quartos, no.5 (edited by G.B. Harrison). Edinburgh: The University Press.

Grosart, A.B. (ed) (1870) *Miscellanies of The Fuller Worthies' Library*. Blackburn. Privately printed.

Grünpeck, J. (1496) *Tractatus de pestilentiali scorra sive mala de franczos*. Augsburg.

Gurr, A. (1987) *The Shakespearean Stage 1574–1642*, Second edition. Cambridge: Cambridge University Press.

Hall, J. (1961) *The Court of Virtue* (edited by R. Fraser). London: Routledge.

Harington, J. (1930) *The Letters and Epigrams of Sir John Harington* (edited by N.E. McClure). Philadelphia: The University of Pennsylvania Press.

Harington, J. (1962) *The Metamorphosis of Ajax* (1596) (edited by E. Story Donno). London: Routledge.

Harrison, W. (1586) 'The Description of England.' In R. Holinshed *Holinshed's Chronicles of England, Scotland and Ireland*, vols.1–6 (edited by H. Ellis). London. Reprint: New York, 1965. AMS Press.

Harrison, W. (1877) *Harrison's Description of England* (edited by F.J. Furnivall). The New Shakespeare Society, 1877, series 6, no.1.

Harrison, W. (1878) *Harrison's Description of England* (edited by F.J. Furnivall). The New Shakespeare Society, 1878, series 6, no.5.

Harrison, W. (1908) *Harrison's Description of England* (edited by F.J. Furnivall). The Shakespeare Library, 1908, part 4, supplement 2.

Harrison, W.A. (1880–6) 'Hamlet's Juice of Cursed Hebona.' *The New Shakespeare Society's Transactions*, 1880–6, series 1, nos.8–10, pp.295–321.

Harvey, G. (1884–5) *The Works of Gabriel Harvey DCL*, vols. 1–3 (edited by A.B. Grosart). London: The Huth Library.

Haustein, H. (1930) *Die Frühgeschichte der Syphilis 1495–1498. Archiv für Dermatologie und Syphilis*, vol.161. Berlin.

Hawes, S. (1974) *The Minor Poems of Stephen Hawes* (edited by F.W. Gluck and A.B. Morgan). Early English Text Society, no.271. Oxford: Oxford University Press.

Hemmingway, J. (1831) *History of the City of Chester*, vols. 1–2. Chester.

Henriques, F. (1963) *Prostitution in Europe and the New World*. [Prostitution and Society, vol. 2]. London: MacGibbon.

Hermann, P. (1590) *An Excellent Treatise Teaching Howe to Cure the French Pockes* (translated by J. Hester). London.

Hester, J. (1594) *The Pearle of Practise*. London.

Hester, J. (1596) *A Hundred and Fourteene Experiments and Cures of the Famous Physitian Philippus Aureolus Theophrastus Paracelsus... Collected by John Hester*. London.

Hester, J. (1596) *The Key Philosophie*. London.

Hilarie, H. (1554) *The Resurreccion of the Masse... by Hughe Hilarie*. Strasbourg.

Hirsch, A. (1883–6) *Handbook of Geographical and Historical Pathology*, vols. 1–3 (translated by C. Creighton). London: New Sydenham Society.

Holdsworth, W.S. (1903) *A History of English Law*, vols. 1–9. London: Methuen & Co.

Holingsworth, M.F. and Holingsworth, T.H. (1971) 'Plague Mortality Rates by Age and Sex in the Parish of St. Botolph's without Bishopsgate, London, 1603.' *Population Studies, 25*, 131–46.

Holmes, K.K. (ed) (1990) *Sexually Transmitted Diseases*, second edition. New York: McGraw-Hill.

Honigmann, E.A.J. (1982) *Shakespeare's Impact on His Contemporaries*. London: Barnes & Noble.

Horman, W. (1926) *William Horman's Vulgaria* (edited by M.R. James). Roxburghe Club. London.

Hosking, G.L. (1952) *The Life and Times of Edward Alleyn*. London: Jonathan Cape.

Howes, J. (1904) *A Brief Note of the Order and Manner of Proceedings in the First Erection of the Three Royal Hospitals of Christ, Bridewell, and St. Thomas the Apostle*. Manuscript edited by William Lempriere. London.

Humphreys, A.R. (ed) (1966) *The Second Part of King Henry IV*. The Arden Shakespeare. London: Methuen & Co.

Hurstfield, J. (1979) *The English Common-Wealth 1547–1640*. Essays to Joel Hurstfield. London.

Hurstfield, J. and Smith, A.G.R. (1972) *Elizabethan People*. London: Edward Arnold.

Hutchinson, R. (1842) 'The Image of God or Layman's Book' (1550). *The Works of Roger Hutchinson* (edited by J. Bruce). The Parker Society, vol.4. Cambridge.

Hutten, U. von (1519) *Ulrichen von Hutten eins teutschen Ritters von der wunderbarlichen artzney des holtz Guaiacum genant... durch dem hochgelerten herren Thomam Murner... geteutschet und verdolmetschet*. Strasbourg.

Hutten, U. von (1525) *L'expérience et approbation Ulrich de Hutem notable chevalier touchant la médecine du boys dict Guaiacum... traduicte et interpretée par maistre Jehan Cheradame*. Paris.

Hutten, U. von (1533) *De Morbo Gallico*, (translated by T. Paynel). London.

Ingram, W. (1978) *A London Life in the Brazen Age: Francis Langley, 1548–1602*. London: Harvard University Press.

Isle, HMC. (1925–66) *Historical Manuscripts Commission Report*. Report of the Manuscripts of Lord de L'Isle and Dudley Preserved at Penhurst Place, vols. 1–6 (edited by C.L. Kingsford). London.

Jacobi, J. (1959) *Complex, Archetype, Symbol in the Psychology of C.G. Jung*. Princeton, N.J.: Princeton University Press.

James I. (1604) *A Counterblaste to Tobacco*. London.

Jaques, E. (1965) 'Death and the Mid-Life-Crisis.' *The International Journal of Psychoanalysis, 46*, 502–13.

Jeaffreson, J.C. (ed) (1886–8) *Middlesex County Records*, vols. 1–3. London.

Jeanselme, E. *et al.* (1931) *Histoire de la syphilis. Tome I. Traité de la syphilis* (edited by E. Jeanselme and E. Schulmann). Paris: G. Doin.

Johnson, D.J. (1969) *Southwark and the City*. London.

Jones, E. (1949) *Hamlet and Oedipus.* London: Victor Gollancz.

Jones, J. (1566) *A Diall for All Agues.* London.

Jonson, B. (1925–52) *Ben Jonson,* vols. 1–11 (edited by C.H. Herford and P. Simpson). Oxford: Clarendon Press.

Judges, A.V. (1965) *The Elizabethan Underworld.* New York: Octagon Books.

Jung, C.G. (1960) *The Psychogenesis of Mental Disease.* The Collected Works of C.G. Jung (edited by Sir H. Read, M. Fordham and G. Adler, vol.3). London: Routledge and Kegan Paul.

Jung, C.G. (1973) *Experimental Researches.* The Collected Works of C.G. Jung (edited by Sir H. Read, M. Fordham and G. Adler, vol.2). London: Routledge and Kegan Paul.

Junius, A. (1585) *The Nomenclator, or Remembrancer of Adrianus Junius.* London.

Keil, H. (1949) 'The Evolution of the Term Chancre and Its Relation to the History of Syphilis.' *Journal of the History of Medicine, 4,* 407–16.

King, A. and Nicol, C. (1975) *Venereal Diseases,* third edition. London: Bailliere.

Kumar Sen, S. (1958) 'What Happens in Coriolanus.' *Shakespeare Quarterly, 9,* 331–45.

Kökeritz, H. (1953) *Shakespeare's Pronunciation.* New Haven: Yale University Press.

Lacey, R. (1971) *Robert, Earl of Essex: An Elizabethan Icarus.* London: Weidenfeld.

Lane, J. (1876) 'Tom Tel-Troths Message, and His Pens Complaint.' In F.J. Furnivall (ed) *Tell Trothes New Yerres Gift.* Shakespeare's England, series 6, no.2. London.

Larkin, J.F. and Hughes, P.L. (eds) (1964–9) *Tudor Royal Proclamations,* vols. 1–3. New Haven and London. Yale University Press.

Larkin, J.F. and Hughes, P.L. (1973–83) *Stuart Royal Proclamations,* vols. 1–2. Oxford: Oxford University Press.

Latimer, H. (1844) *Sermons by Hugh Latimer* (edited by G.E. Corrie). The Parker Society, vol. 16. Cambridge.

Lenton, F. (1629) *The Young Gallant's Whirligigg.* London.

Lenton, F. (1631) *Characterismi.* London.

Lodge, T. (1883) *The Complete Works of Thomas Lodge* (edited by E.W. Gosse), vols. 1–4. Glasgow: The Hunterian Club.

Lowe, P. (1596) *An Easie, Certain and Perfect Method, to Cure and Prevent the Spanish Sicknes.* London.

Lupton, D. (1632) *London and the Countrey Carbonadoed.* London.

Lupton, J.H. (1909) *A Life of John Colet.* London.

Luther, M. (1907) *D. Martin Luthers Werke.* Kritische Gesamtausgabe, 10. Band, Zweite Abteilung. Weimar: Hermann Böhlaus Nachfolger.

Lyly, J. (1902) *The Complete Works of John Lyly* (edited by R. Warwick Bond), vols. 1–3. Oxford: Clarendon Press.

Macht, D.I. (1918) 'A Pharmacological Appreciation of Shakespeare's Hamlet: On Instillation of Poisons into the Ear.' *Johns Hopkins Hospital Bulletin, 29,* 165–70.

Magno, A. (1983) 'The London Journal of Alessandro Magno 1562' (edited by C. Barron, C. Coleman and C. Gobbi). *The London Journal, 9,* no.2, 136–52.

Major, R.H. (1939) Classic Descriptions of Disease. Illinois: C.C. Thomas.

Manly, J.M. (ed) (1897) *Specimens of the Pre-Shakespearean Drama,* vols. 1–2. Boston: Ginn & Co.

Manningham, J. (1976) *The Diary of John Manningham of the Middle Temple 1602–1603* (edited by R.P. Sorlien). New Hampshire: University Press of New England.

Marston, J. (1965) *The Dutch Courtesan* (edited by M.L. Wine). Regents Renaissance Drama Series. London: Edward Arnold.

Marston, J. (1966) *The Scourge of Villanie (1598).* Elizabethan and Jacobean Quartos, no.11. Edinburgh: The University Press.

Martyr, P. (1612) *De novo orbe or The Historie of the West Indies* (translated by R. Eden). London.

Massinger, P. (1976) *The Plays and Poems of Philip Massinger* (edited by P. Edwards and C. Gibson), vols. 1–5. Oxford: Oxford University Press.

McCray Beier, L. (1987) *Sufferers and Healers: the Experience of Illness in Seventeenth-Century England.* London and New York: Routledge and Kegan Paul.

Meres, F. (1938) *Palladis Tamia* (1598). Scholars' Facsimiles and Reprints. New York.

Middleton, T. (1885–6) *The Works of Thomas Middleton,* vols. 1–8 (edited by A.H. Bullen). London: John C. Nimmo.

Moëll, H. (1984) *Ulrich von Hutten, Guajak och Franska Sjukan.* Sydsvenska Medicinhistoriska Sällskapets Årsskrift, Supplementum 3. Lund.

Monardes, N. (1580) *Joyfull Newes out of the Newe Founde Worlde* (translated by J. Frampton). London. Reprint 1970 in The English Experience, no.251.

Montaiglon, M.A. de (ed) (1874) *Le Triumphe de trés haulte et puissante Dame Vérolle.* Paris.

Montgomery, M. (1920) '"Cursed Hebona" as *Guaiacum officinale* (or *Lignum vitae*) in Shakespeare's *Hamlet,* I, V, 62.' *Proceedings of the Royal Society of Medicine* (Sect. Hist. M.), *14,* 23–6.

More, T. (1962) *Thomas More's Utopia,* introduction by John Warrington. London and New York: J.M. Dent & Sons.

More, T. (1968) *Utopia* as printed in *The Norton Anthology of English Literature* (edited by M.H. Abrams). New York: Norton.

Morton, R.S. (1962) 'Some Aspects of the Early History of Syphilis in Scotland.' *British Journal of Venereal Diseases, 38,* 175–80.

Moulton, T. (1539) *Mirrour of Glasse of Helth.* London.

Muir, K. (ed) (1982) *Troilus and Cressida / Shakespeare.* Berkeley: University of California Press.

Munger, R.S. (1949) 'Guaiacum, the Holy Wood from the New World.' *Journal of the History of Medicine and Allied Sciences, 4,* 196–229.

Nashe, T. (1910) *The Works of Thomas Nashe,* vols. 1–5 (edited by R.B. McKerrow). London: Sidgwick & Jackson.

Newman, G. (1895) 'On the History of the Decline…of Leprosy…in the British Islands.' *Leprosy Prize Essays, New Sydenham Society, 157,* 1–150 (houses listed in the Appendix).

Nicholson, B. (1880–6) 'Hamlet's Cursed Hebenon.' *The New Shakespeare Society's Transactions,* series 1, nos.8–10, 21–31.

Nicolas, N. (ed) (1830) *Privy Purse Expenses of Elizabeth of York.* London: Pickering.

Nielsen, G. and Schmidt, H. (1985) *Hud- og kønssygdomme.* København: Nyt Nordisk Forlag, Arnold Busck.

*Nova reperta* (c. 1600) *9 copper engravings by Theodor Galle after an original design by Jan van der Straet.*

Nutton, V. (ed) (1990) *Medicine at the Courts of Europe, 1500–1837.* London and New York: Routledge.

Ogden, M.S. (ed) (1938) *The Liber de Diversis Medicinis.* Early English Text Society. Original Series, no.207.

O'Shea, J.G. (1990) '"Two minutes with Venus, two years with Mercury" – Mercury as an Antisyphilitic Chemotherapeutic Agent.' *Journal of the Royal Society of Medicine, 83,* 392–5.

Overbury, T. (1936) *The Overburian Characters* (edited by W.J. Paylor). The Percy Reprints, no.13. Oxford: Basil Blackwell.

Ovid (1961) *The Metamorphoses of Ovid* (translated and with an introduction by M.M. Innes). Harmondsworth: Penguin.

Packard, F.R. (1924) 'References to Syphilis in the Plays of Shakespeare.' *Annals of Medical History, 6,* 194–200.

Paracelsus (1922–33) *Theophrast von Hohenheim genannt Paracelsus Sämtliche Werke.* Erste Abteilung: Medizinische, naturwissenschaftliche und philosophische Schriften, vols. 1–14, edited by Karl Sudhoff and Wilhelm Matthiessen. Munich and Berlin.

Parran, T. (1937) *Shadow on the Land: Syphilis.* New York: Reynal and Hitchcock.

Partridge, E. (1968) *Shakespeare's Bawdy: A Literary and Psychological Essay and a Comprehensive Glossary.* London: Routledge and Kegan Paul.

Paynel, T. (1534) *A Moche Profitable Treatise against the Pestilence.* London.

Pelling, M. (1985) 'Healing the Sick Poor: Social Policy and Disability in Norwich 1550–1640.' *Medical History, 29,* 115–37.

Pelling, M. (1986) 'Appearance and Reality: Barbersurgeons, the Body and Venereal Disease in Early Modern London.' In A.L. Beier and R. Finlay (eds) *The Making of the Metropolis: London 1500–1700,* pp.82–112. London.

Pendry, E.D. (ed) (1967) *Thomas Dekker.* The Stratford-upon-Avon Library, no.4.

Pennington, D. and Thomas, K. (eds) (1978) *Puritans and Revolutionaries.* Oxford: Oxford University Press.

Platter, T. (1937) *Thomas Platter's Travels in England 1599* (edited by C. Williams). London: Jonathan Cape.

Pope, A. (1871–89) *The Works of Alexander Pope,* vols. 1–10 (edited by W. Elvin and W.J. Courthope). London: John Murray.

Pound, J.F. (1971) *Poverty and Vagrancy in Tudor England.* London: Longman.

Prest, W.R. (1972) *The Inns of Court under Elizabeth I and the Early Stuarts, 1590–1640.* London: Longman.

Prouty, C.T. (ed) (1952–70) *The Life and Works of George Peele,* vols. 1–3. New Haven.

Pusey, W.M.A. (1933) *The History and Epidemiology of Syphilis.* London: Baillière, Tindall and Cox.

Quaife, G.R. (1979) *Wanton Wenches and Wayward Wives.* London: Rutgers University Press.

Randolph, T. (1638) *Cornelianum Dolium.* London.

Randolph, T. (1875) *Poetical and Dramatic Works of Thomas Randolph,* vols. 1–2 (edited by W.C. Hazlitt). London: Reeves and Turner.

Rastell, J. (1979) *Three Rastell Plays* (edited by R. Axton). Cambridge: D.S. Brewer.

R.C. (1871) *The Times' Whistle* (edited by J.M. Cowper). Early English Text Society. Original Series, no. 48.

Read, C. (ed) (1962) *William Lambard and Local Government.* New York: Cornell University Press.

Read, J. (1588) *A Most Excellent and Compendious Method of Curing Woundes,* etc. London.

Reitter, C. (1508) *Mortilogus.* Augsburg.

Remembrancia (1878) *Analytical Index to the Series of Records Known as Remembrancia Preserved among the Archives of the City of London A. D. 1579–1664.* London.

Rendle, W. (1877) 'The Bankside, Southwark and the Globe Playhouse.' In F.J. Furnivall (ed) *Harrison's Description of England in Shakespeare's Youth.* The New Shakespeare Society, 1878, series 6, no.5, appendix 1.

Rich, B. (1614) *The Honestie of This Age.* London.

Rich, B. (1616) *My Ladies Looking-Glasse.* London.

Rich, B. (1617) *The Irish Hubbub, or the English Hue and Crie.* London.

Rimbault, E.F. (ed) (1842) *Cock Lorell's Bote.* Early English Poetry. Percy Society, vol.6. London.

Rolleston, J.D. (1934) 'Venereal Disease in Literature.' *British Journal of Venereal Disease, 10,* 147–82.

Rosebury, T. (1971) *Microbes and Morals.* New York: The Viking Press.

Rowlands, S. (1880) *The Complete Works of Samuel Rowlands,* vols.1–3. The Hunterian Club. London.

Rowse, A.L. (1974) *Simon Forman: Sex and Society in Shakespeare's Age.* London: Weidenfeld and Nicolson.

Roxburghe Ballads, The. *The British Library,* vols.1–4. Microfilm 7526–7527.

Roy, W. (1812) *Rede me and be nott wrothe.* The Harleian Miscellany. London, vol.9.

Rubinstein, F. (1984) *A Dictionary of Shakespeare's Sexual Puns and Their Significance.* London: Macmillan.

Rueff, J. (1587) *De conceptu et generatione hominis.* Frankfurt.

Rye, W.B. (1967) *England as Seen by Foreigners in the Days of Queen Elizabeth and James I.* New York: Benjamin Blom.

Salgãdo Gãmini (1977) *The Elizabethan Underworld.* London: Rowmann and Littlefield.

Salisbury, HMC. *Historical Manuscripts Commission.* Calendar of the Manuscripts of the Marquis of Salisbury (Cecil Manuscripts), vols.7–10. London, 1899–1904.

Schoenbaum, S. (1975) *William Shakespeare: A Documentary Life.* Oxford: Oxford University Press.

Schütz, M. (1565) *Holtzbüchlein.* Strasbourg. Quoted after Montgomery, 1920, p.26.

Scot, R. (1930) *The Discoverie of Witchcraft (1584)* (edited by M. Summers). London: John Rodker.

Seymour-Smith, M. (ed) (1963) *Shakespeare's Sonnets.* London: Heinemann.

Shakespeare, W. (1951–82) *The Arden Edition of the Works of William Shakespeare* (edited by Harold F. Brooks, Harold Jenkins, Brian Morris and Richard Proudfoot). London: Methuen and Co.

Sharpe, J.A. (1980) 'Defamation and Sexual Slander in Early Modern England: The Church Courts at York.' In *Borthwick Papers,* no.58, 1–36. University of York.

Shrewsbury, J.F.D. (1952) 'Henry VIII: A Medical Study.' *Journal of the History of Medicine and Allied Sciences,* 7, no.2, 141–85.

Shrewsbury, J.F.D. (1970) *A History of Bubonic Plague in the British Isles.* Cambridge: Cambridge University Press.

Simon, F.A. (1857–8) *Kritische Geschichte des Ursprungs, der Pathologie und Behandlung der Syphilis, Tochter und wiederum Mutter des Aussatzes.* Hamburg.

Simpson, R.R. (1959) *Shakespeare and Medicine.* Edinburgh and London.

Skelton, J. (1964) *The Complete Poems of John Skelton, Laureate* (edited by P. Henderson). London: J.M. Dent and Sons.

Slack, P.A. (1974) 'Vagrants and Vagrancy in England, 1598–1664.' *The Economic History Review,* second series, 27, no.3, 360–79.

Smith, F. (1914) 'Shakespeare on Syphilis.' *Journal of the Royal Army Medical Corps,* 22, 450.

Spurgeon, C.F. (1931) *Shakespeare's Iterative Imagery (i) As Undersong (ii) As Touchstone, in His Work.* Cambridge: The University Press.

Spurgeon, C.F. (1935) *Shakespeare's Imagery and What It Tells Us.* Cambridge: Cambridge University Press.

Stone, L. (1988) *The Family, Sex and Marriage in England 1500–1800* (Abridged edition). London: Penguin Books.

Stopes, C.C. (1922) *The Life of Henry, Third Earl of Southampton.* Cambridge: The University Press.

Stow, J. (1633) *The Survey of London.* London.

Stow, J. (1908) *A Survey of London,* vols.1–2 (edited by C.L. Kingsford). London: Oxford University Press.

Strausz, D.F. (1895) *Ulrich von Hutten.* Bonn.

Stubbes, P. (1877–9) *Phillip Stubbes's Anatomy of the Abuses in England in Shakspere's Youth.* The New Shakspere Society, series VI, nos.4 and 6. London.

Sudhoff, K. (1912) *Graphische und typographische Erstlinge der Syphilislitteratur aus den Jahren 1495 und 1496.* München: Carl Kuhn.

Sudhoff, K. (1924) *Zehn Syphilis-Drucke aus den Jahren 1495–1498.* Milano: R. Lier and Co.

Summers, M. (1958) *The Geography of Witchcraft.* Evanston and New York: University Books.

Tawney, R.H. and Power, E. (1924) *Tudor Economic Documents,* vols. 1–3. London: Longmans and Co.

Taylor, J. (1630) *The Works of John Taylor the Water Poet Comprised in the Folio Edition of 1630* (reprint). 1973. London: Scolar Press.

Tourneur, C. (1878) *The Plays and Poems of Cyril Tourneur,* vols. 1–2 (edited by J.C. Collins). London.

Turner, W. (1568) *William Turners Herball. The Thirde Parte.* London.

Tyndale, W. (1850) *An Answer to Sir Thomas Mores Dialogue. London 1531–32?* (edited by H. Walter). The Parker Society, no.38. Cambridge.

Vaughan, H. (1957) *The Works of Henry Vaughan* (edited by L.C. Martin). Oxford: Clarendon Press.

Vicary, T. (1888) *The Anatomie of the Bodie of Man by Thomas Vicary* (edited by F.J. Furnivall and P. Furnivall). Early English Text Society. Extra Series, no.53.

Vigo, G. de (1520) *Practica copiosa in arte chirurgica. Liber Quintus.*

Vigo, G. de (1543) *The Most Excellent Workes of Chirurgerye, Made and Set Forth by Maister John Vigon* (translated by B. Traheron). Reprint 1968 in The English Experience, no. 67. London.

Viles, E. and Furnivall, F.J. (eds) (1880) *The Rogues and Vagabonds of Shakespeare's Youth* (edited by E. Viles and F.J. Furnivall). The New Shakespeare Society, 1880, series 6, no.7.

Villalobos, F.L. de (1870) *The Medical Works of Francisco Lopez de Villalobos…translated with commentary and biography by George Gaskoin.* London: John Churchill and Sons.

Vorberg, G. (1924) *Über den Ursprung der Syphilis.* Stuttgart: Julius Puttmann Verlag.

Wager, L. (1902) *The Life and Repentaunce of Marie Magdalene* (edited by F.I. Carpenter). Chicago.

Waugh, M.A. (1973) 'Venereal Diseases in Sixteenth-Century England.' *Medical History, 17,* 192–99.

Webster, C. (ed) (1979) *Health, Medicine and Mortality in the Sixteenth Century.* Cambridge: Cambridge University Press.

Wechter, D. (1928) 'The Purpose of Timon of Athens.' *Publications of Modern Language Association, 43,* 701–21.

Weidenbacher, J. (1926) *Die Fuggerei in Augsburg.* Augsburg: Im Selbstverlag.

Welldon, A. (1650) *The Court and Character of King James.* London.

Wentersdorf, K.P. (1972) 'Imagery as a Criterion of Authenticity: A Reconsideration of the Problem.' *Shakespeare Quarterly, 23,* 231–59.

Werthemann, A. (1930) *Schädel und Gebeine des Erasmus von Rotterdam.* Basel.

Whetstone, G. (1584) *A Mirour for Magestrates of Cyties.* London.

Williams, G. (1968) 'A Sample of Elizabethan Sexual Periphrasis.' *Trivium, 3,* 94–101. Lampeter.

Williams, G. (1971) 'An Elizabethan Disease.' *Trivium, 6*, 43–58. Lampeter.

Williams, R.L. (1980) *The Horror of Life*. Chicago: University of Chicago Press.

Williamson, H.R. (1940) *George Villiers, First Duke of Buckingham*. London: Duckworth.

'Willoby, Henry' (1966) *Willobie His Avisa (1594)* (edited by G.B. Harrison). Elizabethan and Jacobean Quartos, no.9. Edinburgh: The University Press.

Wilson, J.D. (1911) *Life in Shakespeare's England*. Cambridge: Cambridge University Press.

Wither, G. (1635) *A Collection of Emblems, Ancient and Modern*. London.

Wolfe, C.W. (1960) 'Shakespeare Refers to Syphilis.' *Marquette Medical Review, 25*, no.2, 112–4.

Wood, A. (1786–90) *The History and Antiquities of the Colleges and Halls in the University of Oxford*, vols.1–2 (edited by J. Gutch). Oxford: Clarendon.

Woodall, J. (1617) *The Surgeons Mate*. London.

Woods, A.H. (1934) 'Syphilis in Shakespeare's Tragedy of Timon of Athens.' *American Journal of Psychiatry, 91*, 95–107.

Wrigley, A. and Schofield, R.S. (1981) *The Population History of England, 1541–1871*. London: Edward Arnold.

Wriothesley, C. (1875) *A Chronicle of England during the Reign of the Tudors from A. D. 1485 to 1559* (edited by W.D. Hamilton). The Camden Society, New Series, vol.11.

Young, S. (1890) *The Annals of the Barber-Surgeons of London*. London: Blades, East and Blades.

Zimmermann, E.L. (1932) 'The French Pox of That Great Clerke of Almayne, Ulrich Hutten.' *Janus, 36*, 235–55 and 297–310.

Zimmermann, E.L. (1937) 'An Early English Manuscript on Syphilis.' *Bulletin Institute of the History of Medicine, 5*, 461–82.

# Subject Index

# Author Index